A synopsis of
OPHTHALMOLOGY

A synopsis of
OPHTHALMOLOGY

J. L. C. MARTIN-DOYLE
MRCS (Eng) LRCP (Lond) DO (Oxon)

Formerly Senior Surgeon, Worcester Eye Hospital, Senior Ophthalmic Consultant to Worcester Royal Infirmary and Rorkswood Hospital, etc.

and

MARTIN H. KEMP
MB (Dunelm) FRCS (Eng) DO (Eng)

Senior Surgeon, Worcester Eye Hospital

Fifth edition

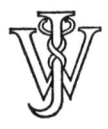

BRISTOL ·
JOHN WRIGHT & SONS LTD

© **John Wright & Sons Ltd. 1975**

All Rights Reserved. No part of this publication may be reproduced, stored in a retrieval system, or transmitted, in any form or by any means, electronic, mechanical, photocopying, recording, or otherwise, without the prior permission of John Wright & Sons Ltd.

First edition: 1951
Second edition: 1961
Third edition: 1967
Fourth edition: 1971
Fifth edition: 1975
   Paperback edition: 1976
   Reprinted: 1980

ISBN 0 7236 0446 0

Reproduced from copy supplied
printed and bound in Great Britain
by Billing and Sons Limited
Guildford, London, Oxford, Worcester

PREFACE TO THE FIFTH EDITION

IN preparing this edition I would like first of all to welcome my colleague Mr Martin Kemp of the Worcester Eye Hospital as joint author. Every ophthalmic surgeon knows the value of consultations with colleagues from time to time especially when confronted with difficult problems. Exactly the same is true when writing a book. When two minds are involved, various viewpoints, problems and theories are looked at from two angles and this is always helpful. I am grateful to him for his co-operation.

We have jointly endeavoured to bring this volume up to date. The chapter on ophthalmic operations has been rewritten and that on recent advances has been enlarged to include such things as operating microscopes and electronic helps for the blind which are being developed but are not yet on the market. Sections on multifocal and tinted lenses have been added. TRIC agent conjunctivitis has been discussed and there is a description of eye damage in the all-too-prevalent 'battered baby' syndrome. A chapter on the personal and social aspects of blindness and partial sight has been added in response to a suggestion by one of the reviewers to whom I am grateful for the idea. Both Mr Kemp and I think this will be fulfilling a real need and neither of us can remember having seen a reference to this in any textbook. Particular attention has been paid to the sections on Treatment and Pathology. The authors gladly acknowledge their indebtedness to Dr C. H. Greer's book *Ocular Pathology* (Blackwell), 2nd ed., 1972. His opinion has been quoted in a few places and Dr Greer's name appears in brackets after quoting his views.

Both authors would like to thank Mrs Beardsell, the orthoptist at the Worcester Eye Hospital, for her kind help in revising the chapter on orthoptics. Lastly, I again thank Messrs John Wright & Sons Ltd, for help and advice concerning various aspects of this edition. No author could have had happier relations with their publishers than I have had with Messrs John Wright over these five editions.

C. MARTIN-DOYLE

1975

PREFACE TO THE FIRST EDITION

IN writing this synopsis of ophthalmology it has been my somewhat optimistic aim to give a comprehensive view of the whole of ophthalmology in one small volume. I have endeavoured to include the rare as well as the common conditions and to give as much attention to pathology and treatment as space permits. It is not for a moment suggested that this work should replace the larger and well-illustrated textbooks, but I hope that it will meet the needs of the following important sections of the medical community:

1. The senior medical student who will appreciate an inexpensive and *multum in parvo* volume to help him when first attending the ophthalmic outpatient department.

2. The busy general practitioner, who lacks the time (and possibly the inclination!) to wade through a larger book, should find this a handy volume for quick reference.

3. The postgraduate student or Ophthalmic House Surgeon working for a higher diploma in ophthalmology, may be glad of a condensed work of this kind when revising for examinations. I have therefore endeavoured to make the work as up to date as possible and to include a number of recently described diseases which have been discussed in ophthalmic periodicals but which have reached few textbooks as yet.

It would be difficult to recall all the textbooks to which I have referred in the preparation of this volume, but I would like to take this opportunity of acknowledging my special indebtedness to the following:

Parsons' *Diseases of the Eye* (the newest edition is by Duke-Elder). This small but complete work has been my constant companion through my professional life and has been of particular help to me in preparing this synopsis.

Duke-Elder's *Textbook of Ophthalmology*, Vols. 1–4. I have made frequent reference to this monumental and exhaustive work and I gladly acknowledge my indebtedness to it.

Wolff's *Pathology of the Eye*. This book has been my chief source of reference on pathological matters.

Without these three textbooks my work would have been much harder.

In conclusion I should like to thank the following individuals for invaluable help: Mr T. G. Shields, the Librarian of the BMA Library, has always upon request posted me up-to-date literature published in all parts of the world dealing with more abstruse and recently described conditions. It is owing to his help that I have been able to include a

viii PREFACE TO THE FIRST EDITION

description of a number of conditions that have not yet appeared in textbooks. My friend Mr C. G. Sinclair, FRCS, of Worcester and the Birmingham Eye Hospital, has kindly read through the proofs and given me constructive and helpful criticism. Miss J. M. Richardson, Secretary of the Worcester Eye Hospital, has in her spare time taken down the whole of this book in shorthand and typed it out with the maximum of efficiency and the minimum of mistakes. Last, but by no means least, it gives me real pleasure to thank the publishers, Messrs John Wright & Sons, for their unfailing courtesy, help and advice in the preparation of this book, and I am especially indebted to their Mr Owens, who has kindly gone through the whole of the typescript with me and advised on typographical details. I am also grateful to the publishers for allowing me to include a number of quotations which, because they are so grossly wrested from their context, add a touch of humour, thus relieving the deadly tedium of an otherwise purely factual book.

C. MARTIN-DOYLE

CONTENTS

	Preface to the fifth edition	*page* v
	Preface to the first edition	vii
I	The routine examination of an ophthalmic patient	1
II	Diseases of the conjunctiva	8
III	Diseases of the cornea	25
IV	Drugs affecting intra-ocular muscles	43
V	Diseases of the uveal tract	45
VI	Diseases of the retina	67
VII	Diseases of the sclera	93
VIII	Diseases of the optic nerve	96
IX	Diseases of the vitreous	104
X	Diseases of the lens	110
XI	Glaucoma	121
XII	Diseases of the orbit	132
XIII	Diseases of the eyelids	141
XIV	Diseases of the lacrimal apparatus	153
XV	Intra-ocular neoplasms	159
XVI	Optical anomalies of the eye	164
XVII	Anomalies of ocular movements	174
XVIII	Subjective visual disturbances	188
XIX	Ocular signs of general disease	196
XX	Ocular side-effects of systemic medication	215
XXI	Contact lenses	218
XXII	The eyes in malnutrition	221
XXIII	Ophthalmic operations	225
XXIV	Sympathetic ophthalmia	234
XXV	Chemotherapy and antibiotics in eye diseases	237
XXVI	Corticosteroids in ophthalmology	244
XXVII	Allergy in ophthalmology	248
XXVIII	Slit-lamp microscopy	250
XXIX	Recent advances in ophthalmic practice	255
XXX	The social aspects of blindness and partial sight	261
	Index	265

Chapter I

THE ROUTINE EXAMINATION OF AN OPHTHALMIC PATIENT

'My method in such cases.' SIR A. CONAN DOYLE, *The Musgrave Ritual*

IN a work that aims at giving a bird's eye view of the whole of ophthalmology in a small volume, space prevents detailed description of the theory and technique of ophthalmoscopy, retinoscopy, etc. The author has, therefore, decided to assume some knowledge on the part of the student of the elementary use of such instruments and to concentrate instead on the various practical points of the routine examination which are frequently forgotten or neglected.

Every good physician has a systematic routine for the examination of every patient, and it is only by carrying this out in the same order that errors and omissions are avoided. The ophthalmologist should be just as precise and businesslike and form his own routine procedure. There is, however, one danger of a routine that must be avoided at all costs: the danger of regarding the patient as a 'case'. He is not. He is a human being, and often a very scared and timid one, and should always be treated accordingly. Kindness and politeness cost nothing and are rewarded by a responsiveness and co-operation that is rarely given to the impatient brow-beating type of surgeon. The patient should never be given the impression that he is regarded as a case. Routine is necessary, but it should not be so inflexible that the patient is aware of it.

Order of Examination: The authors adopt the following order of examination as a routine in almost every case and recognize it as in their experience the best. They in no sense wish to condemn the methods of others who follow a different practice. The important thing for every prospective ophthalmic surgeon to do is to form his own routine order and to stick to it.

History.
Visual acuity.
External examination of:
　Lids;
　Conjunctiva;
　Cornea;
　Sclera;
　Pupil;
　Iris;
　Anterior chamber;
　Lacrimal apparatus.

Refraction.
Lens and media.
Fundus.
Ocular movements.
Muscle balance tests.
Perimetry
Slit-lamp examination
Gonioscopy   } where indicated.
Tonometry
Syringeing of lacrimal passages
Other examinations not directly ophthalmic, e.g. urine, blood pressure, etc.

History: The ophthalmologist will soon find that a careful record of the patient's history is abundantly worth while. In every case the age and occupation should be noted, for very often the power or type of glasses to be ordered will depend upon this. After ascertaining these elementary factors the question: 'What are you complaining of?' should be put to the patient and the answer noted. Care should be taken over these notes. It is not sufficient to write the bald word 'headaches'. Their location, severity, frequency, relationship to close work, whether associated with vomiting or not, should be noted. Lengthy notes are unnecessary, but something trite such as 'pains at the back of the eye after close work' or 'severe right-sided headache with dazzling lights and ending with a bilious attack' is always helpful. Furthermore, on subsequent consultations it is a good plan to inquire about previous symptoms and, rightly or wrongly, it gives the oculist the reputation of having a good memory and therefore of 'taking an interest in my case'. Notes should be taken also of the general health, illnesses, operations and indeed anything else that seems important to the patient and might have a bearing on the case. The oculist who is curt, abrupt and too busy to listen to the patient's history will be a bad oculist and had better give up ophthalmology and try his hand at pathology. He may be quite good at post-mortem examinations, for his patients will be dead!

FAMILY HISTORY: This can be of great importance, as such common complaints as glaucoma, senile cataract, astigmatism, amblyopia, etc. often 'run in families'.

Visual Acuity: Each eye must be taken separately as an invariable routine in every case. This is of fundamental importance and is often most important of all in cases where it seems most superfluous. A record of this is of utmost value in subsequent consultations. More than once the author has come across patients who make claims for compensation for very trivial injuries such as corneal foreign bodies, etc., and who have grossly exaggerated their symptoms. A record of the visual acuity at the time the injury was treated is of obvious value in such cases.

In Britain, the visual acuity is always tested by Snellen's types (*Fig.* 1), which are based upon the assumption that the minimum visual angle is 1 minute. Each letter is shaped so that it subtends 5 minutes of arc at a given distance, while the width of each constituent

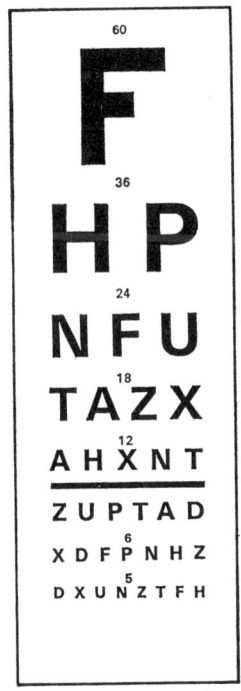

Fig. 1.—Snellen's test types. (*By courtesy of Messrs. Hamblin Ltd.*)

arm of the letter subtends 1 minute. This type is placed 6 m from the patient's eyes (or 3 m if a reverse type is used and it is viewed in a mirror).

The normal patient should be able to read the seventh line at a distance of 6 m, the sixth line at 9 m, the fifth at 12, the fourth at 18, the third at 24, the second at 36 and the top at 60 m, because from each of these distances the respective lines subtend 5 minutes. Normal vision is expressed by the fraction 6/6; if a patient can only read the sixth line his vision is 6/9, and so on, 6/12, 6/18, 6/24, 6/36 and if he can read the top only it is 6/60. If the patient can only read some letters of a certain line this should be recorded, e.g. 6/18 partly or 6/12−2. If a patient cannot see the top letter he should be asked to count fingers at 1 m, and if he cannot do this he should be tested as to his ability to see a hand moving at the same distance. If the vision is too poor even for this, tests should be made as to whether he can perceive light. These last three measures of visual acuity are recorded as CF, HM and PL, respectively. Time will be saved in vision taking if a 1-cm strip of red cellophane or *passe-partout* is stuck on the test type to underline the 6/12 line (A H X N T) and the patient is asked to read below the red line. If the visual acuity is not good enough for this, the patient should be asked to start at the top and read downwards.

In America and some Continental countries, vision is recorded in terms of the 20-ft table. The following is the conversion table:

Snellen's 6-metre Table	*20-foot Table*
6/6	20/20
6/9	20/30
6/12	20/40
6/18	20/70
6/24	20/80
6/36	20/120
6/60	20/200

External Examinations: All examinations of the external eye should be made in the first instance without a magnifier but with a good light. Two methods of illumination are excellent:
1. OBLIQUE ILLUMINATION WITH BRIGHT DAYLIGHT focused on the eye by means of a high-powered convex condensing lens.
2. OBLIQUE EXAMINATION WITH FOCUSING HAND-INSPECTION LAMP.

After examination without magnification, the use of a binocular loupe may be very helpful. The monocular loupe has been somewhat outdated by the slit-lamp, which gives a much greater magnification and the additional advantage of stereoscopic vision. Nevertheless, the monocular loupe still plays a useful part in that it gives a fairly high magnification without elaborate apparatus and in a time-saving manner.

LIDS: These should be examined for blepharitis, ectropion, entropion, trichiasis, meibomian cysts and other abnormalities.

CONJUNCTIVA: Both bulbar and palpebral conjunctivae should then be examined and note should be taken as to whether the former is injected or oedematous and the latter red or velvety. In such cases the upper lid should be everted, for quite often a case of chronic conjunctivitis that fails to respond to treatment is due to a foreign body under the lid. The tarsal surface should be examined for concretions, cysts, etc.

SCLERA: This should be examined for nodules of episcleritis, blue coloration, areas of pigmentation, etc. Circumcorneal injection ('ciliary flush') may be seen in some cases of deep-seated inflammation. Occasionally staphylomata—the herniation of uveal tissue through thinned-out sclera—is observed in cases of grossly increased intra-ocular pressure.

CORNEA: First note whether this structure is large or small. If small and a shallow anterior chamber is present, glaucoma would have to be ruled out. Then examine with a focusing hand-lamp. A search should be made for any of the following conditions:

Oedema;
Pannus;
Keratic precipitates (KP);
Ulcers;
Scars or nebulae;
Tracks made by foreign body;
Dystrophy;
Loss of sensation, etc.

If conical cornea is suspected, examination should be made in profile from the patient's side while he is looking straight ahead. If any corneal abnormality is found, no examination is complete without the slit-lamp.

PUPIL: The state of the pupils should be examined carefully and note made whether they are regular, equal and react to light and accommodation. If irregular, cyclopentolate 1 per cent should be instilled and the patient seen a little while later to ascertain whether the irregularity is due to posterior synechiae or to congenital abnormalities. If doubt exists as to whether it reacts or not, the matter can be decided with the slit-lamp. In every case the consensual reaction should be noted.

IRIS: The iris and ciliary region should then be examined for:

Colour: Whether both irides are the same (*see* HETEROCHROMIC IRIDOCYCLITIS, p. 58) and particularly whether either appear 'muddy'.
Ciliary flush (circumcorneal injection);
Synechiae;
Atrophy;
Nodules;
New vessels;
Iridodonesis.

If any of the above abnormalities are found, examination with the slit-lamp is imperative. The delicate structure of the iris is the easiest part of the eye for slit-lamp examination. The beginner is much encouraged and really feels he is 'seeing something' at this examination. It is well worth practising this before going on to the anterior chamber and the lens which are much more difficult examinations.

ANTERIOR CHAMBER: Should be noted particularly with regard to its depth. If very shallow it is suggestive of closed angle glaucoma. In certain cases of chronic iridocyclitis it is deeper than normal.

LACRIMAL APPARATUS: If epiphora is present, either the punctum is not in apposition or there is some obstruction to the drainage. A careful examination will reveal whether the former is the case. Pressure with the forefinger should be placed upon the sac to test for regurgitation and later in the examination the passages may be syringed through the lower punctum in order to test for patency or in an endeavour to relieve an obstruction.

Note: The *tension* can be conveniently estimated digitally at this point, but if an accurate tonometric investigation is required it is best left until later.

Refraction: A careful written note should be made of the findings. It is impossible to attempt any description of the detailed technique of this examination here. The student is referred to textbooks on the subject, but is at the same time reminded that an ounce of practice is worth a pound of theory. Nothing can take the place of patient practice in the outpatient department. Subjective tests are then made based upon the refraction findings and the appropriate prescription is ordered.

Opinions differ as to whether refraction should be estimated under a mydriatic or with an undilated pupil. All, however, are agreed that in the case of children a mydriatic is highly advisable, if not absolutely necessary. With regard to adults its use has one great drawback: for accurate subjective results a post-mydriatic test is necessary, and this necessitates a second visit and often a second day off work. The following routine is, therefore, recommended with regard to mydriatics:

Children under 5	Atropine
Young people, 5–12	Cyclopentolate
Over 12	Undilated

It must be remembered that the lighter the colour of the iris, the quicker the mydriatic works. In children with deeply pigmented irides, it may be necessary to instil further mydriatic drops at 4-hourly intervals until full dilatation is obtained.

Lens and Media: At this stage the ophthalmoscope comes into its own. Always begin the examination with the +12 lens up; this brings into focus the cornea and anterior segment of the eye and will reveal lens opacities at a glance. Furthermore, begin the examination at a distance of about 30 cm from the eye and gradually bring the ophthalmoscope nearer (distant direct ophthalmoscopy). This is a most helpful clinical technique and is neglected by many oculists. The lens system should be rotated until 'O' is reached. This method will reveal any abnormality anywhere between the cornea and the retina. In the case of very short-sighted persons ophthalmoscopic examination is best done by looking through the patient's own glasses. Slit-lamp examination of the lens is helpful but much practice is required to become efficient. A mydriatic is essential for this.

Fundus: Here again, examination should begin with the +12 lens up and working downwards. Make this an invariable technique, not merely for the purpose of impressing examiners, but because, if it is not done, sooner or later a shallow detechment of the retina is certain to be missed. First, examine the disc region for cupping, papilloedema, etc., then follow up one or two of the vessels until an arteriovenous crossing is found. This should be examined for the pinching of arteriosclerosis. Careful attention is paid to the arteries for irregular calibre, tortuosity, sheathing, etc. At the same time the rest of the fundus should be searched for haemorrhages, exudates, choroiditis or other abnormalities. The patient should be told successively to look up, down, to the right and to the left, and various parts of the fundus explored. Lastly, the macular area requires a particularly careful examination. For this the patient should be told to look directly into the light. A mydriatic should always be used if a thorough search of the fundus is indicated, and for an adequate examination of the macula it is absolutely indispensable.

Ocular Movements, including the cover test, can now be investigated and notes should be taken of any nystagmus, defective movement, squint, etc.

Muscle-balance Tests: Maddox rod and wing tests should be carried out if there is any indication. If squint or heterophoria is present and circumstances permit, it is always wise to obtain an orthoptic report.

Special Examinations: At the close of these routine examinations special instrumental examinations can be undertaken if necessary. These include *perimetry, tonometry, slit-lamp examination* and *gonioscopy*, and each has been touched upon under their respective headings. Occasionally *tonography, ultrasonography* and *fundus photography* are required. These more elaborate examinations are best left until this stage, when all the simple routine has been completed.

General Examinations: Finally, if desired, certain general investigations can be undertaken which are not directly ophthalmic but which are often necessary as the result of examination of the eye. These include blood pressure, urine tests, blood tests, etc. It has been the practice of the author, if these investigations are indicated, to refer the patients back to their own general practitioner or physician, who is better able to carry out these and any other necessary examinations.

Chapter II

DISEASES OF THE CONJUNCTIVA

'Holding his pocket handkerchief before his streaming eyes.' LEWIS CARROLL, *The Walrus and the Carpenter*

THE ANATOMY AND PHYSIOLOGY OF THE NORMAL CONJUNCTIVA

THE conjunctiva is divided into the bulbar and tarsal portions. The bulbar portion covers the anterior third of the eyeball, and is loosely attached to the sclerotic except at the limbus, where it merges with the corneal epithelium. Advantage is taken of this looseness by the surgeon in covering wounds. Medially it runs beneath the semilunar fold (the remains of the nictitating membrane) and at the fornices it is especially loose—hence permitting wide range of movements. The tarsal portion is very firmly adherent. The blood supply comes from the vessels to the skin of the eyelids. The nerve supply of the tarsal portion is from the nerves of the lid, that of the bulbar portion is from the ciliary nerves. The lymph drainage goes to the pre-auricular gland and to a gland in the submaxillary region near the lower border of the mandible. The function of the conjunctiva is twofold: (1) to moisten the lids; and (2) to assist the lids in the cleansing of the cornea.

Bacteriology: The conjunctiva is hardly ever sterile, but most organisms present are not pathological, neither do they multiply very freely owing to the antibacterial action of the lysozyme and the relatively low temperature and the poor blood supply. The following conditions may cause bacteria to multiply, and previously innocuous ones to become pathogenic: (1) Trauma of conjunctiva; (2) Presence of a foreign body; (3) Wearing of a celluloid eye-shield.

Pneumococci, gonococci and *Ps. pyocyanea* are the most dangerous organisms in ocular infections. After these come the *Staph. aureus*. *Esch. coli* and Proteus infections occur less commonly.

The *Corynebacterium xerosis* closely resembles the *C. diphtheriae* and is a frequent inhabitant of the conjunctival sac, as also is *H. influenzae*. Virus infections occur frequently, especially the herpes virus and adenoviruses. It has been shown by Ainley and Brenda Smith at the Oxford Eye Hospital that fungal infections of the human eye occur more frequently than is supposed, and work by Buschmann and others in Humboldt University has been successful in treating these with amphotericin B.

DISEASES OF THE CONJUNCTIVA 9

ACUTE CONJUNCTIVITIS

There are seven distinct clinical variations of acute conjunctivitis: (1) Simple acute conjunctivitis ('pink eye'); (2) Mucopurulent conjunctivitis; (3) Purulent conjunctivitis; (4) Ophthalmia neonatorum; (5) Membranous conjunctivitis; (6) Phlyctenular conjunctivitis; (7) Photophthalmia.

1. **Simple Acute Conjunctivitis:** The affected eye becomes red and the conjunctiva grossly hyperaemic. There is profuse lacrimation and a burning or pricking feeling in the eye. The patient complains of a sensation of 'something in it'. Acute pain is rare and, if present, iritis should be suspected. In severe cases there may be marked oedema. Every care should be taken to examine the affected eye for a foreign body either in the cornea or under the upper lid. After a course of 3–4 days the condition usually subsides, and about this time similar symptoms may commence in the unaffected eye. If the condition is prolonged and remains in one eye only, especially if it affects mainly the lower fornix, malingering may be suspected.

    PATHOLOGY: The condition is very contagious and is inclined to cause epidemics in schools and institutions. A variety of organisms cause these diseases, including *H. influenzae*, diplococci, staphylococci and *H. aegyptius* (or Koch–Weeks bacillus). The conjunctival vessels become enlarged and wavy, transudation or serum occurs, and there is cellular infiltration of the subepithelial tissues.

    TREATMENT: The ideal method would be to isolate the causative organism, and, if this were found to be sensitive to penicillin, chemotherapy or one of the broad-spectrum antibiotics, to institute the appropriate remedy. In practice, however, this involves time and expense, and often by the time the result is known the condition has improved, since simple conjunctivitis tends to correct itself with or without treatment.

    The best treatment is sulphacetamide or chloramphenicol drops four times a day. Eye lotions and irrigations are not indicated since they reduce the lysozyme contents of the conjunctival sac. If there is gross hyperaemia or chemosis, adrenaline drops 1–1000 can be instilled. If photophobia is present, dark glasses are indicated.

2. **Mucopurulent Conjunctivitis:** This differs from simple conjunctivitis only in degree, and is often preceded by it. It is especially common in cases of acute fevers such as measles, scarlet fever, etc. The signs and symptoms are identical with those of acute conjunctivitis, but there is mucopurulent discharge. Pathology is the same as that of acute simple conjunctivitis. When pneumococci are present, there tends to be more exudation and chemosis than with other organisms.

    TREATMENT: Saline irrigations may be used if there is much purulent discharge. Gutt. chloramphenicol 0·5 per cent or Ung. Chloramphenicol 1 per cent may be instilled. Some surgeons have been using antibiotic *ointments* on the supposed grounds that drops become immediately diluted with tears and hence lose their effective concentration. This view has been negatived by work done by F. Ridley, whose experiments do not suggest that ointment is more effective than drops. The eye should *not* be bandaged. Dark glasses or a loose fitting shade may be worn. Great care must be taken to wash after handling, and special precautions must be taken with towels, handkerchiefs, etc., otherwise the disease will spread.

3. **Purulent Conjunctivitis:** This is a much more serious condition and occurs usually in babies (ophthalmia neonatorum, *see* (4) *below*) or in adults. It is frequently, but by no means invariably, due to the gonococcus, and in these cases the eyes are often infected direct from the urethral discharges. When the conjunctivitis is frankly purulent, there is a real chance of corneal involvement. The epithelium becomes devitalized and ulceration, with all its attendant risks, is the result. The condition is acutely painful and the patient is often very ill, with a raised temperature and enlarged pre-auricular glands. In cases of corneal involvement there is a risk of iritis or iridocyclitis. In the worst cases gonococcal arthritis or even septicaemia may supervene.

   TREATMENT: The utmost care must be taken to prevent the spread of infection to the other eye, and likewise the greatest care exercised by the surgeon and nurses to prevent an infection of their own eyes. The following steps should be taken:
   a. First protect the unaffected eye by a Buller's shield.
   b. Take a smear and culture to isolate the causative organism.
   c. Before awaiting the result of the smear and culture, use Gutt. chloramphenicol 0·5 per cent every 2 hours, or one of the newer broad-spectrum antibiotics.
   d. Commence intensive chemotherapy treatment internally and give penicillin injections.
   e. One per cent atropine drops should be used in the affected eye twice a day.
   f. Frequent saline irrigations give relief.
   g. Give careful attention to general health, state of bowels, etc. Sedatives may be given as required.

4. **Ophthalmia Neonatorum:** This is officially defined as a 'persistent discharge from the eyes of an infant commencing within twenty-one days of birth'. It used to be a most serious disease and was responsible for large numbers of blind children. Many cases are preventable and are due to lack of appropriate attention at birth and the failure to instil 1 per cent silver nitrate drops in the eyes of a newborn infant. Fortunately nowadays severe ophthalmia neonatorum is a rare complaint and its serious effects are seldom seen.

SIGNS: Both eyes are usually involved. The lids may be swollen and the conjunctiva is red and often chemosed. Oedema of the cornea may be present and there is mucopurulent or purulent discharge.

PATHOLOGY: Sixty per cent of cases of ophthalmia neonatorum are due to a gonococcal infection and the remainder are usually due to the pneumococcus, the coliform bacillus, *Str. pyogenes* or, rarely, to the *Staph. aureus*. A less serious infection is sometimes seen due to *Chlamydia oculogenitalis* which is a virus infection, venereal in nature, derived from the maternal passage which gives rise to intracellular inclusion bodies.

TREATMENT: It should be remembered that this is a notifiable disease and cases should, therefore, be notified immediately when diagnosed. The best treatment of all is preventive, as mentioned above. All cases seen may be treated in the following manner as a routine:
  a. Take a smear and culture or conjunctival scrapings to isolate the organism.
  b. Antibiotic drops or ointment such as chloramphenicol 0·5 per cent should be instilled 4-hourly, and injection of long-acting penicillin should be given.
  c. Some form of chemotherapy in mixture form may be given in severe cases but this is rarely necessary now.
  d. One per cent atropine drops or ointment should be used three times a day if the cornea is involved.

5. **Membranous Conjunctivitis:** Occasionally in the course of a severe conjunctivitis the tarsal surface of the conjunctiva may become covered with a fibrinous membrane (in exactly the same way as a membrane may appear on the throat). This condition occurs chiefly in children and most commonly during the course of an acute specific fever. Any degree of severity may be found. In a slight case there is a mucopurulent discharge with swelling of the lids associated with a thin membrane that can be pulled off easily. In a severe case there is gross brawny oedema of the lids and the conjunctiva may be covered with exudates. On eversion of the lids (if this is possible) a thick and firmly adherent membrane may be found. The patient may have a high temperature and the pre-auricular gland may be swollen. In unfavourable cases necrosis of the cornea and even of the lids may result. During the process of healing after the membrane has spread there is a risk of symblepharon forming.

PATHOLOGY: It may be stated at once that membranous conjunctivitis is not necessarily diphtheritic. The gonococcus, pneumococcus, streptococcus and Koch–Weeks bacillus have all been found in cases of membranous conjunctivitis. In scarlet fever cases the streptococcus is usually the infecting organism. The bacteriological diagnosis of diphtheritic conjunetivitis is difficult, since the

C. diphtheriae bacillus is morphologically identical with the xerosis bacillus which is a frequent inhabitant of the conjunctival sac. No information can be gained as to the nature of the organism by the severity or otherwise of the attack. The brawny oedema often seen is caused by the fibrinous exudate leaving the vessels and invading the tissues of the lid. The membrane itself is a fibrinous mass, in which are enmeshed necrotic cells, leucocytes and bacteria.

TREATMENT:

   a. Treat every case as diphtheritic until definitely proved otherwise. Therefore, give full doses of antitoxin.
   b. Oral doses of chemotherapeutics must be given. A very convenient form is known as sulphamethoxypyridiaze or sulphadimethazine. Dose: 2 g stat. then 0·5 g daily.
   c. Penicillin injections are required in severe cases. One of the long-acting type is most convenient where a single injection gives prompt and prolonged antibacterial action lasting for 3–4 days. Procaine penicillin is very effective.
   d. Gutt. atropin. 1 per cent three times a day in cases of corneal involvement.
   e. Gutt. chloramphenicol 0·5 per cent or a broad-spectrum antibiotic should be used 3-hourly.

6. **Phlyctenular Conjunctivitis:** This disease is commonest in children of school age and is rarely seen in infants or adults. Generally the patient is an undernourished, weak or ailing child, and very frequently suffers from nasal or respiratory catarrh. It commences with a mild mucopurulent conjunctivitis and on examination one or more small nodules are found, especially near the limbus. The conjunctiva immediately surrounding the phlycten is intensely red and congested and there is often marked photophobia, and occasionally severe blepharospasm may be present. There is sometimes an excoriation of the skin of the lids and cheek, due to irritation by the discharge. This accounts for the former misnomer applied to the condition—'eczematous conjunctivitis'. It is seldom seen in Great Britain today.

PATHOLOGY: Section of a phlycten shows a subepithelial triangular area of cellular infiltration containing large quantities of mononuclear lymphocytes. Smear and culture reveal many of the organisms which are present in mucopurulent conjunctivitis. Phlyctens have never been produced experimentally.

The modern view favours the allergic theory and possibly that of allergy to a tuberculous toxin. Evidence in favour of this is: (1) The poor general health of the average patient; (2) The fact that injections of tuberculin have sometimes been followed by phlyctenular conjunctivitis.

The occasional association of this disease with eczema of the skin may indicate an allergic origin.

TREATMENT:
  a. Local prednisolone is very beneficial.
  b. Gutt. atropin. 1 per cent if there is any corneal involvement.
  c. Local corticosteroid ointment is useful for excoriated areas of the skin.
  d. Dark glasses should be worn for photophobia. The eye must not be bandaged.
  e. Careful attention to general health, sunshine, fresh air, vitamins, tonics if necessary and no school.
7. **Photophthalmia:** For convenience this is included under diseases of the conjunctiva. It is a violent conjunctival reaction secondary to oedema of the corneal epithelium caused by exposure to ultra-violet light. The following are found more or less commonly:
  a. WELDERS' CONJUNCTIVITIS: Those who are indiscreet enough to watch the welding light without appropriate dark glasses.
  b. ELECTRIC FLASHES, from short-circuits, brilliant arcs, etc.
  c. SNOW BLINDNESS, from exposing the unprotected eye to sunlit snowfields.
  d. ULTRAVIOLET LIGHT (UVL): Accidental or careless exposure is common now as numerous patients treat themselves in their homes. Dark goggles (not merely glasses) are essential for these UVL lamps.

In all these cases, there is a delay of about 6 hours between the exposure to the light and the onset of symptoms. These consist of intense burning pain with severe lacrimation and photophobia. In the worst cases the pain may be so severe that the opening of the lids is impossible.

TREATMENT:
  a. The severity of the condition can be greatly reduced if treatment with antihistamine or steroid drops is instigated as soon as exposure to UVL occurs. Initially drops are instilled every 5 minutes for $\frac{1}{2}$ hour, every $\frac{1}{4}$ hour for 2 hours then four times a day for 48 hours.
  b. If necessary, instil local anaesthetic drops to facilitate examination.
  c. A mydriatic gives great relief from photophobia and ciliary spasm.
  d. Double pads and bandaging with the instillation of steroid ointment may be necessary in severe cases; otherwise prescribe antihistamine or steroid drops frequently for 48 hours.

These conditions usually clear up very quickly.

CHRONIC CONJUNCTIVITIS

The following clinical types may be observed: (1) Simple chronic conjunctivitis; (2) Angular conjunctivitis; (3) Follicular conjunctivitis; (4) Trachoma; (5) Spring catarrh; (6) Conjunctivitis due to irritants; (7) Seborrhoea.

14 A SYNOPSIS OF OPHTHALMOLOGY

1. **Simple Chronic Conjunctivitis:** This may be due to a variety of causes such as: (*a*) Irritation from concretions; (*b*) Trichiasis; (*c*) Irritation from a dusty or smoky atmosphere; (*d*) Eye strain from reading in poor light or with an uncorrected refractive error; (*f*) The rheumatic diathesis—the type of patient who suffers from chronic gout, rheumatism or arthritis is particular liable to chronic conjunctivitis; (*g*) The presence of seborrhoea in the scalp often causes a troublesome blepharoconjunctivitis. In this condition the scalp condition must be tackled before local treatment can be successful; (*h*) Working in heat, e.g. cooks, furnace men, etc.

    SYMPTOMS: There is no actual pain, but a sense of grittiness and burning of the eyes. It is often described as feeling 'as though sand is in it'. The discharge is negligible and often there is little to be found to account for the symptoms. At the most there is a slight engorgement of the vessels and the palpebral conjunctiva may resemble red velvet.

    PATHOLOGY: The following changes have been noted: (*a*) Increase in number of the goblet cells; (*b*) Formation of papillae on the tarsal conjunctiva; (*c*) Sometimes follicles are formed.

    TREATMENT:
    a. Aim at eliminating the cause.
    b. Sulphacetamide and other forms of chemotherapy are of doubtful value and if there is no improvement after a short course they should be discarded.
    c. Astringent drops such as zinc sulphate 0·25 per cent often help.
    d. Occasional painting of the lids with 1 or 2 per cent silver nitrate is often beneficial after a preliminary cocainization.
    e. Protective glasses for those working in heat.

    Very often the condition is found to be resistant and troublesome and many remedies may be tried. It is good treatment to 'ring the changes' and not to keep to any one medicament for too long. When the symptoms are alleviated it is wise to discard treatment and not to use any drops during quiescent intervals. Relapses, unfortunately, are common.

2. **Angular Conjunctivitis:** This is a chronic infection which, as its name implies, affects the conjunctiva overlying the angles of the eye at the inner and outer canthi. The remainder of the conjunctiva usually appears healthy. The patient complains of discomfort, slight discharge and sometimes excoriation of the skin of the lids. Chronic blepharitis may be present, and patients with angular conjunctivitis often suffer from nasal infections.

    PATHOLOGY: This disease is almost invariably due to Morax–Axenfeld bacillus. In fact, it is the only type of conjunctivitis where the causative organism can be diagnosed from the clinical appearance. These diplobacilli may be found in nasal secretions

DISEASES OF THE CONJUNCTIVA

from cases of angular conjunctivitis. In older patients this trouble can be caused by prolonged medication of the eyes with certain chemicals and alkaloids such as eserine, pilocarpine or DFP.

TREATMENT: Tetracycline or bacitracin with neomycin ointment locally is the best treatment for these infections. Less effective (but less expensive) is zinc which used to be regarded as a specific for this condition. It is best used as zinc sulph. drops 0·25 per cent. Boric acid may be added to this in the same strength if desired. It is not known how zinc acts in these cases, but it is quite certain that it is helpful even if it is less rapid in its action than the antibiotics.

3. **Follicular Conjunctivitis:** This is a teenage and children's complaint and is most commonly found in catarrhal and debilitated types. Both eyes are affected, but the symptoms are rarely severe and sometimes there are none at all. The characteristic of the complaint is the occurrence of parallel rows of follicles which are nearly always confined to the palpebral conjunctiva of the lower lid. Follicles rarely occur on the upper lid and never on the plica or bulbar conjunctiva.

PATHOLOGY: The follicles are small, round, translucent bodies the size of a pin's head. They consist of aggregations of lymphocytes and are indistinguishable from the lymph patches of the intestines.

TREATMENT: Local treatment is seldom indicated. Attention should be paid to the general health, and nose or throat treatment instituted where indicated. In the few cases where local treatment is required, that advised for chronic simple conjunctivitis should be tried.

4. **Trachoma:** In England this is a rare disease, but less rare than formerly owing to immigration. In many hot climates it is exceedingly common and is the cause of blindness of countless thousands of people in tropical countries. It is endemic in countries where there is a low standard of hygiene and where sand and dust abound and flies are prevalent.

The disease runs a very long and chronic course. In the earliest stages it resembles a severe bilateral chronic conjunctivitis with rather more irritation than normal, and accompanied by photophobia and profuse lacrimation. Examination at this stage reveals the presence of follicles in the conjunctiva. At first these follicles resemble those found in cases of follicular conjunctivitis, but the trachoma follicle is somewhat larger and resembles 'sago grains'. These follicles may form anywhere, and if they appear on the plica or bulbar conjunctiva they are diagnostic of trachoma. The conjunctiva covering the lower tarsal plate is first affected.

Later, the upper portion of the cornea becomes infiltrated and this infiltration slowly spreads downwards. Trachoma pannus develops deep to Bowman's membrane, which eventually disappears and the substantia propria becomes involved. Once this has happened all hope for the cornea is lost. The vessels infiltrating the cornea develop connective-tissue sheaths, hence the cornea that has been thus affected is completely useless from the point of view of vision. Painful corneal ulcers are a common complication.

Next to the corneal conditions the most severe after-effects of trachoma are due to involvement of the lids. The follicles become invaded by blood vessels and fibrosis and scarring is the ultimate result. This scarring causes drooping of the lids and distortion from their normal shape, with resulting ectropion or entropion and trichiasis. This further irritates an already damaged cornea and adds to the misery of the patient.

PATHOLOGY: Trachoma is an infection by a large-sized virus of the *Chlamydia* group recently known as TRIC agents. Included in this group is the virus of lymphogranuloma venereum and psittacosis which cause cytoplasmic inclusions. Inclusions were first discovered (but not named) in 1907 by Halberstaedter and Prowacek who described intracellular inclusions in the conjunctival epithelial cells in trachoma. These inclusions are (mercifully!) called 'HPK' bodies for brevity. These virus inclusions fill the cells they invade by dividing and cause degeneration of their nuclei. They are not entirely pathognomonic of trachoma, being occasionally found in other conditions, thus no characteristic pathology can be described. Gross infiltration of the adenoid layers of the conjunctiva with lymphocytes is present and these aggregations form follicles not dissimilar to those found in follicular conjunctivitis. Late in the disease these follicles become gelatinous, hence the 'sago grain' appearance described above. Secondary infection occurs, leading in time to fibrous changes and the formation of scar tissue. Wolff describes three stages of the disease: (*a*) Infiltration of the adenoid layer with cells; (*b*) Appearance of vascular granulation tissue; (*c*) Resultant fibrosis and scarring.

CAUSE OF PANNUS: The modern view is that the cornea is affected at the same time as the conjunctiva, for some degree of pannus is visible by the slit-lamp in very early stages. It is no longer considered to be due to mechanical inoculation by the affected lids. A continuous process from fornix to limbus and involving the conjunctiva has been made out (Wolff).

DIAGNOSIS: Clinically, this depends upon a variety of signs: conjunctival follicles, pannus in upper corneal segment, and at a later stage scarring of tarsal conjunctiva, distortion of lids, infiltration of corneal stroma, etc. If 'HPK' bodies are found in epithelial scrapings the diagnosis is confirmed.

DISEASES OF THE CONJUNCTIVA

TREATMENT:
- *a.* It must always be borne in mind that trachoma is a highly contagious disease and that the utmost precautions should be taken to ensure that all soiled dressings, etc., should be burned and that the hands of surgeons and nurses who treat the case should be scrubbed immediately afterwards.
- *b.* Remember that treatment with the copper stick and other strong caustics is a relic of barbarism and should rarely if ever be used.
- *c.* Sulphonamides internally and sulphacetamide drops are helpful in the early stages. If the disease is well established and secondary infection is present a broad-sprectrum antibiotic such as terramycin, aureomycin or neomycin should be used in ointment form and should be continued for a considerable time. As some cases are very resistant, other antibiotics should be tried if the response is slow.
- *d.* When secondary infection has disappeared the mechanical treatment should be undertaken. Nothing can replace this. Expression with one of the specially designed instruments for this purpose should be done; all follicles should be squeezed out and in severe cases treatment with carbon dioxide can be tried. In the very worst cases excision of some of the conjunctiva at the fornix may be indicated.
- *e.* Pannus does not require treatment in the ordinary way, but if any is indicated peritomy may be undertaken and the vessels destroyed by the cautery just behind the limbus to cut off their blood supply.
- *f.* When the cornea is involved gutt. atropin. 1 per cent should be used.
- *g.* In severe and late cases with gross lid deformities, plastic surgery and such operations as tarsectomy will be required. The student is referred to textbooks on eye surgery for details.

5. **Spring Catarrh:** This is a rare complaint and its chief symptom is a persistent conjunctivitis which recurs each year in the early summer and persists through the hot months. It regresses as soon as the cooler weather comes. It is a disease of young people, affecting boys much more often than girls, and there may be much burning and irritability of the eyes. There are two chief types: (*a*) the tarsal type; (*b*) the bulbar type.
- *a.* The tarsal conjunctiva covering the upper lid is seen on eversion to be thickened and areas of hypertrophy resembling 'crazy paving' are seen. This must not be confused with the 'sago grains' of trachoma which are different in appearance and much smaller. The general colour of the tarsal conjunctiva suggests a 'milky' hue.
- *b.* Bulbar: This is not typical except at the limbus, where a circle of milky thickening is visible.

PATHOLOGY: The 'crazy paving' and limbal thickenings are both due to cellular infiltration and proliferation of connective tissue. Eosinophilia is present and eosinophil cells are found in the hypertrophied areas and in the conjunctival secretions. The milky appearance is due to hyaloid changes in connective tissue. The presence of eosinophils suggests an allergic origin.

TREATMENT:
   a. Dark glasses.
   b. Local prednisolone in ointment form usually gives prompt relief.
   c. Gutt. adrenalin. 1–1000 helps considerably.
   d. Some good results have been reported from radium treatment when given early in the year, but modern corticosteroid therapy is likely to render this unnecessary.

6. **Conjunctivitis due to Irritants:** Some patients have an idiosyncrasy to various drugs which in normal persons produce no adverse symptoms at all. In these cases there appears great swelling and redness of the lids, accompanied by a painful conjunctivitis. The area of the swelling is more or less confined to the lids and the orbicularis muscle, the remainder of the face being unaffected. The following drugs often cause this:
   a. Atropine.
   b. Pilocarpine.
   c. Eserine.
   d. Boracic—patients are often careless with this. A teaspoonful to a pint is the usual strength for ophthalmic purposes, but it is by no means uncommon for patients to use a tablespoonful to a teacup!

   In addition to the above drugs, there is a long list of allergic substances which can produce an irritant conjunctivitis, e.g. primulas (especially *Primula obconica*), exposure to horses, cats, etc.

   Finally, it must be remembered that the use of mascara on eyelashes often causes a very irritant reaction—sometimes when it has been used for years.

   Malingering is a not infrequent cause of chronic unilateral conjunctivitis. It is caused by putting some foreign substance (such as tobacco ash) into the conjunctival sac, usually at the lower fornix.

TREATMENT:
   a. Remove the cause. If this is atropine, try lachesine, duboisine, scopolamine, hyoscine or mydricaine instead.
   b. Local steroid drops to the conjunctiva and ointment to the surrounding skin are most helpful.
   c. Antihistamine drops such as Benedryl or Otrivine-Antistin are worth a trial.

DISEASES OF THE CONJUNCTIVA 19

d. Cremor zinci to the surrounding skin is a less expensive alternative to steroids.

OPHTHALMIA NODOSUM

This is due to irritation from the hairs of caterpillars and is, therefore, found in the summer months only. Small grey nodules are formed anywhere on the conjunctiva and on section these are found to consist of lymphocytes and giant cells surrounding a caterpillar hair. This condition can be accompanied by severe iridocyclitis if hairs enter the anterior chamber.

SYNDROME CONJUNCTIVITIS

In this section are included various syndromes in which chronic conjunctivitis is one of the main symptoms: (1) Parinaud's syndrome; (2) Sjögren's syndrome; (3) Reiter's syndrome.

1. **Parinaud's Syndrome:** Is usually uniocular. The patient runs a slight temperature and, in addition, there is a severe chronic conjunctivitis often with polypoid granulations resembling tuberculosis. There is enlargement of the pre-auricular and submaxillary glands. Its total duration is of about 4 months. The pathology of this condition is unproven. There are different theories: (1) a leptothrix, (2) a tuberculous infection and (3) a virus infection such as *Lymphogranuloma venereum*. Treatment is symptomatic.

2. Sjögren's Syndrome ('keratoconjunctivitis sicca')

'Never a tear bedims the eye.' BRET HARTE, *The Lost Galleon*

Keratoconjunctivitis sicca has been described for a number of years, but it is comparatively recently that Sjögren discovered that this was part of a much more complex and widespread syndrome. Broadly speaking, the symptoms consist of a drying up of most of the secretions of the body. The lacrimal glands are first affected and the conjunctivae and corneae become lustreless, dry and eventually resemble parchment. There is intense irritation of the eyes but no lacrimation. The nasal and buccal mucous membranes are dry and the tongue is red and cracked. Owing to lack of salivary secretion food cannot be swallowed without water. The voice becomes hoarse from dryness of the vocal cords and there is a harsh unproductive cough. Sometimes there is a complete achlorhydria, with consequent digestive complaints. The syndrome is much more common in women than men and is rarely seen in patients under 40 years of age. Most patients with Sjögren's syndrome suffer from chronic arthritis. A. Whaley and his colleagues at Glasgow have studied 171 cases. They report that 100 of these had rheumatoid or other arthritic conditions, 37 had enlarged salivary glands—usually the parotid. The mean age of the patient was 57 and 89 per cent were females. Many gave a history of increased fluid intake owing to 'dryness'. Artificial tears helped most.

PATHOLOGY: The essential lesion of Sjögren's syndrome is found in the lacrimal and salivary glands. These show round-celled infiltration, with connective-tissue formation which eventually invades the entire gland thus replacing the secreting acini. Glandular changes are present before the ocular symptoms commence.

TREATMENT: Is palliative only. No known treatment helps the glands.
  a. Seal off the puncta with the cautery to preserve the little moisture which is present.
  b. Frequent use of 'artificial tears' helps early cases.
  c. Hydrophilic (= soft) contact lenses give great relief if worn reasonably early in the disease.
  d. Sorsby recommends a daily dose of 300 mg of ascorbic acid.

3. Reiter's Syndrome: This is an uncommon disease characterized by the triad: urethritis, polyarthritis and conjunctivitis, accompanied by pyrexia. In a few cases iritis may develop late. The syndrome occurs chiefly in young male adults, but it is in no way connected with gonorrhoea. When conjunctivitis occurs during an attack of gonorrhoea the symptoms are very much more severe (*see* PURULENT CONJUNCTIVITIS). Reiter's syndrome is a much less serious illness and complete restitution to normality without corneal involvement is the rule. The total duration of the illness is 4–6 months, and the conjunctivitis is the first of the triad to clear up. The pathology is still uncertain but some authorities consider this may be a TRIC agent infection.

TREATMENT: Is symptomatic only. It is a self-limiting disease and does not respond to any known treatment. General or local chemotherapy is useless.

PEMPHIGUS OR ESSENTIAL SHRINKAGE OF THE CONJUNCTIVA

Pemphigus is a very rare disease of the conjunctiva. It commences with the appearance of vesicles (which are often present in the mouth, throat, and nose as well). These lesions cicatrize, causing a shrinkage of the conjunctiva, the disappearance of the fornices and the formation of symblepharon. Xerosis of the cornea is the ultimate result.

TREATMENT: Contact lenses with liquid paraffin sometimes help. Local corticosteroid treatment is indicated.

TUBERCULOSIS OF THE CONJUNCTIVA

This always was a rare disease and in these days when TB has almost disappeared from Great Britain it is very rare indeed. Some of its

DISEASES OF THE CONJUNCTIVA

manifestations are clinically difficult to diagnose from syphilis. It may occur in any of the following differing forms:
1. *Nodular*: The nodules sometimes resemble trachoma.
2. *Ulcerative*: The most common form. The usual position for the ulcer is on the palpebral conjunctiva.
3. *Cock's-comb*: Polypoid prolongations from the tarsal conjunctiva are sometimes produced by the frequent movement of the eyelids. Occasionally small pedunculated tumours are formed in this type.
4. *Lupus* of the conjunctiva occurs as an extension of lupus of the face.

The pre-auricular gland is almost always enlarged, but there is remarkable freedom from pain except in severe ulcerative cases. The patients are usually young adults.

PATHOLOGY: The lesion is very frequently a primary one and is due to local inoculation with the tubercle bacillus. Typical giant-cell systems are seen, and sometimes tubercle bacilli can be isolated from the scrapings.

TREATMENT must be drastic: (1) Excise where possible; (2) Failing this, curette and cauterize; (3) Treatment with isoniazid, PAS or other antituberculous antibiotic is essential.

CONJUNCTIVAL SARCOID

This is by no means uncommon. It is usually seen in the form of translucent nodules in the lower conjunctiva.

SYPHILIS OF THE CONJUNCTIVA

Rare. It occurs in two forms: (1) Primary chancre; (2) Gummatous ulceration. Both these forms resemble tuberculosis, but examination of the scrapings for spirochaetes and the Wassermann test will settle the diagnosis.

TULARAEMIA OF THE CONJUNCTIVA

Tularaemia of the conjunctiva is occasionally seen. It is spread from animals, especially rabbits, and is caused by *Brucella tularensis*. The signs are ulcers or nodules on the conjunctiva, enlarged pre-auricular glands, raised temperature and general debility. Diagnosis is confirmed by agglutination tests and the treatment is with streptomycin locally and generally.

DEGENERATIVE CHANGES

Pinguecula is the name given to small triangular nodules which are found in middle-aged people, especially in those patients who live an open-air and exposed life. These nodules occur on either side of the cornea, the base towards the cornea and the apex towards the palpebral angle. They are symptomless and require no treatment.

PATHOLOGY: Pingueculae consist of connective-tissue fibres showing hyaline changes and the formation of elastic fibres. The yellow

22 A SYNOPSIS OF OPHTHALMOLOGY

colour resembles fat but in fact none is present. The modern view is that they are a form of degeneration due to exposure to sunlight.

Pterygium: Duke-Elder considers pterygium to be an invasion of the cornea from the limbus due primarily to a degenerative process affecting the superficial layers of the stroma and Bowman's membrane. Fuchs considers it to be the continuation of a pinguecula which causes the conjunctiva to encroach on the cornea. The pterygium is a triangular or wing-shaped structure, its base directed towards the palpebral angle and its rounded apex towards the cornea. It occurs in middle life or later and is commonest in those engaged in exposed occupations or who have lived in the tropics. It causes no symptoms and is a serious complaint only when it invades the pupillary area, hence seriously interfering with vision.

PATHOLOGY: A pterygium consists of vascular connective tissue covered with conjunctival epithelium. As it advances the apex passes between the corneal epithelium and Bowman's membrane. This membrane is eventually damaged, causing permanent corneal scarring. It must be carefully distinguished from pseudo-pterygium, which is due to a fold of conjunctiva becoming adherent to a corneal ulcer; in these cases a probe can be passed beneath it, which is impossible in a true pterygium. Greer considers that UVL plays a major part in the causation, especially solar radiation when reflected from water, sand or snow.

TREATMENT: Unless the pupillary area is in danger of invasion it is best to do nothing. If treatment is indicated it must be operative. The head of the pterygium should be shaved off the cornea and the whole pterygium dissected towards its base and completely removed. The cut edges of healthy conjunctiva should be approximated. Care must be taken to ensure complete removal or a recurrence is inevitable.

CONJUNCTIVAL CYSTS

Except for small cysts due to dilatation of lymph space, conjunctival cysts are very rare in England. Implantation cysts can occur following injuries, and very rarely cysticerci or hydatids may be seen.

TUMOURS OF CONJUNCTIVA

Innocent Tumours:
1. DERMOIDS: These usually occur at the junction of the cornea and sclera and both these structures may be involved. A dermoid is an ovoid, flesh- or yellow-coloured tumour with a convex surface. They usually occur at the outer side and consist of fibro adipose tissue with epidermis, hair and sebaceous follicles. Sweat lacrimal glands and cartilage may also be present (Greer).

DISEASES OF THE CONJUNCTIVA

Removal should be undertaken, for, although innocent, it is very unsightly.
2. PIGMENTED NAEVUS: This is usually situated near the limbus and is light to dark brown in colour. It is freely movable with the conjunctiva.

Removal is advised, for there is always the risk of a pigmented tumour developing malignant changes.
3. GRANULOMATA: These usually occur as polypoid outgrowths from the site of a conjunctival wound, a chalazion, etc.

Snip off with scissors and touch the base with a cautery.
4. PAPILLOMATA: These may resemble cock's-comb tubercle. They are most frequent in the region of the caruncle or in the upper fornix.

Treatment as for granulomata.

Malignant Tumours:
1. MALIGNANT PAPILLOMA OF THE LIMBUS: This tumour is sessile and presents a 'raspberry' appearance. It is highly vascular and tends to invade the cornea and sclera, and eventually the globe. In its early stages it resembles an innocent tumour, but it soon becomes obviously malignant, invading the pre-auricular and submaxillary glands and eventually leaving secondary deposits in various parts of the body.
2. EPITHELIOMA: The limbus is the usual site for this growth as it is the junction between the epithelial surfaces of the conjunctiva and cornea and these growths show a preference for such junctions. This growth has a 'cauliflower' appearance and tends to ulcerate early. It infiltrates the cornea and sclera and eventually involves the globe. Glandular enlargement and secondary deposits follow.
3. SARCOMA: This is rare and usually originates from a pigmented naevus. It is most frequently situated at the limbus and is a pedunculated growth tending to cover the cornea, but not to infiltrate it. Secondary deposits are frequent.
4. RODENT ULCER (*see* DISEASES OF THE EYELIDS, p. 141): These may involve the conjunctiva by direct extension from the lids.

TREATMENT:
 a. If seen in an early stage local removal with a shaving of the underlying sclera is indicated. The base should be treated with radium.
 b. If the growth is moderately developed the eyeball should be removed.
 c. In advanced cases nothing but removal of the eyeball and exenteration of the orbit should be undertaken.

CONJUNCTIVAL WOUNDS

In the absence of infection conjunctival wounds heal rapidly. It is a safe rule to suture all except very minute wounds with fine silk. Foreign bodies should be removed and dirty or jagged edges trimmed and approximated as in the case of skin wounds; gutt. sulphacetamide 10 per cent or chloramphenicol 1 per cent should be applied, and no bandage.

CONJUNCTIVAL BURNS

Lime and Other Caustic Burns: Lime burns are the most common of the accidental burns but in these days of 'mugging' and other forms of violence, ammonia and acid burns are increasingly common. These cause great ocular damage by symblepharon or ulceration and necrosis of the cornea. All cases must be regarded with gravity and admission to hospital is advised.

TREATMENT: Cocainize first, then irrigate with normal saline or tepid water for 15 minutes followed by oc. chloramphenicol with hydrocortisone. To prevent symblepharon forming a well-greased glass rod should be swept round the fornices three times daily.

Chapter III

DISEASES OF THE CORNEA

Anatomy and Physiology: The cornea is a transparent structure forming a window in the most anterior portion of the sclerotic. It is somewhat elliptical in shape, with its longer axis horizontal. Its approximate measurements are 12 mm × 11 mm × 1 mm in depth. At its periphery the cornea is slightly overlapped by the sclerotic in the same way as a watch glass is overlapped by the rim. Section of the cornea reveals the following layers:

1. STRATIFIED EPITHELIUM.
2. BOWMAN'S MEMBRANE: A structureless but important membrane, since once it is destroyed regeneration never occurs and a permanent opacity results.
3. SUBSTANTIA PROPRIA: Although perfectly transparent, this consists of laminated fibrous connective tissue, microscopically almost exactly resembling the sclerotic.
4. DESCEMET'S MEMBRANE: This also is structureless.
5. ENDOTHELIUM: This is a single layer of cells which is prolonged backwards to cover the pectinate ligament and on to the iris. It is owing to this continuity that pathological processes in the deeper layers of the cornea tend to spread and lead to such complications as iritis, iridocyclitis and even choroiditis.

Since the healthy cornea is completely avascular, its nutrition is carried out by diffusion from the vascular arcades at the limbus. Owing to this rather inadequate blood supply, the cornea possesses a unique respiratory mechanism whereby oxygen passes through the cornea in one direction only from the air to the anterior chamber, and the carbon dioxide similarly travels in the reverse direction only. The epithelium and endothelium, by some method unknown, effect this interchange of gases, which is known as transpiration.

Pathology: Owing to continuity of tissue, spread of disease from other ocular tissues to the cornea and vice versa is comparatively common, e.g. conjunctival phlyctens near the limbus can cause a localized keratitis; and similarly deep corneal injuries and infections can spread by the endothelium to the uveal tract. Hence the importance of using atropine in these circumstances, as every such case is a potential iritis patient; also it must be remembered that the bacteriology of the cornea is exactly the same as that of the conjunctiva (*see* p. 8), hence pathogens are not infrequently present.

THE USE OF EYE DROPS: In view of the delicate nature of the eye tissues and the presence of organisms in the conjunctival sac, it follows that it is easy to spread infection from eye to eye by the careless use of drops. An annotation in the *Br. med. J.* (1959), **1**, 1028, sums up the situation in these words: 'Infections carried to the eye from drops used in ophthalmic out-patient departments is a chronic problem with acute recrudescences.' All drops used should be sterile, especially when there is a break in epithelium due to trauma, ulceration, etc. Unfortunately this ideal is not easy to attain. It is simple enough to get a perfectly sterile bottle of drops but with the removal of the stopper and the use of a dropper only the first dose is really sterile. Happily it is now possible to get ophthalmic drops in single-dose containers. Messrs. Smith & Nephew have produced these in the form of MIMIMS in which the drops, container and applicator unit give guaranteed sterility and are discarded after use. These are a boon in the outpatient department and the general practitioner's surgery. The range available as MIMIMS include all mydriatics, miotics, local anaesthetics, that are likely to be required. In addition sulphonamides, neomycin, fluorescein, castor oil and sodium chloride can be obtained in MIMIM form.

CORNEAL OPACITIES: There are three degrees of opacities: (1) Nebulae; (2) Scars; (3) Leucomata.

These three differ in degree only, varying from a faint clouding effect imperceptible to the naked eye, to a dense thick white mass completely preventing any rays of light from entering the eye. If the lesion is epithelial only, complete regeneration takes place and a perfect visual result can be expected. If, however, the lesion extends to Bowman's membrane or deeper, a greater or lesser degree of permanent opacity results. Broadly speaking, the deeper the destruction of tissue the denser and more permanent is the resulting opacity. Many opacities tend to improve with the lapse of time, and this is specially true in the case of young people and those cases which are accompanied by vascularization.

CORNEAL VASCULARIZATION: Although the normal cornea contains no blood vessels, in certain conditions vascularization from the periphery may take place. This invasion by blood vessels takes place at the level of the lesion in the tissue, i.e. a superficial lesion may cause vascularization at the level of Bowman's membrane, or a deep one may cause vessels to appear deep in the corneal substance. Superficial vessels tend to branch dendritically and the deeper ones dichotomously. Superficial vascularization occurs in any case of superficial keratitis, e.g. corneal ulcer, acne rosacea, phlyctenular disease, trichiasis, etc., whereas a deeper vascularization is more commonly seen in interstitial or tuberculous keratitis and other diseases which tend to involve the uveal tract. When corneal vascularization is accompanied by the formation of granulation tissue, it is called a 'pannus'.

CORNEAL OEDEMA: Any of the following conditions may cause increase in the normal fluid content of the cornea: (1) Trauma; (2) Inflammation; (3) Increase of intra-ocular pressure.

1. TRAUMA: Normally the epithelium and endothelium are impervious to fluids. In the case of trauma of either of these layers fluid may enter the corneal substance and oedema result.
2. INFLAMMATION: In nearly all acute corneal inflammations oedema occurs early. It may be a localized oedema in the form of vesicles or bullae, or it may consist of a widespread 'bedewing' involving the whole of the cornea.
3. INCREASED INTRA-OCULAR PRESSURE: In these cases fluid is forced into the substance of the cornea by the abnormally high pressure. As soon as the pressure is relieved the cornea returns to normal, with an enormous improvement in the visual acuity.

Classification: Diseases of the cornea can be conveniently grouped under the following headings: (1) Ulcerations; (2) Infiltrations; (3) Virus diseases; (4) Degenerations; (5) Dystrophies; (6) Congenital abnormalities; (7) Wounds; (8) Burns.

I. ULCERATIONS

1. **Simple Corneal Ulcers** are by far the most common of all corneal diseases and are almost always of exogenous origin. In view of the high bacterial content of the normal conjunctival sac, it is rather remarkable that corneal ulceration does not occur more often. This is explained by two facts: (1) the corneal epithelium is very resistant to infecting organisms and (2) the antibacterial content of the lysozyme in the tears is moderately high.

   Corneal ulceration is liable to result if the epithelium is damaged by trauma or its resistance lowered by drying (xerosis), exposure (neuroparalytic keratitis) and desquamation (too frequent use of cocaine or similar drops).

   SIGNS AND SYMPTOMS: During the active stage of a corneal ulcer there is intense pain, lacrimation and photophobia. Toxins reach the intra-ocular fluid in the anterior chamber, causing iris inflammation, ciliary congestion and, in the worst cases, the pouring out by the iris vessels of leucocytes into the anterior chamber, forming a hypopyon (*see below*). The symptoms last for a number of days (or weeks in the absence of proper treatment), after which healing takes place, leaving some degree of opacity. Other cases may progress and lead on to perforation, with all the dire consequences involved.

It should be remembered that a corneal ulcer is not always easily seen and may be confused with a pre-existing scar. This mistake need never be made if the cornea is 'stained' in the following manner: (1) Instil a drop of 2 per cent fluorescein. (2) Immediately wash this out with a little water or normal saline. If an active ulcer is present it will stain a brilliant green. If there is no staining, no ulcer is present.

PATHOLOGY: A corneal ulcer is saucer shaped, with its edge somewhat swollen and oedematous. It may vary in depth from just the epithelial layers to almost the whole corneal thickness. Necrosis of the base takes place and the surrounding area is packed with leucocytes. When healing takes place vessels grow in from the limbus and the neighbouring epithelium, covering the floor of the ulcerated area. Although at first slightly depressed, this area is lifted eventually to the normal level by multiplying spindle cells.

TREATMENT:
- *a.* Heat in the form of hot bathing with a wooden spoon draped with cotton-wool is helpful when there is much pain. Alternatively, rubber hot-water bottles can be applied to the affected eye with the lid closed.
- *b.* Gutt. atropin. 1 per cent should be instilled twice a day, as every corneal ulcer is a potential case of iris inflammation.
- *c.* Local antibiotics such as ung. chloramphenicol should be used.
- *d.* If the condition hangs fire, local steroid therapy combined with antibiotics may be tried. Steroid therapy must be used with caution and rather as a last resort since there is a risk of delaying fibrosis necessary for healing.
- *e.* A flap (*not* a close-fitting shade) should be worn to exclude the light, or the patient may wear dark glasses.
- *f.* Attention should be paid to the patient's general health, and particularly to any disorder tending to lower the resistance of the cornea.

COMPLICATIONS OF CORNEAL ULCERS.
- *a.* HYPOPYON: In discussing the signs and symptoms of corneal ulcers it was mentioned that in the worst cases toxins from the ulcer enter the anterior chamber and cause hyperaemia of the iris and a large-scale migration of leucocytes from the iris and ciliary body into the anterior chamber. These gravitate to the bottom forming a fluid level which varies according to the position of the head. A hypopyon may be of any degree of severity from an almost invisible yellow line at the bottom of the cornea to a complete filling of the anterior chamber. The usual level is about one-third of the way up the iris. Sometimes a thin fibrinous exudate remains and may result in an adherent leucoma, ring synechiae, and occlusion of the pupil.

DISEASES OF THE CORNEA

Pathology: The following points should be remembered:
  i. A hypopyon is always sterile. It is therefore not produced by bacteria spreading inwards from the ulcer. The impermeability of Descemet's membrane renders this impossible anyhow.
  ii. It is produced by the action of irritant toxins which cause an effusion of leucocytes as described above. Pigment has been found in some cases, proving the uveal origin of these cells.
  iii. In many hypopyon ulcer cases the invading organism is the pneumococcus or *Ps. pyocyanea*, the most serious of all eye infections.

Treatment:
  i. Hypopyon is a very serious disease and should always be treated in hospital.
  ii. Since hypopyon is sterile, evacuation is unnecessary.
  iii. Gutt. atropin. 1 per cent three times a day should be instilled.
  iv. General chemotherapy or penicillin treatment sufficient to keep a reasonably high blood concentration should be given in all severe cases, and a broad-spectrum antibiotic such as chloramphenicol should be instilled in the eye at frequent intervals.
  v. Broad-spectrum antibiotics, preferably Soframycin, should be applied locally at 1-hourly intervals and if *Ps. pyocyanea* is suspected, Soframycin must be given.
  vi. When the infection is under control with antibiotics, local steroids can be used in addition.
  vii. If these measures fail and if the tension is raised, paracentesis or Saemisch's section should be considered.

b. ECTATIC SCAR: Sometimes an ulcer may increase greatly in depth and during the process of healing the cornea may become so thin that it is unable to stand the normal intra-ocular pressure, and a permanent bulge results. Rarely the ulcer extends, involving the whole corneal thickness except Descemet's membrane (which is very resistant to infection). In such a case a watery bleb called a *keratocele* (or *descemetocele*) appears on the cornea. Such a condition may be present for some time but eventually ruptures and may leave a corneal fistula.

c. PERFORATION: It is easy to imagine what happens when this occurs. There is a sudden fall to zero of the intra-ocular pressure and a consequent rush of intra-ocular fluid to escape. As this rush occurs the iris and the lens are pushed forwards in contact with the back of the cornea. Part of the iris may even prolapse, and the lens may be dislocated if the pressure was very high.

30 A SYNOPSIS OF OPHTHALMOLOGY

Result: The immediate effect of perforation on the ulcer is good and the lessening of the intra-ocular pressure permits a freer flow of lymph through the corneal tissues, with consequent improvement in its nutrition and powers of resistance. The ulcer may heal very rapidly. It is, however, the remote effects of perforation that make it an extremely serious complication. These effects may be as follows:

   i. *Prolapse of Iris*: The more rapid the escape of intra-ocular fluid the more likely is the iris to be carried into the wound. The prolapsed portion of iris becomes acutely inflamed, is covered with lymph and eventually becomes overgrown with epithelium. Contraction tends to draw up the iris against the back of the cornea.
   ii. *Anterior Staphyloma*: This is the end-result of the pressure just described. The staphyloma is not the cornea but is a bulging scar consisting of iris partly converted into scar tissue and covered with corneal epithelium.
   iii. *Anterior Synechiae* may be formed by the iris becoming adherent to the posterior corneal surface. This often seals off the perforation and allows the anterior chamber to re-form.
   v. *Anterior Capsular Cataract*: If the perforation is central and the lens comes into contact with the ulcer for any length of time a localized central cataract results. This is not a lenticular opacity but a proliferation of the subcapsular epithelium due to its contact with the inflamed cornea.
   v. *Corneal Fistula* is a rare result. The track may become lined with epithelium.
   vi. *Intra-ocular Haemorrhage*: The sudden diminution of the intra-ocular pressure may cause a rupture of any of the vessels in the eye, causing choroidal or vitreous haemorrhage. This may sometimes be profuse enough to expel the contents of the globe.
   vii. *Purulent Iritis* or even panophthalmitis may result if the organism causing the ulcer reaches the interior of the eye.

2. Ulcus Serpens: This is the name given to a characteristic type of ulcer which tends to spread across the cornea in a serpiginous manner. It is often due to the pneumococcus and is accompanied by a marked iritis and usually a hypopyon. There is great pain and marked ciliary injection. Its advancing edge is crescentic in shape and it tends to progress across the cornea, increasing both in area and depth. Perforation is a very common occurrence.

TREATMENT: As for hypopyon, with special emphasis on carbolization of the ulcer. Saemisch's section is sometimes necessary in unresponsive cases.
3. **Phlyctenular Ulcer:** Very commonly occurs as a grey nodule near the limbus. It has already been given a detailed description under DISEASES OF THE CONJUNCTIVA, but when phlyctenular disease affects the cornea the following clinical types can be seen:
   a. FASCICULAR ULCER, which starts at the limbus and sweeps across the cornea, leaving a leash of vessels in its train.
   b. INFILTRATING PHLYCTEN when the deep corneal layers become involved.
   c. MULTIPLE PHLYCTENS, very small in size and always around the limbus.
   d. RING ULCER, when multiple phlyctens coalesce.

   Severe phlyctenular ulceration causes a marked pannus affecting any part of the cornea. There is reasonable hope of phlyctenular pannus regressing and eventually disappearing. For pathology and treatment, *see* PHLYCTENULAR CONJUNCTIVITIS, p. 12.
4. **Marginal Ulcer:** Although this occurs at the limbus, it is in no way connected with phlyctenular disease, being most frequently seen in old people and often associated with debility, rheumatism, etc. Its treatment in no way differs from that of simple ulcer. This type of ulceration is said frequently to be caused by the Morax–Axenfeld bacillus.
5. **Mooren's Ulcer:** This is a rare and serious ulcer occurring in elderly people, tending to run a prolonged course, and spreading over the entire cornea. It advances with a characteristic overhanging edge and leaves marked vascularization in its wake. It may last for many months, but scarcely ever perforates or forms a hypopyon. It is accompanied by a low-grade iritis. The cause is unknown, but its effects on vision are dire in the extreme, especially since 25 per cent of cases are bilateral.

   TREATMENT: In addition to the usual treatment for corneal ulcers, the following measures may be taken:
   a. Removal of the overhanging edge; this is essential.
   b. Cauterization with the electric cautery.
   c. Covering with a conjunctival flap or a tarsorrhaphy.
   d. Radium treatment (beta rays) in severe cases.

   The results are often disappointing.
6. **Neuroparalytic Ulcer:** This condition can develop as the result of Gasserian ganglion lesions, including surgery of the ganglion. It is very rarely seen as a complication of fractured skull and of intracranial tumours. The cornea becomes anaesthetic, hence reflex blinking no longer occurs and small foreign bodies remain unnoticed. In this way the resistance of the cornea is lowered and

pathogenic organisms multiply. The epithelium desquamates and there is great liability to involvement of the corneal stroma, which breaks down and ulcerates. There is no pain in these cases for the cornea is anaesthetic, but there is a real risk of perforation and of gross corneal scarring.

TREATMENT: It is of prime importance to keep the eye protected, hence tarsorrhaphy is indicated in the first instance. This often causes a marked improvement and it is nearly always possible to instil atropine or other drops near either canthus if the tarsorrhaphy is a median one.

7. **Exposure Keratitis:** This can occur whenever a condition arises which prevents the lids from covering the cornea. It is most frequently seen in severe exophthalmos in Graves' disease, orbital tumours, exophthalmic ophthalmoplegia, facial paralysis, etc. The treatment is the same as that outlined for neuroparalytic ulcers.

Dendritic Ulcer is discussed under VIRUS DISEASES (p. 35).

II. INFILTRATIONS

It must be realized that the distinction between infiltrations and ulcerations is somewhat artificial, because it is not always possible to say where the one begins and the other ends. In the following diseases the main sign found is a deep infiltration, but ulceration may be present as well.

1. **Acne Rosacea:** This disease usually affects women in the 45–65 years age group. Many patients develop an infiltrating keratitis with much lacrimation and mucopurulent conjunctival discharge. Grey-coloured isolated patches of infiltration occur. These sometimes break down and form small ulcers. Often iritis is present as well. These cases always run a chronic course, and there is a marked tendency for relapses to occur.

    TREATMENT:

    a. General and local treatment for the skin condition is essential, and the patient should consult a dermatologist. Without the skin treatment, local treatment of the eye is of little avail and even with adequate general and skin treatment some cases are inclined to be intractable.

    b. The most helpful treatment is local corticosteroids. Many cases respond dramatically when treated in this way.

    c. X-ray treatment has been of advantage in some of the worst cases, but such treatment is rarely called for since the introduction of corticosteroids.

    d. Tarsorrhaphy should be undertaken if the disease is inclined to get out of control.

2. **Keratitis Profunda:** A deep infiltration of unknown pathology. It usually occurs after trauma, exposure and other causes which lower

the resistance of the cornea. It consists of a central opacity composed of irregular striations and it tends to improve spontaneously, but may leave some degree of permanent opacity.

TREATMENT: Local steroid therapy is worth a trial.

3. **Disciform Keratitis:** This is a central grey infiltration in the middle layers of the corneal stroma. It is nearly always unilateral. It often has a 'target' appearance with a very dense 'bull's-eye'. Sometimes it is associated with a small hypopyon. It runs a chronic course without very much irritation, but it always leaves a permanent opacity with corresponding visual impairment. It is not amenable to treatment.

PATHOLOGY: Uncertain, but there are two theories:
  a. It may be a virus infection, probably a late stage of superficial punctate keratitis, or herpes corneae.
  b. Some authorities think it is due to neuroparalytic changes in the fifth nerve.

Both these theories, however, must be regarded as unproven.

4. **Interstitial Keratitis:** The name given to a deep and vascularizing keratitis due to congenital syphilis. It is a disease of childhood, usually appearing between the ages of 5 and 15.

SIGNS AND SYMPTOMS: The first symptom is irritation, lacrimation and photophobia, with marked conjunctival inflammation and ciliary congestion. At this stage a few greyish areas of infiltration may appear anywhere in the cornea, and these areas tend to coalesce until the whole cornea appears to be affected. After a few weeks the cornea may resemble 'ground glass' and sometimes becomes so opaque that a view of the iris is difficult or impossible. While these changes are going on, vascularization of the grey areas occurs, giving the appearance of 'salmon pink' patches. In severe cases the vascularization extends almost to the centre of the cornea. After the peak of the disease is reached the cornea begins to clear from the periphery inwards, and as the haziness clears up the vessels become obliterated, but they can always be seen by the slit-lamp as grey lines tending to run radially. If this picture is found it is a positive proof of the presence of congenital syphilis. The disease is always bilateral, but there is often a lapse of a few weeks before the second eye is affected. The acute stage may last for months. Rarely a unilateral interstitial keratitis occurs in adults, and still more rarely interstitial keratitis may occur as a manifestation of acquired syphilis.

PROGNOSIS: Interstitial keratitis shows a marked tendency to improvement, and this must always be borne in mind when treating what might well appear to the uninitiated to be a hopeless case. It is not uncommon in the acute stage for the vision to be down to hand movements only, but when complete recovery occurs it may be 6/18 or even 6/12. Not every case runs this favourable course. In some, a marked permanent opacity remains with great impairment of vision. The point to be remembered is that no given case should be regarded as hopeless until eighteen months or two years have elapsed. In slight cases there may be no visual disability remaining. Patience is necessary, for the process of improvement may take a very long time.

PATHOLOGY: The cornea in interstitial keratitis is not the real seat of the disease. The condition is really an anterior uveitis affecting the iris, ciliary body and choroid—hence posterior synechiae and 'KP' are present, but these are not apparent clinically until the keratitis begins to subside, for the corneal infiltration prevents a good view of the inner structures of the eye. Interstitial keratitis should always be thought of as an anterior uveitis with corneal manifestations. The parts of the cornea most infiltrated are the deeper layers just anterior to Descemet's membrane.

AETIOLOGY: Girls are affected more often than boys, and nearly all cases, as previously stated, are due to congenital syphilis. The following additional stigmata of syphilis should be looked for:

a. Flatness of the nose.

b. Deafness.

c. Hutchinson's teeth. The two upper central incisors of the permanent dentition are deformed. There may be a central notch and the teeth may be peg-shaped and unduly small. The milk teeth are not affected.

d. Glandular enlargement, especially in the posterior triangles of the neck.

e. The limbs should be examined for periosteal nodules and synovitis of joints.

The Wassermann reaction will settle the diagnosis.

Note: It must be remembered that very rarely a tuberculous iritis may be associated with a keratitis closely resembling interstitial keratitis.

TREATMENT:

a. Antisyphilitic treatment is most disappointing in interstitial keratitis and does not influence the course of the disease owing to the non-vascularity of the cornea.

b. Atropine treatment should be started at the earliest moment and persisted in throughout the duration of the disease.

c. Local steroid treatment is invaluable and often results in improvement that is little short of dramatic. It should be started at the earliest moment and continued until long after the eye is white.

d. Hot bathing or short-wave diathermy is helpful if there is pain during the acute stages.

e. Dark glasses are essential.

DISEASES OF THE CORNEA 35

 f. Everything possible for the general health of the patient should be done—good food, vitamins, fresh air, etc.

 g. Late visual defects due to corneal scarring may be improved with contact lenses or corneal grafting but there is often an associated chorioretinitis.

5. **Filamentary Keratitis:** This is not strictly an infiltration of the cornea. During the course of a superficial keratitis dying filaments, consisting of shreds of epithelium, become partly detached from the cornea. Movement of the lids causes these movable shreds to become elongated while still remaining attached at one end. A fully developed filament resembles a minute tadpole with the tail attached and the head free. The condition is found in subsiding corneal oedema and in any condition which has produced a drying or desquamation of the cornea. It can be intensely irritating.

 TREATMENT: Local removal of the filaments wherever possible and carbolization of their bases of attachment is recommended. Atropine should be used and dark glasses worn while the eye remains irritable. Local steroid therapy can be tried.

III. VIRUS DISEASES

There are five types of virus infection of the cornea: (1) Herpes febrilis; (2) Dendritic ulcer; (3) Superficial punctate keratitis; (4) Herpes ophthalmicus; (5) TRIC.

1. **Herpes Febrilis:** In this disease, tiny vesicles form on the cornea. It is commonly seen in febrile conditions or even after a severe common cold. The vesicles vary in size from the point to the head of a pin, and are often placed in groups. They rupture, but usually heal spontaneously without scar formation, although successive crops may appear and in the more severe cases they may break down and form a dendritic ulcer *(see below)*. The condition is usually unilateral and accompanied by much irritation, lacrimation and photophobia.

 PATHOLOGY: The essential lesion of herpes febrilis lies in the nuclei of the epithelial cells. These are swollen and the chromatin fibrils run together and adhere to the thickened nuclear membrane. Eosinophil bodies appear first in the nucleus and later in the cytoplasm as well. The nucleus breaks down and so does the whole cell after swelling and vacuolation (Wolff).

2. **Dendritic Ulcer:** The advanced stage of herpes febrilis of the cornea. The vesicles have broken down and tiny ulcers appear. These are so small that in the early stages they are difficult to detect. They spread dendritically, and on staining give a characteristic appearance, branching in any or all directions. It is a very painful condition with much lacrimation and photophobia, and in the absence of proper treatment tends to last for weeks or even months, and to produce dense scarring. It is believed that in some untreated cases the deeper

corneal tissues become involved leading eventually to disciform keratitis (q.v.).

TREATMENT:

a. Atropine 1 per cent in oil twice a day should be used.

b. In superficial lesions, the use of 5-iodo-2'-deoxyuridine (IDU) gives dramatic improvement. The drops, however, have the disadvantage of requiring frequent application and do not remain stable above a temperature of 40 °F. MacKenzie of Manchester considered his results with this treatment to be less favourable than those obtained by carbolization. This view is shared by Davidson and Jameson-Evans of Birmingham, who found iodization the most helpful treatment. IDU is now available in ointment form 0·25 per cent or 0·50 per cent.

c. Attention should be paid to the general health and some surgeons have found salicylates helpful; also full doses of vitamin C 1 g daily.

d. Dendritic ulcer is a positive indication for cauterization, which may be done with carbolic, iodine or even the electric cautery if the other two fail. The importance of cauterization cannot be too strongly stressed, for the majority of cases respond very quickly, but if not undertaken the ulcer may go on branching and lead eventually to an opaque cornea. Cryogenic cauterization of the ulcer by means of an applicator frozen with solid carbon dioxide or liquid nitrogen has given good results according to Krwawicz of Lublin.

e. Steroid therapy is generally regarded as contra-indicated, but the authors have tried it in several unresponsive cases with encouraging results. It must, however, be used with caution and reserved for exceptional cases.

f. One of the authors (C. M.-D.) has used alphachymotrypsin drops in resistant cases with encouraging results, but some American observers state that in experimental lesions in rabbits this treatment is harmful. More work remains to be done in this field.

g. Cryotherapy is a recent treatment that promises a reasonable proportion of success.

3. Superficial Punctate Keratitis: An infrequent form of virus infection. It commences as a painful acute conjunctivitis, during the course of which groups of raised grey dots appear towards the centre of the cornea. These remain unchanged for some weeks, but tend to spontaneous resolution eventually. A few cases, however, are said to develop into disciform keratitis. The disease is usually unilateral, liable to attack young people, and associated with pain and lacrimation. Some eventual visual defect is common. It occurs in epidemic form in some hot climates, especially in India.

TREATMENT: As for dendritic ulcer, but there is no need for cauterization.

4. **Herpes Ophthalmicus:** This is a disease of middle-aged or elderly people, and in a surprising number of cases there is a history of contact with chicken-pox. One or more branches of the ophthalmic division of the fifth nerve are affected. The disease is unilateral and is accompanied by malaise, fever and much pain. The pain follows the course of the nerve so typically that it is often possible to diagnose herpes ophthalmicus before the skin eruption appears. Shortly after the onset of the pain skin vesicles appear as in herpes zoster in other parts of the body. The skin over the affected areas is swollen and erysipeloid. Vesicles appear, which often suppurate leaving depressed scars. Some anaesthesia of the skin area is often present. When these symptoms begin to subside the eye troubles appear. Tiny spots appear on the cornea, which soon develops a deep-seated infiltration, and a troublesome and persistent iridocyclitis commences. The cornea is anaesthetic, and in rare cases a transient paralysis of one or more cranial nerves occurs, lasting for many weeks or even months. Severe pain may continue for a very long time after all the skin lesions have healed. In the elderly herpes ophthalmicus must be considered as a major illness. There are three serious manifestations of herpes ophthalmicus:

a. Iridocyclitis, with all its attendant risks, especially that of increased tension.

b. Anaesthetic cornea may persist for months, impairing its nutrition and rendering it liable to further damage by minute foreign bodies, abrasions, etc.

c. Corneal scarring may be severe and permanent.

PATHOLOGY: The headquarters of this disease is in the Gasserian ganglion itself. The virus spreads downwards from the Gasserian ganglion along one or more of the branches of the ophthalmic division of the fifth nerve. Section of the affected ganglion shows haemorrhages and thromboses similar to those found in the anterior horns of the spinal cord in cases of infantile paralysis. Serological evidence indicates that the zoster and varicella viruses are identical and there is considerable support for the view that zoster is a re-infection of a partially immune person by varicella virus which has remained dormant (Greer).

TREATMENT:
  a. Calamine lotion or similar application for the skin lesion.
  b. Physeptone or other analgesics may be necessary and morphine may sometimes be required for the relief of severe pain.
  c. Short-wave diathermy is often helpful.
  d. Atropine must be used to prevent synechiae.

e. In cases with marked corneal anaesthesia, tarsorrhaphy should be performed.
f. Antibiotic treatment is ineffective.
g. Steroid treatment is indicated in event of uveal complications.

5. **TRIC Agent Keratoconjunctivitis:** TRIC (name coined from the first letters of *TR*achoma *I*nclusion *C*onjunctivitis) agents belong to the *Chlamydia* group of virus which cause trachoma, 'inclusion' conjunctivitis and inclusion blenorrhea—a purulent conjunctivitis which occurs in the newborn between the fourth and tenth day. It can also occur as a follicular conjunctivitis in adults. TRIC agents also cause chronic inflammation in the cervix and urethra which can, in turn, infect the eyes. TRIC agent infections are sensitive to sulphonamides.

IV. DEGENERATIONS

There are eight principal degenerative conditions: (1) Band opacity; (2) Arcus senilis; (3) Arcus juvenilis; (4) Marginal atrophy; (5) Pannus degenerativus; (6) Fanconi's syndrome; (7) Saltzmann's nodular degeneration; (8) Wilson's disease.

1. **Band Opacity:** The name given to characteristic changes which appear in the interpalpebral gap of old, blind, shrunken eyes. These changes progress right across the centre of the cornea but leave the limbus moderately clear. It is due to hyaline degeneration followed by calcareous deposits. When fully developed, these deposits appear as a chalky band across the centre of the cornea. Malnutrition and exposure are the chief factors in the commencement of this degeneration. Rarely this condition may occur in younger persons with otherwise healthy eyes. This may be bilateral.

2. **Arcus Senilis:** This is the name given to a grey line of fatty degeneration which encircles the cornea just inside the limbus. It is $\frac{1}{2}$–1 mm broad and is separated from the limbus by a small area of clear cornea. Its presence is of no significance.

3. **Arcus Juvenilis:** Very rarely an exactly similar condition to arcus senilis is found in children. This, too, is without significance and requires no treatment.

4. **Marginal Atrophy:** A rare degeneration found in old people. A 'gutter' forms in the region of the arcus senilis, and if the gutter deepens ectasia will result and Descemet's membrane may rupture. The gutter is formed by the absorption of the fat present in the arcus senilis. The disease may be bilateral.

5. **Pannus Degenerativus:** This occurs in degenerate blind eyes and develops between Bowman's membrane and the epithelium. It is a granulation tissue which spreads inwards from the limbus, and at a later stage fibrous and hyaline changes occur and the epithelium becomes thickened. Bowman's membrane is completely destroyed.

DISEASES OF THE CORNEA

6. **Fanconi's Syndrome (Cystine Disease)**: This rare complaint is due to dysfunction of cystine metabolism which first manifests itself in infants about 9 months of age. The signs and symptoms are renal dwarfism associated with thirst, vomiting, glycosuria and photophobia. Cystine deposits occur in various organs of the body and they appear comparatively early in the disease in the eye. They may occur in the conjunctiva, the lens, the iris and especially the cornea. The lesions are usually too small to be seen with the naked eye, but are characteristic when viewed with the slit-lamp. Masses of tiny cystine crystals are seen in the corneal substance with the narrow beam. These sparkle like minute diamond studs with a powerful polychromatic lustre. Similar deposits are seen in the conjunctiva and lens, and when the iris is affected a particularly beautiful picture is seen, the iris glistening with tinsel-like crystals looking as though it had been decorated for a Christmas party. It may be mentioned that slit-lamp examination of infants is comparatively easy with the aid of rectal chloral hydrate. A similar disease occurs in young children. It is known as Lignac's disease.
   TREATMENT is by the injection of 200 000 units of calciferol per day.
   PROGNOSIS is not good, for the condition usually affects the kidneys and other organs.
7. **Salzmann's Nodular Degeneration**: Occurs in patients who have previously suffered from corneal disease. It consists of rounded areas of a bluish colour which appear in the superficial corneal layers involving Bowman's membrane. Lamella keratoplasty may be required.
8. **Wilson's Disease** is an inborn metabolic disorder of childhood. Copper deposits occur in the liver, kidneys, brain and corneae. The Kayser–Fleischer ring in the corneae is diagnostic of the disease: A complete brown ring at the corneal periphery in the situation of the common arcus senilis. 'Sun-flower' type of cataracts is sometimes seen. Diagnosis is confirmed by estimation of copper content of urine and serum.
   TREATMENT: J. M. Walshe has found that if treatment is started early and continued long enough, penicillamine causes the ocular signs to regress and the body stores of copper to become depleted. This alters the prognosis of what was previously a fatal disease.

V. DYSTROPHIES

Three varieties are described: (1) Epithelial (Fuchs); (2) Endothelial; (3) Familial.

1, 2. **Epithelial (Fuchs) and Endothelial**: These are uncommon and obscure conditions of a degenerative nature. They occur in elderly people and show a diffuse opacity of the cornea with some grey dots. The epithelium becomes oedematous and vesicles occur. It is probable that the essential lesion is an endothelial degeneration which permits access of the intra-ocular fluid to the corneal stroma; thus endothelial and epithelial dystrophies are really one and the same disease in different stages.

No treatment helps epithelial or endothelial dystrophies.

3. **Familial:** Nodular (Groenouw) and lattice-like (Biber) opacities appear bilaterally as a familial disease. Males are the usual victims and the trouble manifests itself at puberty. There is a very slow and progressive increase in the opacities, spreading over many areas, eventually leading to blindness.

Optical iridectomy can be performed if there is sufficient clear area of cornea left.

VI. CONGENITAL ABNORMALITIES

1. **Conical Cornea** is believed to be due to a congenital weakness which rarely manifests itself before puberty. The centre of the cornea is thin and bulges forwards to assume a cone-shaped appearance. This bulging causes marked myopia and a high degree of astigmatism, with consequent gross impairment of vision. Sometimes the bulging cornea pulsates with the arterial pulse, and this has been demonstrated on a Schiötz tonometer. In a suspected case of conical cornea examination should be made with the patient in profile, when the corneal protrusion often becomes obvious. Reflections seen in Placido's disc will be distorted if the cornea is conical. The condition is frequently bilateral, but one eye is usually more affected than its fellow.

PATHOLOGY: In the bulging area the cornea is thinned to about a quarter of its normal thickness and Descemet's membrane is either ruptured or absent. Slit-lamp examination shows a brown ring (Fleischer's ring) at the base of the cone. This ring is due to deposits of haemosiderin.

TREATMENT:
   a. In slight cases spectacles should be provided to correct the astigmatism and myopia, and periodic examinations made.
   b. In more severe cases contact lenses are an ideal treatment. These abolish the astigmatism and the visual result is often excellent. Unfortunately, it frequently happens that they cannot be worn for long at a time.
   c. Modern operative treatment consists in removing the entire central area of the cornea and replacing it with a penetrating donor graft (*see* p. 227).

2. **Megalocornea (and Keratoglobos):** A bilateral hereditary enlargement of the cornea which affects males only and, unlike buphthalmos, is not associated with increased tension or cupping of the disc. It is a congenital overgrowth and does not normally affect vision. No treatment is needed. This condition is sometimes associated with arachnodactyly.

VII. WOUNDS OF THE CORNEA

The treatment of corneal wounds depends upon three factors: (1) Extent of the wound; (2) Site of the wound; (3) Presence or otherwise of complications.

1. *Extent of the Wound* may vary from a puncture to a severe laceration involving the whole cornea and even extending to the sclera.
2. *Site of the Wound*: It is obvious that a central lacerated wound would produce a more severe visual impairment than one in which the pupillary area is left intact. Also, wounds that involve the corneoscleral junction, and especially any that extend to the ciliary body, are most serious from the point of view of sympathetic ophthalmia. This area is known as the 'danger area'.
3. *Complications*: The prognosis depends largely upon these. Iris prolapse may involve sepsis, which may spread throughout the eye, causing panophthalmitis, and a punctured lens in the vast majority of cases leads to serious loss of vision. However, very high velocity or hot foreign bodies tend to be sterile.

TREATMENT:

SMALL WOUNDS can be treated expectantly. Atropine and antibiotic ointment should be instilled into the eye. In very small wounds a miotic should be used (instead of atropine) to prevent iris prolapse.

WOUNDS INVOLVING IRIS PROLAPSE: In a large wound there are nearly always some complications, the commonest of all being iris prolapse. The prolapse should be excised and never replaced owing to the risk of carrying infection into the eye. If the iris is adherent to the posterior surface of the cornea an attempt should be made at freeing it with an iris repositor inserted through the corneal wound. Atropine and penicillin should be instilled.

WOUNDS INVOLVING THE LENS: These are dealt with under DISEASES OF THE LENS.

WOUNDS INVOLVING THE CORNEOSCLERAL JUNCTION:

1. Excise any prolapsed uveal tissue.
2. Suture the wound with an eyeless corneoscleral needle, suturing first the sclera and then the cornea.
3. Instil atropine and an antibiotic.

Great care must be taken to avoid vitreous loss, which is very common in these cases. It should always be remembered that this type of wound is liable to produce sympathetic ophthalmia in the uninjured eye. If after 10–14 days the injured eye does not appear to be settling down, and especially if any 'KP' occur, the eye should be excised forthwith. This is a complication that may arise following a perforating injury of the cornea in spite of the best treatment. Thanks to steroid therapy and modern suturing techniques this complication is less dreaded than formerly.

Panophthalmitis: Any severe corneal wound (including cataract sections) can lead to this extremely grave condition in which the eye becomes to all intents and purposes an abscess cavity which eventually forms granulation tissue and is vascularized from the choroidal vessels. Later on fibrosis takes place with consequent contraction and with the following results:

1. The retina becomes detached.
2. The choroid and ciliary body are detached and the latter no longer secretes intra-ocular fluid.
3. As the result of these changes the eye becomes shrunken and the condition known as 'phthisis bulbi' is apparent.
4. Calcified areas may appear, particularly in the cornea.
5. Actual bone formation sometimes occurs in old shrunken eyes.

Hypopyon ulcer can also result in panophthalmitis.

VIII. BURNS OF CORNEA

See CONJUNCTIVAL BURNS (p. 24).

Chapter IV

DRUGS AFFECTING INTRA-OCULAR MUSCLES

The ophthalmic surgeon is frequently called upon to prescribe drugs in order to dilate or constrict the pupils or to paralyse accommodation. Pupil dilators are called mydriatics. Pupil constrictors are miotics and those which paralyse accommodation are cycloplegics. All these drugs are to some extent interacting, e.g. pupil dilators cause some degree of paralysis of accommodation and the constrictors increase accommodation. These drugs act in different ways and are classified according to their action.

1. **Parasympatholytic Drugs:** These block the action of acetylcholine, thereby causing pupil dilatation by making it impossible for the sphincter muscle to contract. The characteristic example of this drug is atropine which is a very powerful dilator, slow in action but lasting a long time and causing complete paralysis of accommodation. Hyoscine and duboisine act similarly but are much less powerful. Homatropine is similar in action but transitory in effect and causes only partial paralysis of accommodation.

2. **Parasympathomimetic Drugs:** This group acts as parasympathetic stimulants, thus causing miosis. They act in one of two ways:
    a. CHOLINERGIC: These drugs stimulate the myoneural junctions thereby increasing the effect of acetylcholine. The characteristic example of this type is pilocarpine. Its action is not very long—about 3 hours.
    b. ANTICHOLINESTERASE: These drugs neutralize the enzyme cholinesterase which limits the action of acetylcholine. Eserine is the most used drug in this group. It is very powerful in action and can cause spasm of accommodation. Prostigmin has a similar action but is less powerful. DFP and phospholine iodide are also in this group.

3. **Sympatholytic Drugs:** These are not very frequently used. They produce miosis by antagonizing the sympathetic nerve-endings. The best examples of these drugs are priscol and ergotamine which are used for various purposes in ophthalmology, but their miotic action is only incidental.

4. **Sympathomimetic Drugs:** These act on the sympathetic at the myoneural junctions, producing a substance similar to adrenaline, which is eventually destroyed by enzymes. This type of drug either suppresses the enzyme or stimulates directly the myoneural junctions.

Drugs under this heading include adrenaline, epinephrine, ephedrine and phenylephrine. All these have a mydriatic action by stimulating the dilator muscle. Cocaine has a similar but much less marked action by preventing the destruction of adrenaline.

Chapter V

DISEASES OF THE UVEAL TRACT

ALTHOUGH the iris, ciliary body and choroid are each distinct anatomical entities, it is of utmost importance to remember that these structures bear a close and continuous relationship one with the other—hence the frequency with which we see an inflammation involving the whole of the uveal tract. If all pathological processes were visible to clinical examination it would probably be found that iritis never exists without cyclitis and vice versa, and whenever either of these conditions occurs, there is probably some choroiditis as well. The uveal tract, therefore, may be pictured as a continuous and uninterrupted tract extending from the pupil margin to the optic disc.

ANATOMY

The uveal tract is the middle vascular coat of the eye, internal to the sclerotic and external to the retina. It is composed of three parts: (1) Iris; (2) Ciliary body; (3) Choroid.

Iris: This is the most anterior portion of the uveal tract and is situated in contact with the lens capsule. Peripherally it is attached to the ciliary body and to the ligamentum pectinatum iridis. It separates the anterior from the posterior chambers of the eye. In its centre is a round diaphragm, the pupil. The anterior surface is coloured and the colour depends upon the amount of pigment present in the stroma. The iris shows the following layers from the front backwards:

1. Endothelium.
2. Stroma—consisting of connective tissue, pigment cells, blood vessels and nerves.
3. Muscular layer. Two muscles are seen: (*a*) The sphincter close to the pupillary margin; (*b*) The radial dilator fibres.
4. The pigment epithelial layer.

The Ciliary Body is an asymmetrical girdle. It is triangular in section with its apex towards the choroid and its base towards the centre of the cornea. Its outer edge is attached to the scleral spur and its inner edge lies just anterior to the equator of the lens. Its external surface is separated from the sclera by the perichoroidal space. Its interior surface faces the vitreous and is continuous with the internal surface of the retina, which ends in the scalloped margin, the 'ora serrata'. Posteriorly, next to the ora serrata, is a dark pigmented zone with narrow radial striae running from the ora serrata into the valleys between the ciliary processes. Anteriorly is the pars plicata, which is overlapped by the lens and continuous with the posterior surface of the iris. This has prominent pale radiating stripes, the ciliary processes, 70–80 in number, each measuring about 1–2 mm in length and $\frac{1}{2}$–1 mm in height. These ciliary processes are almost entirely vascular. The anterior surface of the ciliary body is hidden.

CILIARY MUSCLE: A few unstriped muscle fibres are found in the epichoroid near the equator. These increase greatly in the ciliary region both in number and size. Three distinct series of muscle fibres are present:
1. MERIDIONAL FIBRES lie most externally and are attached to the scleral spur—sometimes called the 'tensor choroideae'. When these fibres contract they pull on the scleral spur and exert a pumping action on the canal of Schlemm.
2. RADIAL FIBRES are internal and anterior. With them is the connective tissue forming the basis of the iris.
3. CIRCULAR FIBRES are inseparable from the radial ones. The ciliary muscle is well developed in hypermetropia and very feebly developed in myopia.

Choroid: The choroid is a highly vascular pigmented structure extending from the ora to the optic disc. It is separated from the sclera by the suprachoroidal lymph space. Internally, it is separated from the pigment epithelium by a structureless membrane. The choroidal blood vessels are largest externally and get smaller as they reach the inner layers, eventually forming a fine capillary network, the choriocapillaris. The function of the choroid is nutritive only.

Blood Supply: The blood supply of the posterior part of the uveal tract is through the short posterior ciliary arteries. The anterior part of the tract derives its supply from the anterior ciliary arteries and the two long posterior ciliary arteries. The ciliary body is supplied by the long posterior arteries which form a circle at the root of the iris, called the greater arterial circle of the iris. The anterior ciliary arteries reach the globe by the recti muscles passing through the sclera posterior to the corneosclerotic junction. These join the greater arterial circle of the iris just short of the pupil. The uveal venous blood returns by the vortex system of four large veins which are formed by the union of the many smaller choroidal veins.

Nerve Supply: The nerve supply of the uveal tract is by the long ciliary nerves which contain sympathetic fibres to supply the dilator muscle, and the short ciliary nerves which carry sensory fibres from the fifth nerve, also some fibres from the third nerve to the ciliary muscle and the constrictor pupillae. At this stage, the reader is advised to refresh his knowledge of the physiology of the intra-ocular muscles and the pharmacology of the chief drugs that act upon them (*see* p. 43).

DISEASES OF THE UVEAL TRACT

GENERAL REMARKS ON UVEAL INFLAMMATION

Before discussing diseases of the individual parts of the uveal tract it will be convenient here to consider some affections of the tract as a whole.

Views on the aetiology of uveitis have changed with the passage of time, but it must be admitted that even now the aetiology in the majority of cases is a matter of speculation. Towards the end of the past century, it was considered to be of chronic bacterial origin, e.g. tuberculous, gonococcal, syphilitic, etc., in spite of the fact that the bacteria were seldom if ever demonstrated. Early this century the concept of focal infection emerged and this was considered to be the causative factor. This theory, however, was never proved. More recently, with the advent of high-power magnification, viruses are under consideration and the past decade has seen the emergence of protozoan infections (such as toxoplasmosis) as the chief cause of posterior uveitis. It is now believed that an auto-immune or hypertensive allergic reaction is the most likely cause of many cases of anterior uveitis and that this may be a contributory factor in posterior uveitis also. This cannot be proved in many cases but it is the most likely theory so far advanced. There is a close association between uveitis and a number of articular or rheumatic diseases, e.g. Behçet's syndrome, Reiter's syndrome, Still's disease, spondylitis, etc. There is tremendous scope for research into the aetiology of uveitis.

Acute Suppuration: Acute suppuration of the tract may be either exogenous or endogenous. It starts in some part of the tract and spreads in all directions, eventually involving every structure of the eye, when the condition is known as 'panophthalmitis'.

SIGNS AND SYMPTOMS: In cases of trauma there is very severe pain in the region of the eye, with photophobia and lacrimation. Endogenous cases are often painless, unless the iris becomes inflamed or the tension rises. There is marked redness of the lids and chemosis of the conjunctiva, with marked ciliary injection. The cornea becomes hazy, the iris muddy, the intra-ocular fluid is cloudy, later frankly purulent. By this time, sight in the eye is lost and the purulent infection involves the vitreous, the eye thus becoming a bag of pus.

PATHOLOGY: Exogenous infections enter through perforated wounds, especially those which have a prolapsed iris, the vitreous acting as a culture medium. Endogenous infections are usually through the bloodstream in septicaemic conditions and occasionally by local spread from cellulitis of the orbit, meningitis, etc. In untreated cases the eyeball bursts and the pus escapes. There is an immediate relief from pain, but the final result is a small shrunken eye (or phthisis bulbi). Pneumococci are the commonest organisms found in this condition, and after this streptococci, staphylococci, *Esch. coli* and *Ps. pyocyanea*. Prognosis is bad, but in cases of frank suppuration sympathetic ophthalmia is very unlikely.

48 A SYNOPSIS OF OPHTHALMOLOGY

TREATMENT:
1. Energetic and immediate general and local antibiotic and/or chemotherapeutic treatment is indicated, the choice of drugs depending upon the causative organism.
2. Until the organism is isolated, subconjunctival injections of penicillin or framycetin should be given, a broad-spectrum antibiotic ointment instilled into the eye 1-hourly, and sulphonamide treatment given systemically.
3. Removal of a few minims of aqueous and its replacement with penicillin solution may be tried. This is best done with a fine hypodermic needle. It is, however, doubtful whether this is more effective than less drastic methods.
4. In hopeless cases intravitreous penicillin injections have been tried, but the published results are very unconvincing.
5. If the above methods fail evisceration of the eyeball should be undertaken. Enucleation in these cases involves an element of risk of spread of the infection to the meninges via the subdural sheath of the optic nerve.

Chronic Inflammation of the Uveal Tract: This group, for reasons which will be appreciated later, is best studied under the headings IRITIS. IRIDOCYCLITIS and CHOROIDITIS.

DISEASES OF THE IRIS

Acute Iritis:
PATHOLOGY: A brief review of the anatomical relations to the iris will throw much light upon the pathology of some of the complications which arise when the iris becomes inflamed. When this occurs its numerous blood vessels dilate and albuminous lymph is poured out. These changes result in a narrowing of the pupil due to irritation and spasm of the sphincter and a tendency for the iris to adhere to the lens capsule. At the same time, the albuminous lymph tries to make its way out of the anterior chamber via the filtration angle in the normal manner, but owing to its high viscosity it is more difficult for it to escape. The iris becomes full of sticky fluid, hence its movement is impaired and the pupil reaction is sluggish or abolished. Furthermore, the inflammation causes much pain and this tends to a reflex spasm of the sphincter muscle, which tends still further to contract the already small pupil. The presence of quantities of lymph permeating the iris causes an alteration in its appearance. The iris pattern, instead of being sharp and well defined, becomes blurred and 'muddy' in appearance, and the colour is seen to be of a somewhat different hue when compared with that of the unaffected eye.

Bearing in mind the continuity of the uveal tract, one would expect in cases of iritis to find some inflammation of the ciliary

DISEASES OF THE UVEAL TRACT

body (cyclitis) as well. Such indeed is the case, and this is evidenced by the 'ciliary flush' which is universally found. This is due to hyperaemia of the anterior ciliary vessels supplying the ciliary body, and when this sign is present it is proof of the presence of cyclitis. There is, of course, an accompanying congestion of the conjunctival vessels as well, but when ciliary flush is well defined it cannot be mistaken for mere conjunctivitis. It appears as a dusky red corona surrounding the limbus.

The more the ciliary body is involved the more fibrinous exudate is poured out. Inflammatory cells may make their appearance in the anterior chamber and form a hypopyon (without any corneal ulcer being present). If the exudate is exceptionally fibrinous, strands may appear in the front of the iris and they may even spread over and completely fill the pupil (occlusio pupillae). This fibrin may cause the posterior surface of the iris to adhere to the anterior lens capsule (posterior synechiae). In the most severe cases the whole pupil may become bound down to the lens capsule. This is known as 'ring synechiae' or 'seclusio pupillae'. It is a serious condition, for it prevents the intra-ocular fluid from circulating from the posterior chamber through the pupil to the filtration angle. The iris in these cases is ballooned forwards by the accumulation of fluid (iris bombé), and a serious secondary glaucoma results. In this condition the peripheral margin of the iris is in contact with the cornea, thus obliterating the filtration angle and the inflamed iris may adhere to the cornea at its periphery (peripheral anterior synechiae). In very severe cases the anterior endothelium of the iris may be shed, and pigment may wander from the epithelium. Sometimes the contraction of the exudates on the surface of the iris may cause the pigment epithelium to be pulled forwards over the pupil margin (ectropion uveae). Hyphaema may in rare cases occur spontaneously in severe iritis.

AETIOLOGY: The following factors often play a part in the causation of acute iritis:

1. SYPHILIS.
2. GONORRHOEA.
3. FOCAL SEPSIS.
4. TUBERCULOSIS.
5. DIABETES.
6. ANKYLOSING SPONDYLITIS.
7. RHEUMATISM.
8. BEHÇET'S SYNDROME.
9. TOXOPLASMOSIS (q.v.).
10. SARCOIDOSIS (q.v.).
11. ULCERATIVE COLITIS.

An endeavour should be made to exclude all these factors in any given case, but it must be admitted that in many cases all investigations made to exclude the above conditions have proved negative.

SIGNS AND SYMPTOMS: Severe pain in and around the eye, with photophobia and lacrimation. The conjunctiva is congested and ciliary flush is present. There is impairment of vision. There then appears the train of signs mentioned in the section headed PATHOLOGY: 'muddy' iris, sluggish pupil reaction, small irregular pupil, and in untreated cases all the pathological processes mentioned above, and the eye may finish up as a painful blind one due to secondary glaucoma. It will be convenient at this stage to consider the different types of iritis as outlined under the heading AETIOLOGY. Several of these have characteristic signs of their own.

1. SYPHILITIC IRITIS: This can be divided into two headings: (*a*) Congenital; (*b*) Acquired.

    a. Congenital: Iritis due to congenital syphilis is of two distinct clinical types. The commonest is that seen during an attack of interstitial keratitis (q.v.), which has already been dealt with under that heading. The second type is much rarer and appears to be present either at birth or very soon afterwards. It is the result of intra-uterine inflammation. In this condition, gummatous nodules may be present in the iris. Many of these cases are unilateral and it is supposed to be more common in females than in males.

    b. Acquired Syphilis: Iritis may occur in either the secondary or tertiary stages. Nodules sometimes appear at the pupillary or ciliary margins. They are usually multiple and about $\frac{1}{2}$–1 mm in diameter. Much lymph is present and synechiae occur in these gummatous cases. Areas of atrophy appear in the iris.

    Care must be taken not to confuse gummata with nodules due to tuberculosis, sarcoma or sarcoid. It must be remembered that sarcoma is nearly always a single tumour and that signs of iritis are absent in this condition. Furthermore, sarcoma of the iris is a very rare disease. The Wassermann reaction will settle the diagnosis.

2. GONOCOCCAL IRITIS: This is a blood-borne infection and usually occurs during or after an attack of gonococcal arthritis. So far as the eye signs are concerned it does not differ from any other iritis, but this particular type is very liable to recurrences and is nearly always bilateral.

3. IRITIS DUE TO FOCAL SEPSIS: Follows the same course as any other iritis. In every case when the aetiology is doubtful a careful watch should be made for a septic focus in some part of the

body. The teeth should be examined for pyorrhoea and if necessary the roots should be radiographed for absorption. Special care should be taken to exclude this in cases where crowned or dead teeth are present. After the teeth, a search should be made for sepsis in the tonsils, nasal sinuses, etc. Sometimes the focus may be found in the intestinal or genito-urinary tracts. If any possible source is found anywhere in the body, it should be removed if practicable.

4. TUBERCULOUS IRITIS occurs in two distinct clinical varieties: owing to diminishing incidence of TB these are rarely seen now:

   a. *Miliary Form*: In this type small yellow nodules appear which tend to congregate on either the pupillary or the ciliary margins of the iris, leaving the middle portion clear. 'KP' are usually present and a hypopyon of caseating tuberculous products may be found.

   b. *Conglomerate Form:* Here a large solitary yellowish tumour is seen which may resemble either gumma or sarcoma. The accompanying iritis is much less pronounced in this type than in the miliary one. In this form of tuberculosis the tumour tends to erode the cornea, which in due time collapses, leading to prolapse of the iris and loss of the eye. Wassermann reaction will exclude gummatous origin.

   In any possible cases of tuberculous iritis, tuberculin should be used with the greatest caution (if it is used at all), for a violent local and general reaction may be set up.

5. DIABETIC IRITIS: This is rare, but it has one almost diagnostic characteristic: the appearance of visible new vessels on the surface of the iris (diabetes rubeosis). Plastic exudates are always formed and occasionally a hypopyon, but on the whole the prognosis in treated cases is fair.

6. ANKYLOSING SPONDYLITIS is very frequently associated with iritis, as also are other forms of articular disease. It is a particularly frequent complication of cases of arthritis that are associated with non-specific conditions. Nearly one-third of these cases develop iritis.

7. 'RHEUMATIC' IRITIS: There is no doubt whatever that in a number of pathological eye conditions, and iritis among them, the so-called 'rheumatic diathesis' is a definite factor in their aetiology. In many cases where all the previously mentioned causes have been excluded, a careful inquiry into the history will reveal a story of attacks of chronic fibrositis, arthritis, gout, etc. The link between these rheumatic conditions and the iritis has yet to be discovered, but such a proportion of cases manifest the double symptoms that little doubt exists that there is a link. Possibly both conditions may have a common cause. 'Rheumatic'

iritis has no special clinical features to distinguish it from other types. The diagnosis is based on the history alone.

8. BEHÇET'S SYNDROME: A rare condition. The signs are buccal ulceration, followed by iritis with hypopyon. Work by Mortada and Imam in Cairo has proved this to be a virus infection of the neuro-epithelium of the iris, ciliary body and retina. The virus has been isolated from the anterior chamber from buccal and genital ulcers, also from the patient's blood during febrile stages.

9. TOXOPLASMOSIS: Recently recognized as the cause of some unexplained iritis cases. Retinal lesions are usually present, but the diagnosis depends upon serological investigations.

10. SARCOIDOSIS, *see* p. 58.

11. ULCERATIVE COLITIS is sometimes complicated by iritis.

TREATMENT: In considering this it is of utmost importance to bear in mind much of what has been written on the pathology of this condition. It will at once be evident that most of the serious after-effects and complications arise from one factor alone, viz. the tendency of the inflamed iris to cause adhesions. To combat this tendency is the chief aim of treatment. Unless full dilatation of the pupil can be obtained there will almost certainly be adhesions forming. The first and most important step in the treatment is:

1. Atropine, 1 per cent, either as drops or ointment three times a day, or even 4-hourly in severe cases. Atropine tends to produce a marked dilatation of the pupil and therefore often breaks down synechiae which have already formed, and it also tends to prevent the formation of fresh adhesions. Furthermore, atropine possesses another important property—it keeps the iris and ciliary body at complete rest. In addition, therefore, to the important function of breaking down adhesions it gives the internal muscles of the eye some degree of freedom from movement in the same way that a splint gives rest to skeletal muscles. As previously mentioned in the chapter on DISEASES OF THE CONJUNCTIVA, atropine sometimes produces a severe and unavoidable irritation in certain persons who have an idiosyncrasy to the drug. If this occurs it should be replaced by lachesine 1 per cent, scopolamine 1 per cent or duboisine 1 per cent. Mydriatic treatment should be continued until the eye is white and all symptoms have gone. This may take weeks or even months.

2. If atropine fails to dilate the pupil, subconjunctival injection of 4 minims of mydricaine is sometimes effective.

3. Local steroid therapy is often remarkably effective in reducing the intra-ocular inflammation and preventing the more serious

DISEASES OF THE UVEAL TRACT

complications. It is best given locally as ointment, or by subconjunctival injection. If the response is delayed, prednisolone tablets should be given internally. Corticosteroids are of doubtful value in chronic cases.

4. Heat, either dry or wet, in the form of short-wave diathermy, electric pad, rubber hot-water bottles, hot saline bathing or hot fomentations should be applied frequently in the acute and painful stage.
5. Analgesics or narcotics may be given if required.
6. Special attention should be paid to the general health, and attention should be given to the bowels during the acute stage.
7. Antibiotics and chemotherapy are disappointing in cases of allergic non-granulomatous iritis, the disease being an *inflammation* rather than an *infection*.

TREATMENT OF PARTICULAR FORMS OF IRITIS: This treatment is in addition to that outlined above which should be used in every case.

1. SYPHILITIC IRITIS:
    a. *Acquired*: Anti-specific treatment should be instituted at once, in addition to the local treatment mentioned above.
    b. *Acute Infantile Iritis* is very rare and the advice of a venereologist should be sought.
    c. *Iritis in Congenital Syphilis*: See INTERSTITIAL KERATITIS, p. 33.
2. GONOCOCCAL IRITIS: Full doses of chemotherapy should be commenced forthwith and continued for 14 days.
3. TUBERCULOUS IRITIS: Some good results have been obtained with tuberculin injections, but these should be used with the utmost caution and starting with minute doses.
4. 'RHEUMATIC' IRITIS: Salicylates sometimes are effective not only in rheumatic cases but in others of doubtful aetiology. It is always worth giving them a trial.
5. BEHÇET'S SYNDROME: Injection of 50 000 units of calciferol twice a day. In some cases aureomycin has been beneficial. Being of possible virus origin the condition is likely to prove resistant to treatment. Sometimes intramuscular gamma-globulin has been tried.
6. TOXOPLASMOSIS: In addition to local therapy, daraprim 25 mg per day should be given.
7. ULCERATIVE COLITIS: When coincident inflammation is present in the iris and colon, steroid therapy sufficient to control the colitis is normally adequate to control the iritis also. Local steroid drops and cycloplegics are indicated in addition.

TREATMENT OF COMPLICATIONS: It must always be remembered that in any case of acute iritis operative treatment is to be avoided if humanly possible. The iris is extremely friable and bleeds

54 A SYNOPSIS OF OPHTHALMOLOGY

on the slightest provocation. Both these factors tend to make what is a simple operation in a normal eye one of extreme difficulty in an acutely inflamed one. Furthermore, the trauma caused by handling the inflamed iris will tend to increase the trouble by causing traumatic inflammation as well.

1. IRIS BOMBÉ: In this case something must be done to restore the circulation of the intra-ocular fluid, and the simplest and safest procedure is iridotomy with a Graefe knife.
2. SECONDARY GLAUCOMA: In treating this we are 'between the devil and the deep blue sea'. The iris needs atropine, which in glaucoma is absolutely contra-indicated. What, then, is the right thing to do? Definitely to treat the causative condition by *pushing atropine to the full*. Permanent relief to this form of secondary glaucoma can only come by curing the iritis which is causing it. In cases of recurrent iritis with secondary glaucoma, an iridectomy can be attempted in a quiescent interval, but it is a risky and somewhat uncertain procedure and not to be recommended if avoidable.

CONGENITAL ABNORMALITIES OF THE IRIS

Aniridia is a rare condition. On first sight it appears that the whole of the iris is missing, but 'aniridia' is a misnomer, for slit-lamp examination always reveals some iris tissue present. Occasionally the ciliary processes and always the suspensory ligament of the lens are visible in these cases. It is a bilateral condition and there is marked tendency to glaucoma owing to remnants of the root of the iris blocking the angle. Sometimes associated congenital abnormalities are present, such as cataracts, coloboma of the choroid, etc.

CAUSE OF ANIRIDIA: It is probably due to adhesions between the vascular lens capsule and the mesoderm at the edge of the optic cup, which prevent the growth of the iris.

Persistent Pupillary Membrane occurs in various forms:
1. Probably the most frequent consists of stellate pigmented dust on the anterior lens capsule giving the appearance of 'peppering'.
2. Delicate strands often invisible except by a slit-lamp may arise from the anterior surface of the iris in the region of the lesser arterial circle. These occasionally branch, and may be attached to the lens capsule or to another part of the collarette.
3. Very rarely a persistent pupillary membrane may be attached to the back of the cornea.
4. *Rieger's Malformation*: Very rarely, strands pass from the iris root, across the angle, to the trabecular network to a congenital opacity in Descemet's membrane, known as the posterior embryotoxon. This is known as Rieger's malformation and may lead on to glaucoma. All these conditions are without significance and do

DISEASES OF THE UVEAL TRACT 55

not interfere with vision. They are frequently only discovered during a slit-lamp examination.

Heterochromia is very common and occurs in one of two forms: either the colour of the two irides is completely different or, more commonly, a segment of a different colour is present in either or both irides. It must be remembered that in some cases of iridocyclitis the pigment may be lost owing to degenerative changes, otherwise a wrong diagnosis of congenital heterochromia may be made. In such cases the diseased iris is always the paler one.

Albinism: *See* DISEASES OF THE CHOROID, p. 60.

Ectopia Pupillae: Normally, the pupil is slightly to the nasal side, but in ectopia it may be greatly displaced and in any direction.

Polycoria: This is a very rare condition in which more than one pupil is present.

Coloboma of the Iris: This is a common condition consisting of a pear-shaped gap in the iris extending downwards and inwards, corresponding with the position of the embryonic fetal cleft. The gap extends sometimes as far as the ciliary border. Coloboma of the iris is frequently associated with coloboma of the choroid, zonule and lens and other congenital abnormalities.

TUMOURS OF THE IRIS
See INTRA-OCULAR NEOPLASMS (p. 159).

CYSTS OF THE IRIS
These occur very rarely, but the following may be seen occasionally:
1. **Implantation Cysts:** These result from a perforating wound of the corneoscleral junction involving the root of the iris. Epithelium from the conjunctiva or cornea grows into the wound and on to the root of the iris. Later the corneal epithelium becomes cystic, and this epithelial mass covered with thinned-out iris tissue may fill the anterior chamber and cause glaucoma. Intra-ocular operations may cause this condition.
2. **Serous Cysts** are endothelial and are due to closure of crypts with retention of fluid.
3. **Retinal Epithelial Cysts** occur at the back of the iris and are due to the spontaneous separation of the two layers of the retinal epithelium with accumulation of fluid between them.

DEGENERATIONS OF THE IRIS
Areas of atrophy can occur in the iris in senile cases; also as the aftermath of inflammatory changes. There is, however, another rare but definite clinical entity:

Essential Atrophy of the Iris: This is a progressive unilateral disease of unknown aetiology affecting young adults. Areas of atrophy appear

56 A SYNOPSIS OF OPHTHALMOLOGY

which coalesce and ultimately lead to the disappearance of large portions of iris tissue. Distortions and malpositions of the pupil are present with ectropion uveae. After some years, the iris tissue almost disappears and an intractable glaucoma develops, leading eventually to blindness.

DISEASES OF THE CILIARY BODY

Stress has already been laid upon the fact that there is no sharply defined line between inflammation of the iris and that of the ciliary body. The former occurs sometimes with very few signs of cyclitis, but cyclitis is never present without fairly obvious signs of iritis. It is, therefore, customary to refer to inflammation of the ciliary body as iridocyclitis, which will now be considered.

Iridocyclitis:

AETIOLOGY: The same as that of IRITIS.

PATHOLOGY: Just as there is no sharp dividing line between iritis and cyclitis, so there is no obvious distinction between acute, subacute and chronic iridocyclitis. In all acute cases polymorphonuclear leucocytes (characteristic of *acute* inflammation) put in an appearance and eventually dominate the scene. Collections of these cells sometimes form tiny nodules with masses of bacteria at their centres. In the more severe forms exudates from the ciliary body not only pass through the pupil, forming posterior synechiae in the manner already described (*see* IRITIS), but they also pass backwards behind the lens and into the vitreous, forming the cyclitic membrane. In children these cyclitic membranes may resemble a glioma. Fibrous tissue is thus formed and is sometimes attached to the retina. When this tissue contracts retinal detachment and fibrosis of the ciliary processes may result. This leads to the absence of secretion of intra-ocular fluid, lowered tension, a soft eye, a shrunken globe, degeneration of the choroid and possibly, at a much later date, to bone formation in the choroid.

SIGNS AND SYMPTOMS: This is frequently an insidious disease and is more common in women than in men. The patient notices progressive loss of vision without any very marked symptoms. Occasionally there is pain and photophobia, with ciliary flush and tenderness of the eye. Posterior synechiae may not be present at first, but they are almost always formed sooner or later. A characteristic sign of cyclitis is the presence of 'KP' (q.v.) on the back of the cornea, which are present in every case. Keratic precipitates (KP) and their causation can be briefly summarized as follows: the corneal endothelium becomes swollen in places and desquamates. The cells which are shed tend to adhere to one another and to the epithelium in small deposits. In an early stage they may be very fine and dust-like, sometimes invisible

DISEASES OF THE UVEAL TRACT

without the slit-lamp. The importance of a thorough examination with the slit-lamp in every possible case cannot be over-emphasized. These KP tend to deposit themselves in a triangular manner, with the apex somewhere near the centre of the pupil and the base between the 4 and the 8 o'clock positions. The finer KP are near the apex and the larger ones nearer the base. Sometimes this triangular arrangement is not observed and they are scattered indiscriminately, and in other cases the spots coalesce, giving a 'mutton fat' appearance. Occasionally, pigmented KP are visible, and this is an indication that the inflammation is an old-standing one. In the more severe cases of iridocyclitis opacities appear in the vitreous, the pathology of which is uncertain but is probably in the nature of albuminous exudates. Owing to defective nutrition some vitreous degeneration occurs, resulting in an undue fluidity. Increased tension sometimes occurs owing to the high viscosity of the intra-ocular fluid and this may result in an unusually deep anterior chamber.

In the more chronic cases (especially in tuberculous ones) infiltration of the choroid occurs. This is often seen to be associated with nodules on the iris. The disease runs a protracted course, with great liability to recurrent attacks, each one of which impairs the vision more than previously. It is frequently bilateral and the prognosis (except in slight cases) is bad. Iridocyclitis may be broadly divided into two types: Granulomatous and Non-granulomatous.

GRANULOMATOUS UVEITIS may be the result of an invasion of the eye by micro-organisms which cause a chronic inflammatory proliferative reaction. These cases may respond to antibiotic treatment. This type of uveitis is not always due to an infection. It may be an allergic reaction to a local infection, or it may be entirely allergic, e.g. tuberculous uveitis, sympathetic ophthalmia, etc. A variety of other conditions can cause granulomatous iritis, e.g. toxoplasmosis, *Toxocara canis*, sarcoiditis, etc. It will therefore be seen that with such a diverse aetiology, the actual cause may remain uncertain in many cases.

NON-GRANULOMATOUS UVEITIS is almost always an allergy. Examples of this are anaphylactic and atopic uveitis.

Clinically these two types of uveitis often merge and cases are seen showing features of both types, e.g. sarcoid uveitis is clinically granulomatous but no organisms have ever been demonstrated.

TREATMENT:
1. A thorough overhaul to eliminate any possible aetiological factor, as described under IRITIS.
2. The same local treatment as defined for cases of IRITIS.

3. Local corticosteroid treatment is of utmost value in all non-granulomatous cases and if the condition does not respond rapidly, systemic corticosteroids should be tried in addition. Of the granulomatous types, sarcoid uveitis and sympathetic ophthalmia respond well to this treatment.
4. Protein shock is always worth a trial, and one of the following three methods is recommended:
    a. The simplest form is the intramuscular injection of 4–5 ml of milk. This dose can be increased to a maximum of 10 ml.
    b. TAB vaccines may be used as an alternative.
    c. Autohaemotherapy. This method consists of withdrawing anything up to 10 ml of the patient's own blood and injecting it intramuscularly.

    All these protein shock measures increase antibody formation.
5. Paracentesis is helpful in cases of increased tension and this treatment may be repeated if necessary, but the same remarks *re* operations to be found under IRITIS apply in all these cases: no operative interference if it can possibly be avoided is the safe rule.

Heterochromic Iridocyclitis: This is a low-grade form of iridocyclitis characterized by loss of colour and atrophy of the affected iris with 'KP'. Secondary cataract often supervenes in these cases. Pathology is uncertain, but it is thought to be the result of involvement of the sympathetic nerve-supply causing loss of pigment.

Uveoparotid Fever (Heerfordt's Disease): In this disease there is a bilateral enlargement of the parotid glands associated with iridocyclitis and the paralysis of one or more of the cranial nerves, usually the facial. The patient has a mild pyrexia and occasionally erythema nodosum or other skin rashes. It is usually a complaint of young adult life and it runs a course lasting from 3 to 18 months. It is generally due to sarcoidosis.

Vogt–Koyanagi–Harada's Syndrome is a rare condition characterized by the following signs:
1. Meningeal irritation;
2. Bilateral uveitis leading to detached retinae;
3. Various skin eruptions;
4. Lymphocytosis;
5. Deafness.

Its pathology is unknown, but Greer (*Ocular Pathology*, 1972) points out that both clinically and histologically this disease has much in common with sympathetic ophthalmia. In both conditions there is abnormal response to uveal components, but the significance of this similarity remains unknown.

Sarcoidosis is no longer a rare disease and in about one-third of the cases ocular symptoms are present. It is a systemic granulomatous disease

DISEASES OF THE UVEAL TRACT

DIFFERENTIAL DIAGNOSIS OF ACUTE EYE INFLAMMATIONS

	ACUTE CONJUNCTIVITIS	ACUTE IRITIS	ACUTE NARROW ANGLE GLAUCOMA	ACUTE IRIDOCYCLITIS
HISTORY	Sudden onset. Often history of contact with 'pink eye'	Fairly sudden onset	Very sudden onset often after cold or virus infection. Sometimes history of previous slight attack	Sometimes sudden, but may be insidious
VISION	Normal	Severe impairment, depending upon amount of exudates and presence of adhesions (usually 6/60 to hand movements)	Rapid loss. Often hand movements only	Misty. Depending on amount of 'KP' and exudates
PAIN	Pricking or gritty feeling. Real pain infrequent	Severe	Severe and in region of 5th nerve	Slight. Some tenderness
WHETHER BILATERAL	Second eye involved as first eye improves	Sometimes	Rarely	Sometimes
VOMITING	Absent	Absent	Almost always present	Absent
CILIARY FLUSH	Absent	Present	Present	Usually present
CORNEA	Clear	Clear	'Steamy' or ground-glass appearance	Clear
PUPIL	Normal and reacting	Small, irregular and non-reacting, adhesions present	Oval, dilated, non-reacting	Small, irregular, adherent, non-reacting
IRIS	Normal	'Muddy'	Difficult to see owing to corneal haze	Occasionally lighter colour than other pupil
TENSION	Normal	Normal, unless complicated by secondary glaucoma	Greatly increased	Usually normal

of uncertain aetiology and pathology. It presents a wide range of symptoms affecting a multiplicity of tissues, accompanied by little general disturbance but a marked tendency to relapse. Lesions are chiefly found in lymph nodes, lungs, skin, salivary glands and the eyes. Histologically the appearance resembles that of tuberculosis, but the tubercle bacillus has never been demonstrated, the lesions never caseate, and animal inoculations have proved negative. It is generally regarded as a benign form of tuberculosis, but it is difficult to accept a brief for this theory in the absence of any definite evidence to support it. The tuberculin reaction is usually negative but the Kveim test is often positive. False positives to this test are almost unknown, but a negative result does not entirely exclude sarcoidosis. The eye manifestations usually consist of a low-grade anterior uveitis with marked synechiae, and 'mutton fat' KP nodules are often found on the iris, especially in the pupillary region (Koeppe's nodules). Varying degrees of corneal involvement may be found, and, provided there are no corneal opacities, the prognosis for vision is reasonably good. Ocular sarcoidosis can also affect the conjunctiva as translucent nodules in the lower fornix. When there is ocular involvement systemic steroid treatment is always indicated.

DIAGNOSIS requires some temerity but can be presumed if other systemic changes are found in the lungs or elsewhere.

TREATMENT: As for other forms of uveitis. Steroid therapy is helpful in mild cases, but in all chronic cases the outlook even with steroids is far from good.

Sympathetic Iridocyclitis: A very dangerous form following injury. It is dealt with under EYE INJURIES.

DISEASES OF THE CHOROID

The continuity of the various parts of the uveal tract has already been pointed out and the fact that inflammation of one part of the tract never occurs alone. It is always affected *as a whole*. Similarly, the intimate relationship between the choroid and the retina will at once be obvious. The outer layers of the retina receive their nutrition from the choroid and it will, therefore, follow that when any choroidal disease is present the retina is certain to be affected. Diseases of the choroid may conveniently be studied under the following headings: (1) Congenital abnormalities; (2) Inflammations; (3) Degenerations; (4) Detachments; (5) Tumours.

Congenital Abnormalities:

1. COLOBOMA OF THE CHOROID: A congenital mal-development of part of the choroid and retina. It is commonly seen as a bright white patch shaped like the stump of a cigar, with clearly defined almost punched-out edges which are usually dotted with small patches of pigment. The white appearance is due to the fact

that the sclera is visible, since the choroid and retina are missing. Various vessels are seen crossing the colobomatous area. These are retinal, choroidal and posterior ciliary vessels. Sometimes the sclera may be thinned out and ectatic over the area. In coloboma of the choroid it is nearly always the lower part that is involved, the part which occupies the position of the fetal cleft. Imperfect closure of this cleft is the cause of coloboma. Not infrequently other congenital abnormalities (such as coloboma of the iris) are associated with it.

TOTAL ALBINISM: In these cases the pupil appears a pink colour since rays of light are able to pass through the sclera without being absorbed by the pigment in the choroid and retina. The patient is troubled greatly by light, and nystagmus and defective vision are usually present also. The retinal and choroidal vessels are seen with the ophthalmoscope standing out very clearly against the white background of the sclera. These cases are congenital, and in addition to the eye signs they usually show some pigment defects in other parts of the body (white hair, etc.).

PARTIAL ALBINISM: This is commoner than the total condition. The irides may be a light blue colour (i.e. slightly pigmented), but the pigment may be absent from the choroid and retina and the hair light, but not the almost white hair of the total albino.

TREATMENT: (1) Dark glasses; (2) Contact lenses with scleral haptics and clear pupillary areas have helped.

2. CHOROIDEREMIA: The chief sign of this complaint is the absence (except possibly in a very rudimentary form) of the choroidal vessels, with the appearance of an almost pure white fundus except for a red fovea. It is a congenital anomaly. Sorsby considers it to be a sex-linked hereditary condition progressive in nature and inherited from women who present a characteristic fundal appearance. In addition to cases of complete choroideremia, an incomplete form is occasionally seen. McCulloch (*Trans. Am. ophthal. Soc.*, 1969, **67**, 142) traces the origin of this condition to a pig farm in Ireland in 1850 where the owner blinded his pigs before selling them to increase their weight through lack of exercise. The story alleges that he was cursed by an old woman for his cruelty and he later became blind. He had 2 sons and 7 daughters; neither of the sons were blind but 6 daughters married and had large families. McCulloch examined 600 of about 1600 descendants. The male descendants went slowly blind but the females showed incomplete choroideremia with little visual defects but they were carriers of the disease.

In these, the brilliant white fundus of a total choroideremia is intersected by a number of choroidal vessels, and a few patches of pigment may be seen. The ophthalmoscopic picture is suggestive of a partially developed choroidal circulation.

Inflammations of the Choroid:

Occur in two forms: (1) Acute suppurative; (2) Chronic non-suppurative.

1. ACUTE SUPPURATIVE CHOROIDITIS occurs in the form of endophthalmitis or panophthalmitis, when the eye becomes a 'bag of pus'.
2. CHRONIC NON-SUPPURATIVE CHOROIDITIS: Before considering this condition in its different forms, it is well to consider the following factors.

    PATHOLOGY: This form of inflammation is always a chronic one and little fluid exudate is present. In the early stages collections of round cells are present which are either scattered throughout the choroid or form into localized masses. These cell aggregations infiltrate the choriocapillaris and may penetrate Bruch's membrane and enter the vitreous. Chromatophores assemble at these collections of cells and disintegrate, leaving pigment present in the tissues. Scar tissue is formed and granulation tissue sometimes involves the retina. The cells of the pigment epithelium lose their pigment, some of which enters the retina. After a lapse of many years, newly formed connective tissue in the eye may even become calcified.

    AETIOLOGY: By far the most important factor is syphilis, and after this, septic foci. There are, however, numerous cases in which no causative factor can be found.

    SIGNS AND SYMPTOMS: The patient complains of dimness of vision in one eye with gradual onset but progressive loss. Metamorphopsia may be present, also flashes of light, and the patient may be conscious of either a positive or a negative scotoma. There is usually no pain, redness or photophobia. On examination, vitreous haze is often present, which obscures the red reflex and prevents an adequate view of the fundus. Vitreous floaters are very frequently seen. Sometimes small white or yellow-centred areas are visible, which are poorly defined and vary in size from a pin's head to an optic disc. These areas are, in fact, patches of round-celled infiltration of the choroid. The exudates formed by these patches tend to organize, with consequent destruction of normal choroidal and retinal tissues. The pigment epithelium is released from some of the cells involved in these changes and it tends to become heaped up in masses at the edges of the inflamed areas. The white sclerotic is seen in these affected places, hence the pearly white patches lined with dense black pigment which are seen in all cases of old choroiditis. Old choroidal infection can always be differentiated from an active infection by this sharp definition of the affected areas.

DISEASES OF THE UVEAL TRACT

In very severe cases, the ciliary body is involved and vitreous opacities increase. Sometimes cataract may result from malnutrition of the lens. The duration of the disease may be for months, during which time successive areas of choroid are involved. As soon as one area settles down a fresh patch makes its appearance.

TREATMENT:
1. It is of prime importance to treat the aetiological factor when that can be traced.
2. Atropine is essential.
3. Steroid therapy is indicated but the more posterior the inflammation is the more disappointing are the results of *local treatment*. A course of systemic steroid therapy sometimes helps. The earlier it is given the better the prognosis.
4. Close work must be avoided and dark glasses worn.

CLINICAL VARIETIES:
1. *Juxta-papillary*: An exudative form of choroiditis which may involve the macular region occurs in young people. KP are present and vitreous opacities are almost invariably seen. The inflammation eventually settles down, leaving a scotoma of proportionate size to the area involved.
2. *Forster's Areolar Choroiditis*: This is not to be confused with central areolar choroidal atrophy, which is a degenerative lesion. In this disease, the first lesion is in the macula and the trouble spreads outwards, hence the peripheral lesions are the more recent ones. The behaviour of the individual lesions is quite characteristic. The spots are all pigmented at first, but as organization proceeds the pigment is lost from the centre outwards, so that the lesions resemble dark rims with white centres. This is, of course, the reverse of a normal choroiditis, when the pigment increases with the duration of the disease.
3. *Tuberculous Choroiditis*: This occurs in two forms: (*a*) Miliary; (*b*) Chronic or conglomerate.
   a. *Miliary*: This condition is most frequently found in the late stages of tuberculous meningitis, but many cases are never diagnosed because the tubercles only appear a few days before death. Parsons considered that in almost every case of tuberculous meningitis miliary tubercles would be found if a search was made. They occur as rounded pale spots in any part of the choroid, varying in size from the point of a pin to 1 or 2 mm. Their presence is diagnostic of tuberculosis. Each spot seen is a giant-cell system containing tubercle bacilli.

64   A SYNOPSIS OF OPHTHALMOLOGY

- b. *Chronic*: Chronic tuberculous choroiditis affects areas of the choroid similarly to an ordinary non-tuberculous lesion, but it causes extensive formation of granulation tissue and it can even form a large mass resembling a sarcoma. This mass (which is really a tuberculous granuloma containing giant cells) may fill the posterior part of the globe. Eventually, the sclerotic becomes involved, perforation takes place, and the fungating mass may appear. It requires a careful differential diagnosis from glioma.
- c. *Treatment*:
    - i. Streptomycin with PAS is the most promising treatment.
    - ii. Tuberculin injections may be tried with great caution.
    - iii. Enucleation is indicated in severe cases where hope of vision is lost.

4. *Metastatic Choroiditis*: This usually occurs as a manifestation of uveitis of endogenous origin. Bacteria or toxins enter the bloodstream from different parts of the body, such as teeth, tonsils, generative organs, etc. and cause emboli. It may be stated at the outset that these endogenous infections are not nearly so virulent as an exogenous infection with the same organism. Severe cases of metastatic bacterial endophthalmitis are rarely seen in these days, thanks largely to therapeutic results of penicillin and chemotherapy. Apart from such septic foci mentioned, it may occur in the course of an illness such as influenza, pneumonia, typhoid, meningitis, etc.

    Signs: Owing to the haziness of the vitreous little can be seen but occasional glimpses of retinal oedema. A few KP and posterior synechiae may be present. The condition usually subsides leaving some permanent impairment of vision, but in the worst cases a shrunken eye results following involvement of the ciliary processes. In children, a cyclitic membrane with fibrous tissue may be formed in the vitreous and the condition may resemble glioma, conglomerate tubercle or retrolental fibroplasia.

    Treatment: This depends upon two factors: (*a*) The source of the infection; (*b*) The severity of the attack. It varies from rest and atropine with chemotherapy, to evisceration if the eye becomes full of pus.

Degenerations of the Choroid

Before considering details of the different clinical varieties of choroidal degeneration found, it is necessary to make two facts abundantly clear: (1) In any lesion affecting the choroid the underlying retina suffers atrophy, since the means of nourishment to its outer layers has been cut off; (2) Degenerative changes in the choroid cause migration of pigment epithelium to the more superficial parts of the retina.

DISEASES OF THE UVEAL TRACT

These facts account for the loss of function and the appearance of pigment in retinitis pigmentosa, syphilitic choroiditis, etc., and even in the more localized conditions such as senile macular degeneration.

1. TAY'S CHOROIDITIS: In this common condition small discrete yellow spots appear both in the macular region and farther afield. They tend to increase in number but not in size, and there is no pigment disturbance. The condition is bilateral and has sometimes been mistaken for retinopathy due to diabetes. As a rule there is very little visual disturbance and no treatment is indicated.

    PATHOLOGY: The spots are colloid bodies situated on Bruch's hyaloid membrane, with the pigment epithelium and normal retina stretched over them.

2. CENTRAL AREOLAR ATROPHY: This condition must not be confused with Forster's areolar choroiditis (q.v.). The pathology of the two conditions is totally different, the former being an atrophy and the latter an inflammation. Central areolar atrophy is a bilateral condition affecting elderly people. It consists of a large round degenerated area extending from the disc to the macula and beyond. The pigment epithelium atrophies and the choroidal vessels and sclerotic are visible. There is a corresponding absolute scotoma with gross diminution of vision.

3. SENILE MACULAR DEGENERATION: This is a very common condition affecting the fovea only. It is usually bilateral, but one eye is more involved than the other and it results in a serious and progressive deterioration of central vision. It is the commonest cause of grossly defective vision in old people. Examination with a mydriatic should always be undertaken when this condition is expected, for the lesion may be so small as to escape notice unless a thorough examination is made. Amsler's charts (procurable from Messrs. Hamblin) are very useful in detecting this condition in an early stage. A similar appearance is seen in some juveniles in a familial form of macular degeneration known as Stargardt's disease. These changes occur at about puberty.

    PATHOLOGY: The cause of the trouble is a vascular lesion of the choriocapillaris underlying the macula.

    SIGNS: A very fine stippling is visible in the region of the macula. The retina here appears to be lightly peppered with fine dusty pigment. In the more advanced cases it appears 'moth-eaten'. The lesion tends to be circular.

    TREATMENT: Nothing can be done to arrest the progress of the disease, but much can be done to help the patient optically before central vision is lost:

    a. A hand magnifier used in conjunction with the patient's own reading glasses is helpful in many cases.

b. Special glasses of short focal length incorporating prisms (such as the Bishop Harman loupe) sometimes help patients when a hand magnifier fails.
   c. As a last resort some form of low visual acuity aid as made by Messrs. C. Davis Keeler may be tried.
   d. Recently there is a ray of hope in laser photocoagulation in those cases where fluorescein angiography shows vascular breaks, but the hope is very slender indeed.

   In spite of all the above the disease slowly progresses until central vision is lost, when the patient will be unable to read or write. Assurance may be given, however, that peripheral vision will remain reasonably good, so that the patient will be able to get about by himself and not be dependent upon other people.

4. MYOPIC DEGENERATION: Choroidal degenerative changes occur in every case of severe myopia. Patches of atrophy occur usually near the disc and these patches coalesce and may surround it. Choroidal vessels can be clearly seen and sometimes migrated pigment is visible. The sclera is often seen, giving a somewhat whitish reflex when viewed ophthalmoscopically. These degenerated areas alternate in patches with normal retinal tissue.

5. CHOROIDAL SCLEROSIS: This is a rare disease. The choriocapillaris and pigment epithelium atrophy, leaving the fundus a curious chocolate colour. The choroidal vessels are clearly visible and appear to be ensheathed in a whitish membrane. The cause of the condition is unknown.

Detachment of the Choroid

The choroid may become detached from the sclerotic in the following conditions:

1. In old diseased eyes lost through iridocyclitis, old glaucoma, etc.
2. In cases of severe haemorrhage.
3. In cases of intra-ocular neoplasm.
4. Postoperative cases after cataract extraction, trephine operation for glaucoma, etc. This type of case is due to hypotony producing detachment of the ciliary body and subsequent aqueous seepage into the suprachoroidal space. The anterior chamber is shallow or absent in these cases and the detached choroid is visible with the ophthalmoscope as a black mass behind the lens. The choroid usually becomes re-attached spontaneously, the anterior chamber is re-formed, and the prognosis is good. It is our policy to adopt an expectant approach and to treat these cases with full doses of acetazolamide, wide mydriasis and a firm pad and bandage. Persistence of a flat anterior chamber beyond 5 days requires drainage of the suprachoroidal fluid and re-formation of the anterior chamber with air.

Tumours of the Choroid: *See* INTRA-OCULAR NEOPLASMS, p. 159.

Chapter VI

DISEASES OF THE RETINA

Anatomy: The retina is a membrane of highly complex structure that lines the innermost surface of the globe from the ora serrata to the optic disc. It consists of eight layers, which when viewed from within outwards are as follows: (1) Nerve-fibre layer; (2) Ganglion-cell layer; (3) Internal reticular layer; (4) Inner nuclear layer; (5) External reticular layer; (6) Outer nuclear layer; (7) Rod and cone layer; (8) Pigment epithelium.

It should be noted that in the case of these layers the terms 'inner' and 'outer' refer to their positions *in relation to the centre of the ball of the eye*, e.g. the outer layers are those nearest the sclerotic, the inner layers are those nearer the lens. These various layers are separated by neuroglial tissue, prolongations of which form the internal and external limiting membranes. The internal membrane separates the retina from the vitreous and the external membrane forms the basement for the rod and cone layer. Two parts of the retina deserve special description:

1. THE OPTIC DISC REGION: Here the nerve fibres from the retina pass into the optic nerve and the other retinal elements cease. For this reason the optic disc is a 'blind spot'. For a more detailed description of the optic disc, *see* chapter on DISEASES OF THE OPTIC NERVE (p. 96).

2. THE MACULAR REGION: About 3·5 mm to the temporal side of the optic disc is situated the macula, in the centre of which is a tiny depression known as the fovea centralis. In this region cones only are present in the neuro-epithelial layer, and all the other layers are completely absent.

Apart from these two highly differentiated areas of the retina, its structure is the same throughout, with one important exception: in the rod and cone layer, the nearer the macula the more cones are present, and these structures get progressively fewer towards the periphery. The reverse is true of the rods, which are entirely absent at the macula but increase towards the periphery.

The blood supply of the outer or epithelial layers is through the choriocapillaris and that of the inner layers is from branches of the retinal arterial system.

Classification: For the sake of convenience, retinal affections will be dealt with as under-mentioned, but it is readily admitted that these headings are somewhat arbitrary and that in certain instances it is not easy to decide under which classification a particular lesion falls:

68 A SYNOPSIS OF OPHTHALMOLOGY

(1) Vascular lesions; (2) Retinopathies; (3) Retinitis; (4) Degenerations of the retina; (5) The phakomatoses; (6) Toxic amblyopias; (7) Traumatic lesions; (8) Detachments; (9) Retrolental fibroplasia.

I. VASCULAR LESIONS

Retinal Haemorrhages: These may vary in size from a tiny speck which is just visible with the ophthalmoscope to a massive haemorrhage that may infiltrate the whole thickness of the retina and even burst through into the vitreous. The appearance of a haemorrhage varies with its situation:

a. *In the nerve-fibre layer* the blood fills the space between the fibres, which gives it a slightly striated appearance known as 'flame-shaped', which is so commonly seen in arteriosclerosis.

b. *In the nuclear layers*, on the other hand, the blood tends to collect in tiny round spaces as is so typical in cases of diabetes.

c. *In preretinal (subhyaloid) haemorrhage* the blood collects between the retina and the vitreous. These haemorrhages are usually large and hemispherical in shape, the rounded end being downwards owing to gravity. They usually absorb spontaneously and the vision returns to normal. They are often seen in cases of subarachnoid haemorrhage, when it is probably due to pressure on the central vein as it crosses the subarachnoid space.

AETIOLOGY: There are many causes of retinal haemorrhages:
1. Senile vascular degeneration, hypertension, etc.;
2. Blood diseases such as pernicious anaemia, leukaemia;
3. Toxaemic conditions, such as nephritis, diabetes, pregnancy toxaemia, etc.;
4. Deficiency diseases, e.g. scurvy;
5. Trauma, such as contusions of the eye, pressure during birth of infants, etc.:
6. Pressure causing cerebral congestion, e.g. compression of neck or chest, whooping-cough, etc.;
7. Sudden reduction of intra-ocular tension, such as occurs during operative procedures.

Haemorrhages, unless they involve the macula, can cause very little diminution of vision, but in cases of macular haemorrhage the visual acuity, although it may improve with the lapse of time, rarely becomes normal.

TREATMENT is entirely that of the causative condition.

Eales's Disease or Periphlebitis Retinae: This is a form of retinal vascularity leading to serious and recurrent vitreous haemorrhages occurring in young adults, usually males. If the case is seen early the source of the haemorrhage is usually to be found in a vein with perivascular thickening usually towards the periphery of the retina. It is often bilateral and although absorption of the haemorrhage usually occurs, after repeated attacks serious complications may arise, e.g. gross opacities or retinitis proliferans (q.v.) when organization and fibrosis take place with eventual loss of vision.

PATHOLOGY is still uncertain. It has been variously attributed to defective power of coagulation, tuberculous thrombophlebitis and endocrine dysfunction. The modern view is that it is due to a perivasculitis—possibly of tuberculous or septic origin.

TREATMENT: Laser coagulation (*see* p. 90), if applied in early stages to the thickened sheath and the area surrounding it, is the most helpful treatment so far. In cases where tuberculosis is suspected, skin tests should be undertaken and a prolonged course of tuberculin given. The ultimate prognosis is far from good.

Arterial Spasm: In some cases of migraine, spasm of the arteries has been observed ophthalmoscopically during an attack, but it is very doubtful whether this is the rule. It is quite certain, however, that arterial spasm is the earliest retinal sign visible in the case of toxaemia of pregnancy. It is probable that if every case of pregnancy toxaemia were seen early enough this sign would be invariably present.

Arterial Obstruction: If the main trunk of the great central artery of the retina is blocked by an embolism or thrombus an immediate and complete retinal anaemia results, the eye becoming suddenly and permanently blind. Fundus examination shows tiny thread-like arteries with normal-looking veins. The central area of the retina appears a milky-white colour, often making the disc difficult to see. At the fovea, standing out rather strikingly in the middle of the milky retina, is a bright 'cherry-red' spot. In these cases the obstruction occurs almost invariably at the lamina cribrosa. Sometimes this picture is modified when the blockage occurs in one of the smaller branches, and in these cases complete blindness does not result. There is merely a sector defect corresponding to the area involved. The ischaemic necrosis of the retina clears up in some weeks, but it is, of course, useless as an organ of vision since it is quite atrophic. The disc also atrophies later. Very rarely cilio-retinal vessels carry on some degree of circulation, and in these cases a certain amount of vision may remain.

AETIOLOGY:
1. ARTERIOSCLEROSIS: In these cases the actual lesion is usually a thrombosis rather than an embolism. This group is naturally commonest amongst older persons.
2. MITRAL STENOSIS: Sometimes causes emboli in young people. Cases have been reported in all ages varying from 15 to 80 years. It is very rarely bilateral.
3. CAROTID INSUFFICIENCY WITH EMBOLI.

PATHOLOGY: The blockage, whether by embolus or thrombus, occurs at the lamina cribrosa where the vessels are normally constricted. The milky appearance of the central area is due to ischaemic necrosis of its elements with cloudy swelling of the ganglion cells. At the fovea (where there are no ganglion cells) the retina retains its normal colour, and this is the explanation of the cherry-red spot. It is not a haemorrhage, as was originally thought. It will be seen, therefore, that the serious results of a blockage of the central artery are due to atrophy of the nerve fibres and the ganglion cells. The outer layers, including the rods and cones which receive their blood supply from the choriocapillaris, are not affected.

TREATMENT: Is usually ineffective, but a vasodilator such as tolazoline hyd. can be given intramuscularly and orally. It is well worth a trial, provided the case is seen early. Retrobulbar injection of acetylcholine has been tried. Branch occlusion may be relieved in this way. Sometimes paracentesis of the anterior chamber and injection of acetylcholine has been tried.

Venous Thrombosis: Either the central vein of the retina or one of its branches is not infrequently affected by thrombosis and, as in the case of arterial blockage, the thrombus usually occurs where the vein is constricted behind the lamina cribrosa. The patient, usually past middle age and arteriosclerotic, complains of diminution of vision but not so suddenly or dramatically as in occlusion of the artery, neither is the loss of sight so profound, unless, of course, there is complete occlusion of the central vein. There is always a central scotoma and often a contraction of the peripheral field. When a branch vein is involved, the loss of vision is by no means severe and is confined to the area involved. Very rarely is the condition bilateral.

SIGNS: The retinal veins are grossly enlarged and engorged with blood. Haemorrhages occur scattered all over the retina and some of them may be very large, even obscuring the disc. In the case of a branch vein, the haemorrhages and engorgement are confined to the area supplied by that vein. The thrombus in a branch vein usually occurs at an arteriovenous crossing. After a lapse of time, the retina becomes atrophied and pigmentary changes occur. In some cases tortuous vessels develop in the region of the disc and these form a collateral circulation between the retinal and choroidal systems.

THROMBOTIC GLAUCOMA: A curious complication of thrombosis of the central vein is the occurrence of a severe and intractable glaucoma between three and four months after the onset of the thrombosis. Nearly 40 per cent of cases develop this complication and in almost all cases of thrombotic glaucoma, new vessels can be observed on the iris. It is now recognized that in a small proportion of cases such a thrombosis may be the first sign of a primary glaucoma. The moral: always exclude glaucoma in the unaffected eye in every case of central venous thrombosis.

The cause of thrombotic glaucoma is by no means certain. Wolff considered that in many cases the venae vorticosae are either thrombosed or narrowed, thus causing albuminous exudates in the vitreous which push the lens and iris forwards and narrow the filtration angle. The modern view is that it is due to vascular engorgement and new vessel formation in the region of the trabeculae of the anterior chamber resulting in organization of tissues at the drainage angle.

AETIOLOGY: Arteriosclerosis is the chief cause of thrombosis of the retinal veins. In many cases there is associated cardiac or kidney disease and the patient is often elderly and debilitated. It sometimes occurs in younger persons following local sepsis such as orbital cellulitis or during the course of acute infections.

TREATMENT: In the early stage, phenindione, coumarin or some similar anticoagulant may be tried, but in the case of a complete thrombosis all treatment is useless. Its occurrence, however, should always be regarded as an indication for a complete overhaul of the cardiovascular–renal systems. Atropine is contraindicated, since it might precipitate glaucoma in what must be considered as a predisposed eye.

Sautter and Sartani of Hamburg had encouraging results with anticoagulant treatment by coumarin derivatives. They have found considerable improvement in vision and a decrease in the incidence of glaucoma. Treatment is recommended for at least 4 weeks.

Anaemic Amaurosis: Considering the frequent occurrence of severe haemorrhage, this is a very rare condition. When it does occur it is usually the result of medical conditions involving frequent loss of moderate amounts of blood, e.g. haematemesis, melaena, uterine haemorrhage, etc. It is very rare indeed after wounds, even those of a severe nature, when the patient is almost exsanguinated. This blindness is usually bilateral and may be total. In nearly 50 per cent of cases it is permanent. Other cases recover after a lapse of hours or days, but usually some degree of visual impairment remains.

SIGNS: The pupil is non-reacting and dilated. Usually the fundi appear normal, but in some cases a few haemorrhages are seen and occasionally some scattered white patches of oedema. In the worst cases complete optic atrophy follows.

PATHOLOGY: The essential lesion is believed to lie in the ganglion cells. The retinal anaemia causes a degeneration of these cells and their fibres without any evidence of inflammation being present.

TREATMENT is entirely that of the causative condition and must have two aims: (1) To maintain the efficiency of the general circulation (blood transfusion, if necessary); and (2) To remove the cause of the haemorrhage as soon as possible.

II. RETINOPATHIES

In past years it has been the custom of ophthalmologists to refer to the various retinal manifestations of general disease as 'retinitis'. This is another misnomer, even though a time-honoured one, implying as it does that the manifestation in the retina is an inflammatory one. In point of fact, the changes seen are essentially those of a *degenerative* nature, although some slight inflammation may be present as well. The modern term 'retinopathy' is less misleading and should be used instead.

1. **Arteriosclerotic Retinopathy:** It is only comparatively recently that medical practitioners have realized the value of the ophthalmoscope in the diagnosis and prognosis of arterial disease. The central artery of the retina is the only artery in the body that is *visible* and the retina is the only part of the human anatomy where arterial disease can be *seen*. Furthermore, if arterial changes are seen in the retina, it may be assumed that similar changes are present in the arteries of the brain, but the converse is not necessarily true, and cerebral arterial disease can exist in the absence of retinal changes.

    SIGNS: There are no symptoms of retinal arteriosclerosis as such, vision only being affected when some haemorrhage or exudate impinges on the macula or when some catastrophe occurs, e.g. embolism or thrombosis.

    a. The arteries become irregular in calibre, parts of the vessels appear constricted and other parts normal or even slightly dilated.

    b. Changes occur in the light reflexes from the vessel walls giving a copper- or silver-wire appearance in the case of the smaller arteries.

    c. Changes occur at the arteriovenous crossings. The hardened artery causes a marked constriction of the vein at the point of crossing. It obstructs the flow of blood and gives the vein a 'pinched appearance'. In severe cases the vein appears to be pushed off its course by the artery.

    d. Severe changes make the walls of the arteries visible, so that the vessels appear to be lined with white fibrous lines (pipe-clay sheathing).

    e. Tiny aneurysms are sometimes seen.

    All the above changes can be seen in most cases of severe arteriosclerosis. When, in addition to any or all of the above, the following changes are observed, arteriosclerotic retinopathy is said to exist:

DISEASES OF THE RETINA

- *f.* Oedema of the retina may arise either in the macular area or in scattered patches in the region of the vessels. Later these appear as well-defined spots due to exudates of lymph.
- *g.* Flame-shaped striated haemorrhages, the result of increased permeability of the walls of the diseased vessels, may appear. Rounded haemorrhages may occur, but are less frequent.
- *h.* A star-shaped patch of exudate is visible at the macula in very severe cases.

Any of these signs call for an exhaustive examination of the cardiovascular–renal systems because the various retinopathies may resemble each other and the final diagnosis must, in many cases, rest with the physician.

PROGNOSIS: In arteriosclerotic retinopathy the prognosis for sight is good, especially as the disease is sometimes unilateral. Unless the macula is affected by haemorrhage or exudate, good vision may be retained, but it must be remembered that the retinal picture is a small replica of the cerebral one and that quite a number of patients with advanced retinal arteriosclerosis die from cerebral haemorrhage.

2. **Renal Retinopathy:** When this is at all advanced it presents a characteristic appearance:
- *a.* The vessels usually show degenerative changes, but not nearly so marked as in arteriosclerosis.
- *b.* Some haziness and oedema of the retina and disc are present.
- *c.* Scattered haemorrhages are found throughout the fundus, and these are often much larger than those seen in arteriosclerotic retinopathy.
- *d.* In early stages fluffy 'cotton-wool' patches of exudates are visible. Later in the disease these tend to become clearly defined and eventually to coalesce.
- *e.* A well-defined star figure may appear at the macula.
- *f.* Retinal detachments can frequently occur, and in the cases that recover these detachments may replace themselves spontaneously when the exudates are absorbed.
- *g.* In malignant hypertension when renal failure is present, severe general retinal oedema is observed, also gross papilloedema. Massive exudates tend to form throughout the retina and vision is grossly impaired.

It must be stressed that many cases of lesser severity occur with far fewer changes, and this fact emphasizes the importance of a routine test of the urine in every case of retinopathy. So far as symptoms are concerned, progressive dimness of vision is usually the only complaint. Occasionally there may be severe headaches. Any age group can be affected and the condition is invariably bilateral and is always associated with high blood pressure.

PROGNOSIS: In advanced cases prognosis is bad both as regards sight and life, and the younger the patient the graver the outlook. Many cases go quite blind and a large proportion die of uraemia. This very grave condition must not be confused with uraemic amaurosis, which has a sudden transitory loss of vision occurring in the course of an attack of nephritis or uraemia. In these cases no retinopathy is present. The prognosis is less serious in puerperal cases and during an attack of acute nephritis when the vessels are reasonably healthy. In cases that recover some impairment of vision is the rule. The 'cotton-wool' patches clear up first, then the macular star. Partial optic atrophy sets in and some pigmentary changes are common.

PATHOLOGY: The 'cotton-wool' and other white patches are fibrinous exudates. They lie in the external reticular layer but may infiltrate other layers as well. Leucocytes tend to aggregate around these patches. The nerve fibres that have been lying in oedema fluid swell up and form cystic varicosities known as 'cytoid bodies'. Aggregations of these cytoid bodies lying, as they do, superficially in the retina, bulge into the vitreous and are probably the cause of some of the white patches that are visible. The macular star owes its shape to exudates following the course of the nerve fibres. The disc shows the same histological changes as are found in papilloedema (q.v.), but these are less pronounced.

3. **Diabetic Retinopathy:** The actual cause of this complication of diabetes is unknown. It does not depend upon the level of the blood sugar, for it is found alike in cases where the disease is well controlled and in neglected cases. It would seem to depend upon the length of time the patient has suffered from it; thus the elderly who have had diabetes for many years are more prone to retinal complications than are younger patients. Most patients who have had diabetes for more than 20 years show some signs of retinopathy, and some patients develop it considerably earlier than this. Considering the large number of cases of diabetes that occur, retinopathy is definitely an uncommon complication. It is usually bilateral and the typical case presents features which permit a broad classification of *simple* or *malignant*.

SIMPLE RETINOPATHY: When scattered haemorrhages, exudates and micro-aneurysms are present.

MALIGNANT RETINOPATHY: When there is vascular proliferation, vitreous haemorrhage and fibrous tissue invasion.

a. The exudates are of a yellow wax-like appearance, quite different from the 'cotton-wool' patches of arteriosclerotic cases. These exudates form numerous, small, scattered spots often invading the macula, but the familiar star figure is very rare in diabetes.

DISEASES OF THE RETINA 75

b. The haemorrhages are of the punctate type, consisting of small ragged dots and spots scattered anywhere over the fundus. Massive haemorrhages are uncommon, as also are flame-shaped ones.
c. The arteries may appear normal and healthy, but scattered micro-aneurysms are usually present.
d. Very rarely is the optic disc affected.
e. In malignant cases vitreous haemorrhages and vascular proliferation occur.

It must, however, be remembered that in many diabetics coexisting arterial disease and albuminuria are found. It is, therefore, true to say that diabetic retinopathy frequently cannot be distinguished ophthalmoscopically from the arteriosclerotic and renal forms.

PROGNOSIS depends more upon the length of time the patient has had diabetes than upon the severity of the disease. The outlook for sight is good if the macula is not involved, but once retinopathy is present no treatment, even with insulin, is effective. In some cases treatment with a laser beam picking out individual haemorrhagic lesions has been helpful but the eventual prognosis is uncertain. This treatment undoubtedly prolongs vision. Occasionally a retinal haemorrhage will penetrate into the vitreous and may lead to retinitis proliferans (*see* p. 77). Any vitreous haemorrhage in a diabetic adds greatly to the gravity of the prognosis. Diabetic retinopathy has been treated by ablation of the pituitary gland by various techniques but much more work will have to be done before it is possible to assess the ultimate value of this drastic treatment. Some workers have reported regression of haemorrhages and lessening of vascular proliferation after this treatment, but fibrous tissue remains unchanged.

Miss Enid Taylor of St. Bartholomew's Hospital gives encouraging results following treatment with xenon or argon lasers. The aim is to destroy micro-aneurysms which are replaced by scar tissue thus lessening the oedema of the retina. As the oedema lessens the vision improves in some cases but the visual results are not always consistent. Rubinstein and Mysha report improvement in 25 per cent of cases. Geltzer describes 25 such cases treated with ruby laser coagulation where the course of the disease was stabilized, no fresh retinal haemorrhages occurred and some visual improvement resulted when they were followed up for 12 months. Aiello observed 115 cases for 3 years and noted a reduction in angiopathy in 78 per cent of cases.

Lipaemia, though a rare complication, is of grave prognostic import. It occurs in young people with severe diabetes accompanied by acetonuria. In this condition, emulsified fat is present in the circulation and the retinal vessels assume a milky hue. Both

arteries and veins appear to be accompanied on each side by yellowish-white stripes. These changes are most marked in the smaller vessels near the periphery. Lipaemia retinalis responds immediately to insulin treatment.
4. **Leukaemic Retinopathy** occurs in any form of leukaemia, acute or chronic, lymphoid or myeloid, and its appearance is characteristic. The retinal vessels, especially the veins, are grossly engorged and tortuous and they tend to assume a yellowish hue which makes it difficult to distinguish between the arteries and the veins. Scattered haemorrhages, usually rounded ones, appear, and these show a central white area due to accumulation of leucocytes. Small scattered exudates also occur. Retinal micro-aneurysms can be picked out and destroyed by a laser beam, thus prolonging sight in this fatal disease. In the late stages the whole fundus becomes pale and orange-coloured.
5. **Toxaemic Retinopathy in Pregnancy:** This occurs late in pregnancy and closely resembles arteriosclerotic retinopathy in the early stages. Later, retinal oedema resembling that of the renal retinopathy occurs if the blood pressure rises. This leads to massive exudates and even to detachment. Such retinopathy is an indication for the immediate termination of the pregnancy to save the sight and possibly the life of the mother. If the pregnancy is terminated in reasonable time, the prognosis is good and the pathological changes seen in the retina are usually reversed.

III. RETINITIS

In the foregoing section on the retinopathies, we have discussed the retinal manifestations of various general diseases, manifestations that are mostly of a degenerative rather than an inflammatory nature. In this section we will consider some cases of genuine retinal inflammation. As ophthalmic terminology dies hard, included in this section will be a description of certain retinal changes that have been known as 'retinitis' for years, but which are neither degenerative nor inflammatory. They are included here because they are called 'retinitis' and it is more convenient to describe them in this section than to coin new names, or to classify them under other headings.

Syphilitic Retinitis: Syphilis is one of the commonest causes of retinitis. It is usually associated with, and secondary to, a choroiditis (q.v.). Primary retinitis due to syphilis is much rarer and occurs in three forms:
  1. In congenital cases a form of peripheral pigmentation known as 'pepper and salt' fundus is common. The name is apt, for the retina is dotted with a mixture of black and white fine dusty spots. These may be seen in some cases of interstitial keratitis. The Wassermann reaction will settle the diagnosis.

DISEASES OF THE RETINA

2. In acquired cases, retinitis may occur in the form of a cloudy oedema with a few white and yellow spots at the macula and pigment changes may be present in the periphery. Sometimes the condition may resemble an atypical retinitis pigmentosa. Vitreous haemorrhages and opacities occur. Later in the disease new blood vessels are formed, usually near the disc, and coils of vessels project into the vitreous—a condition known as 'rete mirabile'. Connective tissue may be formed and retinitis proliferans (q.v.) results.
3. Sometimes acquired retinal syphilis takes the form of a neuroretinitis. In these cases there is some swelling of the disc with marked oedema of the retina, and a few scattered haemorrhages and exudates. Neuroretinitis does not present any signs in themselves diagnostic of syphilis, and therefore cannot, with the ophthalmoscope, be distinguished from renal neuroretinitis. In every case the Wassermann reaction should be taken, the urine examined and the cardiovascular system overhauled. The symptoms of syphilitic retinitis are visual only and the treatment consists in adequate antisyphilitic measures.

Retinitis Circinata: This disease is a distant aftermath of retinal haemorrhages. It may be bilateral and occurs in old people. It consists of a circular arrangement of bright white patches, sometimes surrounding the macula. Retinal vessels can be seen to cross these spots, and fine pigment changes are visible. It is thought that the patches represent masses of red cells that have degenerated and undergone hyaline changes. It will, therefore, be seen that a better name for the condition would be 'circinate degeneration of the retina', since no inflammatory changes are visible in this disease.

Retinitis Proliferans: In the whole of ophthalmology there can be found no more glaring instance of inaccurate nomenclature than in the term 'retinitis proliferans'. It is quite incorrect to imply that it is an inflammatory lesion as will be seen from the remarks in the following paragraph on its pathology. However, time and generations of oculists have honoured the name 'retinitis proliferans', so we will let it takes its ancient name and place amongst diseases of the retina rather than attempt the difficult task of coining a new name.

Retinitis proliferans is an occasional aftermath of vitreous haemorrhages. When blood leaks into the vitreous, one of two things may happen:
1. It may be absorbed completely without doing any damage or leaving any trace behind;
2. It may be invaded by granulation tissue which, in the course of time, leads to connective-tissue and scar formation.

The former result fortunately describes the vast majority of cases, but when the haemorrhages are severe and recurrent, and especially when they are associated with diseases of the retinal vessels, the latter result may develop, and this produces retinitis proliferans. In these cases the clot organizes and fibrosed bands form in the vitreous. New blood vessels from the retinal system (usually in the region of the disc) grow into these fibrous bands, which are adherent to the retina and as they contract may actually cause a detachment by traction. Retinitis proliferans is particularly liable to supervene in retinal haemorrhages associated with the following conditions: (1) Syphilis; (2) Diabetes; (3) Nephritis; (4) Eales's disease; (5) Traumatic cases.

In this disease preventive treatment can be tried by locating small micro-aneurysms and applying photocoagulation by laser beam before fibrosis occurs. In advanced cases no treatment is of help.

Exudative Retinitis (Coats's Disease): This occurs in young people and is usually bilateral. Boys are affected more frequently than girls. A large white or yellow patch of exudates forms deep in the retina and involves the macular region. Occasionally glistening spots of cholesterol crystals are seen. At first the patch is transparent, but it soon increases in size and depth and becomes opaque. The retinal vessels are seen to pass over it and these vessels, particularly the veins, may be grossly dilated, tortuous and show aneurysmal dilatations. The condition is very similar to *angiomatosis retinae* in clinical appearance but pathologically they are quite different. It must also be differentiated from *retinoblastoma* and *Toxocara canis* (q.v., p. 206). Detachment of the retina is a common end-result and glaucoma or cataract may follow. The causation and pathology are unknown. Photocoagulation or treatment of aneurysms by the laser beam has been reported but the ultimate prognosis is bad.

Photo-retinitis: Occurs as the result of exposure of the unprotected eye to bright sunlight or other source of brilliant illumination, e.g. welding, electric flashes, mercury vapour lamps, etc. Watching an eclipse of the sun has frequently caused this and it has even been known to result from watching an eclipse reflected in a pond. Accidental exposure to laser beam causes a severe retinal burn. The actual lesion is probably a burn of the retina and as the patient is nearly always looking at the source of light, the burn is often bilateral and at the fovea.

SYMPTOMS: An 'after-image' may be present for a very long time, merging into a central scotoma which is permanent, central vision being lost. In slighter cases the prognosis is not quite so bad, but some serious visual defect always results.

SIGNS: Some oedema of the macula is visible soon after exposure and this is followed by pigmentary disturbances. Rarely, a typical 'punched-out' macula hole occurs as a result of a light burn of the retina.

Purulent Retinitis: This is usually the result of a septic perforating wound and ushers in panophthalmitis. Less frequently it is a metastatic manifestation, the result of pyaemia. A septic embolus lodges in the retina producing a severe retinitis, which in its turn spreads to the vitreous, producing panophthalmitis. In these days of penicillin and chemotherapy, the metastatic process may sometimes be arrested, the eye saved, and useful vision result.

Toxoplasmosis (*see* p. 207): Sometimes manifests itself as a choroido-retinitis.

IV. DEGENERATIONS

Retinitis Pigmentosa: The term 'retinitis pigmentosa' is one of the many misnomers in common use in ophthalmology. Much is uncertain about its causation and pathology, but one fact is transparently clear: it is *not* a retinitis. It is a degenerative and not an inflammatory lesion. A far more correct name is that given by Duke-Elder: pigmentary retinal dystrophy.

Retinitis pigmentosa is an insidious and progressive disease with a characteristic symptom of night-blindness. This symptom is often present for years before objective signs can be found. It usually begins in early adult life and sometimes even in childhood. This disease is strongly hereditary. In the majority of cases it is a recessive characteristic. Sometimes it takes a dominant form when it is handed down to several successive generations. Rarely it is sex-linked. The wise oculist will not commit himself as to the probability of passing on the trait unless he has carefully studied the pedigree of the particular patient. There is a history of consanguinity in some cases, and deafness, polydactyly, deaf-mutism and mental retardation may be associated with it. Visual acuity may be good in early stages, but there is some peripheral contraction of the fields of vision which is specially noticeable in poor illumination. In early stages, a ring scotoma may be present. As time goes on, the fields continue to contract until a tiny central field alone remains and the patient is unable to get about. Apart from the contraction of the fields, the visual acuity diminishes slowly over many years and the night-blindness increases so that after dark the patient has literally to be led about.

Refsum's syndrome described by Toussaint (*Am. J. Ophthal.*, 1973, **72**, 342) is an atypical retinitis pigmentosa with field constrictions and pupils which do not respond to mydriatics. Subcapsular cataracts are present. The general signs include anosmia, ataxia and abnormalities of hands and feet. It is probably due to an inborn error of lipid metabolism.

SIGNS: These are quite characteristic. In the peripheral regions of the retina are many black pigmented spots resembling stars or bone corpuscles, and in advanced cases choroidal vessels are visible and the fundus appears 'striped'. Pigmented spots are scanty early in the disease, but they increase in number as it progresses. Furthermore, in early cases the periphery of the retinae are affected only, but later on the pigmented spots approach the centre. As the atrophic process spreads the ganglion cells are destroyed and their axis cylinders degenerate, causing optic atrophy. Late in the disease, the nutrition of the lens suffers and cataract results, beginning in the posterior layers and later spreading throughout the cortex.

CAUSES: Four different views are expressed:
  a. Parsons found that the choriocapillaris is absent in the affected areas and concludes that the disease is primarily a choroidal vascular lesion.
  b. Wolff considered it to be a degeneration of the neuro-epithelium which spreads to the ganglion cells and nerve-fibre layers, the retina and choroid tending to become fused together.
  c. Dax thought the condition to be one of pituitary dysfunction. Blood and urine of patients with retinitis pigmentosa when injected into frogs cause melanophores to show signs of activity, thus proving the presence of a melanosome-dispersing substance, which indicates some pituitary dysfunction.
  d. Duke-Elder presumes it to be an abiotrophy which is genetically determined.

PATHOLOGY: According to Wolff, three distinct pathological changes can be traced in every advanced case of retinitis pigmentosa.
  a. *Disappearance of the retinal elements* due to degeneration of the neuro-epithelium commencing at the periphery and working inwards. Thus the rods are affected before the cones (hence night-blindness). Furthermore, the process affects the outer layers before the inner ones, hence the ganglion cells and nerve-fibre layers are affected late in the disease. As the result of the degeneration of these elements, the optic nerve becomes atrophic and the disc a yellowish-white colour.
  b. *The formation of glial tissue*: When the retinal elements have degenerated glial proliferation occurs, starting at the outer layers and spreading to the inner. The external limiting membrane disappears and the neuro-epithelium is replaced by glial tissue.
  c. *Pigmentation* only occurs in the diseased retina. It comes from the pigment epithelium after the external limiting membrane has been destroyed. Pigment tends to follow the course of the veins and in places may obscure them from the observer's view. The stellate arrangement of the pigment with anastomosing processes is thought to be due to obliterated pigmented arterioles.

DISEASES OF THE RETINA 81

In addition to these main changes the arteries are narrowed and tend to become obliterated. The choriocapillaris is absent and sclerosis of choroidal vessels occurs. Later, doubtless due to impaired nutrition, a stellate opacity appears in the posterior cortex of the lens and this may lead to a complete cataract.

TREATMENT is entirely without avail. Vitamin A may be tried since it is known to be necessary to the formation of visual purple and deprivation of this leads to night-blindness, but it has no permanent effect. Cataract extraction in retinitis pigmentosa cases should not be lightly undertaken, for its results are most disappointing.

RETINITIS PUNCTATA ALBESCENS is a disease closely allied to retinitis pigmentosa, with similar history and symptoms, but the retina is studded with tiny white dots scattered evenly over the fundus. It is thought to be an atypical retinitis pigmentosa with one important difference: it is relatively non-progressive. Leber considers the dots to be colloid bodies and Nettleship has reported a case in which these colloid bodies gave way in course of time to typical pigment changes.

Angeoid Streaks: In certain retinae which have been the victims of degenerative conditions, curious dark-brown streaks are visible in the neighbourhood of the optic disc. These bear a superficial resemblance to veins, but careful examination shows marked differences both in depth and distribution. They are deeper than the retinal vessels and they tend to run both radially from and concentrically with the optic disc like the strands of a spider's web. The modern view is that they are splits in Bruch's membrane due to degeneration of its elastic tissue, and the tearing of this membrane resulting from movement of the ocular muscles pulling against the fixed site in the region of the optic nerve. Angeoid streaks are often associated with *Pseudoxanthoma elasticum*. Choroidal degeneration at the macula often develops.

Circinate Degeneration of the Retina: See RETINITIS CIRCINATA (p. 77).

Amaurotic Family Idiocy (Tay–Sachs Disease): Most commonly affects Jewish children. It shows itself in infancy and is frequently familial and always bilateral. The child becomes mentally dull, and muscular asthenia and wasting occur. Blindness follows, and death ensues usually within a year of the onset of symptoms.

SIGNS: With the ophthalmoscope the macular area is seen to be a bright white colour with a red rounded spot at the fovea. The periphery of the fundus is normal. Later in the disease, optic atrophy is seen.

PATHOLOGY: Although the ophthalmic picture somewhat resembles that of embolism of the central retinal artery, the actual pathology is totally different. It is a lipoid degeneration of the ganglion cells

82 A SYNOPSIS OF OPHTHALMOLOGY

of the whole body. In the retina, ganglion cells are most numerous in the macular region, and it is these degenerated cells that give the characteristic white appearance. The red spot at the fovea is normal retina (since ganglion cells are absent at the fovea) showing up in sharp contrast with the white degenerated area that surrounds it. Optic atrophy is the inevitable sequel to degeneration of the ganglion cells.

Lipoid Histiocytosis (Niemann–Pick Disease): A widespread lipoid degeneration usually beginning in infancy and involving the liver and spleen. In the late states retinal degeneration occurs resembling that seen in amaurotic family idiocy. The condition is always fatal.

Cerebromacular Degeneration (Batten–Mayou's Disease): This is also a familial disease, but it is not confined to Jewish children and occurs at a later age, usually affecting the 6–8-year-old age group. It is characterized by grossly defective vision with a central scotoma, mental deterioration and convulsions. A similar macular condition has been described by Stargardt which occurs about puberty, with convulsions or mental deterioration. This is also bilateral, familial, and progressive, leading to complete blindness.

SIGNS: The fundi may be normal but the macula shows obvious disturbances with spots and pigmentation. Sometimes there are peripheral pigment changes, rather resembling retinitis pigmentosa.

PATHOLOGY: The essential lesion here is a primary degeneration of the rod and cone and pigment layers of the retina. The choroid is normal, but late in the disease the pathological changes resemble those of retinitis pigmentosa.

V. THE PHAKOMATOSES

This name has been given to four groups of familial syndromes which present a multiplicity of signs, and in many organs of the body, but all of which have two signs in common: (1) the occurrence of tumours or cysts, some of which may become malignant; (2) the presence of ocular lesions, which in each group are most important.

The table given on the opposite page will help to clarify a somewhat complicated symptomatology.

1. Angiomatosis Retinae (von Hippel–Landau's Disease): A rare familial syndrome usually commencing by the third decade. A small pink swelling first appears at the periphery of the retina which communicates with a branch of the central artery and vein. These branches become hugely swollen and tortuous and numerous crimson tufts appear at the ends of arterioles. Often a red tumour resembling a raspberry appears on the retina. Haemorrhages and exudates are present, resembling exudative retinitis, sometimes leading to retinal detachment, glaucoma, cataract and phthisis bulbi. While these ocular changes are going on, cysts occur on the medulla, cerebellum, kidneys, spinal cord, epididymis and elsewhere. The whole course of the disease may take up to 10 years from start to finish. The only ray of hope of prolonging vision in this disease is in photocoagulation of individual lesions by laser beam; alternatively, cryothermy can be tried.

2. **Tuberous Sclerosis (Bourneville's Disease):** In this condition tumours resembling tiny potatoes (hence the term 'tuberous') may occur on the fundus and in many other organs, including the heart, kidneys, thyroid, uterus, etc. The characteristic feature is, however, the occurrence of sebaceous adenomata on the skin and particularly in the region of the face. Patients are frequently mentally defective and sometimes epileptics. It should be noted that tuberous sclerosis can occur without ocular involvement.

3. **Neurofibromatosis (von Recklinghausen's Disease):** A congenital neurofibromatosis associated with the peripheral nerves and with pigmented neuro-ectodermal tumours of the skin. Enlarged nerves can be felt like cords running subcutaneously. Neurofibromata may be found on the iris, and sometimes on the optic nerve. When in this latter position it may even cause an enlargement of the optic foramen, which can be demonstrated radiologically. Occasionally retinal tumours occur in this condition and resemble tuberous sclerosis.

4. **Sturge–Weber's Syndrome:** This consists of a 'port-wine' type of facial naevus usually in the area supplied by the first and second divisions of the fifth nerve. It is sometimes associated with choroidal haemangioma leading to glaucoma. Occasionally calcification of the meninges and underlying cortex occurs, resulting in epilepsy.

	VON HIPPEL	BOURNEVILLE	RECKLINGHAUSEN	STURGE–WEBER
EYE SIGNS	Angiomata, exudative retinitis, choked disc	Potato-like cysts and tumours, choked disc	Tumour of optic nerve, exophthalmos, ? pulsating tumour of iris, choked disc	Glioma of retina, buphthalmos
NERVOUS SYSTEM	Angiomata and cysts of cerebellum and medulla	Tumour and cysts of brain, especially ventricles	Tumours of cranial and sympathetic nerves	Calcification of cerebellum, cerebrum and arachnoid
OTHER ORGANS	Cysts of kidneys, suprarenals, pancreas, epididymis, ovaries and skin	Cysts of tumours of kidney, thyroid, uterus, breast and skin	Tumour of throat, bones, endocrine organs and skin	'Port-wine' naevus of face

VI. TOXIC AMBLYOPIAS

For many years oculists have known that certain drugs can, in patients who are sensitive to them, produce a varying degree of defective vision. Toxic amblyopia affects vision in different ways. Some substances directly poison the retinal ganglion cells, others attack the optic nerve and a few cause a pigmentary degeneration of the retina, clinically resembling retinitis pigmentosa. Many of these conditions have been attributed to retrobulbar neuritis (q.v.), but recent evidence suggests that most toxic amblyopias are primarily a retinal condition.

Tobacco Amblyopia: Results from the excessive use of tobacco either by smoking or chewing. The stronger and cheaper the tobacco the greater the liability to produce amblyopia, and it is almost invariably the result of pipe smoking; it is believed that the trouble is due to cyanide contents in tobacco. It is very doubtful whether cigars or cigarettes alone ever cause it. If excessive smoking is associated with excessive consumption of alcohol the liability to toxic amblyopia is greater, since alcohol alone can produce amblyopia even without tobacco. There is, however, no evidence to show that the visual loss in tobacco amblyopia is greater in drinkers than in teetotallers. From observations made during the Second World War, Schepens of Brussels has proved beyond a doubt that the incidence of tobacco amblyopia is far greater amongst those who are suffering from malnutrition, and he attributes this fact to hepatic deficiency, not to any vitamin deprivation, because the addition of vitamins to the diet did not affect the course of the disease.

SIGNS AND SYMPTOMS: The only symptom is that of increasing diminution of central vision affecting both eyes, but not necessarily to the same extent. There is a central scotoma to colour, especially for red and green, but the peripheral fields are full. Generally there are no ophthalmoscopic changes visible, but occasionally some blurring of the disc edges may be noticed. The course is long and chronic, but the ultimate prognosis is good provided the patient refrains from smoking.

PATHOLOGY: The disease is due to a poisoning of the ganglion cells of the papillo-macular bundle.

TREATMENT:
1. Total abstinence from tobacco. Cutting it down is useless. The patient has to choose between his smoking and his sight. Lobeline sometimes helps as a smoking deterrent.
2. A full vitamin intake (including large doses of vitamin B_{12}) should be recommended and the patient should pay special attention to general health, fresh air, exercise, etc.
3. Some observers have found that a copious intake of bland fluids is helpful.

DISEASES OF THE RETINA 85

4. Vasodilators sometimes help, e.g. sod. nitrite, erythrotetranitrate or the injection of acetylcholine.

Alcohol Amblyopia: Very similar to that caused by tobacco, and all that is written under tobacco amblyopia applies to alcohol amblyopia. It would seem that in certain patients alcohol and tobacco have a synergistic toxic effect on the ganglion cells. In such cases total abstinence from both is essential for the recovery of sight.

Methyl Alcohol Amblyopia: Usually occurs as the result of drinking methylated spirits. After a drinking bout the patient becomes deeply comatose and he finds upon waking that his vision has failed, hence the expression 'blind drunk'. The fields are contracted and there is a large central scotoma which sometimes leads on to blindness. In other cases the vision improves somewhat, but optic atrophy sets in later. Ophthalmoscopically little is visible except optic atrophy in the late stages. Fields are constricted and there may be a central scotoma. Treatment is useless.

Quinine Amblyopia: Usually follows a single large dose such as may be taken at the onset of an attack of malaria or with the intention to induce abortion.

SIGNS AND SYMPTOMS: Pupils are dilated and inactive and the patient complains of sudden deafness and distressing noises in the ears. The retinal vessels are seen to be markedly constricted and the discs are pale. The fields show great contraction and in extreme cases 'tubular vision' is present, i.e. a tiny central area alone remains and the patient has to grope about because all peripheral vision is lost. In more favourable cases the fields gradually widen out, but some permanent constriction always remains. Optic atrophy, either partial or complete, may be the end-result.

Similar symptoms may result from poisoning by *barbiturates*, *optochin*, *Filix mas* and *arsenic*. *Aspirin* and *salicylates* cause similar signs and symptoms, but the attack is much less severe.

PATHOLOGY: There are two theories:

1. Quinine causes extreme vascular spasm producing ischaemia of the ganglion cells leading to optic atrophy in much the same way as a blockage of the central retinal artery produces blindness.
2. That quinine acts as a direct poison to the ganglion cells and that vision fails before the vascular spasm occurs.

TREATMENT:

1. Discontinue the drug.
2. Vasodilatation as described in the treatment of tobacco amblyopia.

VII. TRAUMATIC LESIONS

Commotio Retinae: Results from a blow on the eye. Signs are an oedema of the retina visible with the ophthalmoscope as a milky area at the posterior pole. Occasionally scattered haemorrhages are present.

The oedema is localized and the retina appears normal towards the periphery. Recovery with full restoration of vision is the rule, but every case should be treated seriously and one week of complete rest in bed should be ordered. Rarely pigmentary changes supervene and even more rarely a macular 'hole' results which is thought to be caused by cystic degeneration following retinal oedema. If either of these complications occurs great deterioration of vision results.

Detachment of the Retina: Sometimes traumatic, and this is discussed later in this chapter.

Rupture of the Retina and Choroid: Rare except as a wartime blast injury.

Retinal Haemorrhages: May occur as the result of a trauma. This has been fully discussed on p. 68.

VIII. RETINAL DETACHMENTS

It will be remembered that the retina is firmly attached to the pigment epithelium at the disc and at the ora, but that between these points their surfaces are merely in apposition without any structural attachment. It is, therefore, obvious that there is an inherent weakness in this arrangement and under certain conditions it will be possible for these two surfaces to separate. Furthermore (although it is doubtful whether many students remember this for long after they have ceased to study anatomy) embryological studies make it clear that there is a potential space caused by the invagination of the primary optic vesicle, and this space lies between the neuro-epithelium (the rod and cone layer) and the pigment epithelium. This potential space is the weak spot mentioned above, and when a detachment occurs the separation of the retinal layers invariably takes place between the neuro-epithelium and the pigment layer. Thus, a retinal detachment is really a re-formation of the cavity of the primary optic vesicle.

Retinal detachments can be caused by any of the following processes:
1. The retina may be *pulled* off the pigment layer by traction from fibrous bands in the vitreous or scar formation in the retina, e.g. retinitis proliferans.
2. It may be *pushed* off by the accumulation of fluid, neoplasms, etc. behind it.
3. It may be *floated* off by fluid vitreous entering through the hole.

The ensuing paragraphs will show how these different processes operate in various pathological conditions.

Clinically, detachment of the retina is most commonly seen in the following circumstances:
1. In *myopia* of moderate severity. It is not so common in extreme myopes as in those of, say, −6 dioptres to −8 dioptres. This group represents over 50 per cent of detachment cases.
2. Following *trauma*. This may occur in any eye, but it is more common in the case of myopes.

DISEASES OF THE RETINA

3. In *sarcoma of the choroid*. It is of utmost importance to exclude this in every case of detachment (*see* INTRA-OCULAR NEOPLASMS, p. 159).
4. *Secondary to chronic ocular disease*, e.g. iridocyclitis, retinitis proliferans, etc.
5. Degenerative conditions of retina with cyst formation at periphery.

To these must be added a number to which no such cause can be assigned and which for the lack of a better term may be called 'idiopathic'.

SIGNS AND SYMPTOMS: The patient, usually between 45 and 60 years of age, complains that 'a curtain or veil has descended in front of my eye'. This has caused parts of objects to be obscured, i.e. he can usually see the upper or lower parts only. Careful inquiry may elicit a history of occasional flashes of light before the eye for some days or weeks prior to the detachment. Preliminary examination reveals that there is a gross positive scotoma in the visual field, and perimetry confirms that this scotoma corresponds to the detached area. Fortunately, detachments do not usually involve the macula, at any rate in the earlier stages. If they do, almost all vision is lost. In cases without macular involvement central vision is usually present but impaired.

It must be emphasized that detachments vary greatly in severity from a small shallow one (as is seen in early cases of sarcoma of the choroid) to a large balloon-like detachment involving the greater part of the retina. It is quite easy to miss a detachment unless the observer rigidly adheres to a routine technique of examination:

1. With the pupil fully dilated the reflex should be studied with the ordinary retinoscope mirror. If even a slight detachment is present there would be some departure from the normal reflex.
2. Indirect ophthalmoscopy is invaluable in the diagnosis of retinal detachments. Any abnormality can be seen at once far more easily than it can by the direct method.
3. Direct ophthalmoscopy should next be undertaken, starting with the +12 lens and working downwards. This examination should be made in all four quadrants successively. It is never sufficient to make one cursory examination. A detachment may occur in any quadrant, and unless the whole retina is examined as described above, some case will be certain to be missed. When examining the myope it is sometimes easier to see the fundus when looking with the ophthalmoscope through the patient's own glasses.

The following signs will be observed in the fundus:

1. If the detachment is of any size a grey or green bulging mass will be seen, and puckered folds on its surface are sometimes visible. This bulging area is usually noted best with a high convex lens when the normal portion of the retina is out of focus.

2. The vessels appear strikingly different from the normal, indeed sometimes they appear almost black, and it is very difficult to distinguish between the arteries and the veins.
3. Careful search should reveal some sort of 'hole' or 'rent' through which a normal, bright-red, choroidal reflex is visible. It is probable that 'holes' are present in every case of non-malignant detachment, but they are by no means always easy to find and in a very few cases they may be situated so as to be invisible ophthalmoscopically. As will be seen later, the discovery and accurate location of all retinal holes are of paramount importance.

In a late stage, when the retina is completely detached, it assumes the shape of a partially opened umbrella fixed at the ora and optic disc and hanging in loose folds between these attachments. Later still, it lies behind the lens like a crumpled ball of paper. While these changes are taking place, a low-grade iridocyclitis may set in with KP, posterior synechiae and secondary glaucoma, and as the final end-result the lens become cataractous owing to malnutrition.

For detachments due to malignant disease see chapter on INTRA-OCULAR NEOPLASMS (p. 159).

RETINAL HOLES may be of any shape or size and may occur in any part of the retina. The clinical varieties are:
1. *Dis-insertions* always occur at the periphery and are due to the retinal edge being turned from the ora. They are frequently of traumatic origin and are the commonest form of hole seen.
2. '*Horseshoe*' or '*Arrowhead*' *Rents* can occur anywhere in the retina but are commonest near the periphery. The convexity or the point of the arrowhead always points towards the centre of the retina.
3. *Round Holes* are not nearly so common. They are usually small and well defined and are often present when a detachment is associated with inflammatory changes, e.g. choroiditis, etc.
4. *Irregular Tears or Holes* may be of any size and can occur anywhere in the retina. They are often, but not always, the result of a trauma.

PROGNOSIS: In untreated cases, the prognosis is almost hopeless, but in cases treated by operation it is reasonably good, subject to the following provisos:
1. The eye must be free from disease of the retina or choroid and if myopia is present the retinal degeneration must not be excessive.
2. Operation must be undertaken reasonably soon after the detachment occurs. If 6 months or more have elapsed, surgical intervention will be of doubtful value.

3. A hole or holes must be found and these areas successfully sealed off at operation. Unless this can be done the operation is certain to be a failure.

TREATMENT: Chigwell and Shilling (*Br. J. Ophthal.*, 1973, **57**, 291) use prophylactic treatment before an actual detachment occurs in high-risk cases, e.g. myopes and those with a family history of detachment, also in those who have already had a detachment in one eye. They seal off any form of hole or weak spot found by cryosurgery. Very occasionally this treatment causes retinal puckering with visual impairment so this risk must be taken into consideration and explained to the patient.

In established cases treatment is operative only and, as has already been indicated, the whole result of operation depends upon the exact location of the hole and sealing off this area by a diathermy, cryosurgery or light coagulation. Retinal holes may be very elusive and more than one may coexist, and unless all are adequately treated the operation cannot succeed. It is, therefore, necessary for the patient to be admitted to hospital and for the surgeon to make repeated examinations of the fundus. These should be made with the patient in different positions and a drawing of every fundus detail should be made until the surgeon is familiar with every nook and cranny of the patient's retina. Most particularly, every hole must be exactly located in regard to its position on the outside scleral surface. This is best done by using Cole–Marshall charts, by means of which the fundus is divided into meridians. The distance along the meridian (either from the disc or ora) is calculated in terms of 'disc-diameters'. Once the exact position on the fundus is located, a second Cole–Marshall chart enables the surgeon to work out its position on the outside scleral surface by a system of all surface landmarks and measurements.

The authors have sometimes found it necessary to make six or more examinations, each one lasting up to half an hour, before all holes are found and every fundus detail noted. There is no short cut to charting these details, and the reader is advised never to attempt an operation unless he is prepared to make whatever sacrifice of time and patience may be necessary for these preliminary investigations.

The pioneer of detachment surgery by sealing off the hole by diathermy was Jules Gonin of Lausanne, who first successfully operated upon this condition in 1919.

The operation usually undertaken for slight cases with disinsertion which is not too extensive consists of the application of surface diathermy to the sclera over the immediate area of the hole. Sufficient current should be used to give the sclera a slightly 'toasted' appearance. This causes a coagulation in the choroid which is visible ophthalmoscopically, and its position in relation to the hole should be checked in this way. Recently cryosurgery has been used instead of diathermy. If the charted position has been correct, the neighbourhood of the hole will have been sealed off and the retina and choroid firmly adherent in this area. More recently retinal holes have been sealed off by a laser, *see* Chapter XXIX, p. 255. The sclera should then be punctured with a sharp diathermy needle in one or two places where the operator considers he will find the maximum accumulation of subretinal fluid. This fluid should be removed by suction. Both eyes are bandaged and the patient is returned to bed and placed when possible so that the hole is in the most dependent position. The patient should be kept at absolute rest for 3 weeks. Major advances in the surgical treatment of detachment have been made in the past decade but the ideal technique has not yet been found.

Alternative operations for detachment cases are:
1. LAMELLAR SCLERAL RESECTION AND OVERLAP: After the hole has been localized in the usual manner the globe is virtually shortened by the removal of a 4 × 7 mm strip of sclera behind the recti insertions. Only the superficial scleral layers are removed, the deeper layers being left to minimize risk to the choroid. The deeper scleral layers are treated with cryotherapy and the edges of the resected area are sutured. Due to difficulties in wound closure this procedure has been superseded by scleral overlap. Instead of removing an ellipse of sclera, the sclera is incised down to the deeper layers and dissected posteriorly, cryotherapy is applied to the scleral bed and appropriately applied mattress sutures cause the scleral fringe to slide forwards by the desired amount. A similar procedure of scleral pocketing can be employed to bury silicone sponge implants.
2. GLOBE ENCIRCLEMENT: Arruga in 1962 introduced the operation of globe encirclage using suture material, and this was widely adopted. It has the great advantage of speed, simplicity and effectiveness but unfortunately is prone to complications ('string syndromes'). These complications are largely obviated by using a flat silicone strap either fixed by mattress sutures or let into scleral 'trap-doors'. Greater indentation can be achieved by incorporating localized plastic implants in the areas of retinal breaks. It is of great value in cases with multiple breaks, peripheral degenerative changes, aphakia and in the elderly in that it allows early ambulation.
3. SCLERAL BUCKLING: This is probably the most popular procedure used today. The sclera is indented by the application of a 3 or 5 mm tube of silicone sponge held in situ with mattress

supramid sutures. The indentation coapts the choroid to the retina and seals off the break usually without resorting to drainage of subretinal fluid. To achieve success it is essential that hole and choroid are in apposition with the hole on the apex of the choroidal 'hillock'.

4. LIGHT COAGULATION: The area of the hole can be sealed off by a carefully directed beam from a powerful arc light. This excellent technique was perfected by Meyer Schwickerath of Bonn. The original apparatus was elephantine in proportion and price but the recently introduced portable models bring the scope of light coagulation techniques within the financial resources of most eye departments. The argon lasers, whilst less versatile, are more precise in that they produce small retinal burns (a disadvantage if large areas have to be treated). Light coagulation is of great value in treating macular holes, 'flat' holes, retinoschisis, potential breaks and peripheral degenerations, as well as an adjunct to other methods of detachment surgery. More recently it has been used in treating diabetic retinopathy, vascular lesions and macula degenerations.

5. VITREOUS IMPLANT: This is another recent advance in detachment surgery. It is of most value in the more serious cases and especially in aphakia. Successes have been reported in cases that have failed to respond to diathermy operation. The vitreous (up to 2 ml) is removed by aspiration through a special widebore needle within a few hours of death. The recipient eye is then subjected to the conventional diathermy or scleral reaction operation and as soon as the subretinal fluid is aspirated, the donor vitreous is injected into the inferotemporal quadrant at a point about 7 mm behind the corneal margin. The immediate result of this operation when viewed through the ophthalmoscope is little short of dramatic—the detached area of retina seeming to return to its proper place almost with a click. Vitreous bands can also be divided, using a knife-needle or vitreal membrane scissors. Giant dialysis with contracted, rolled edges can be reposited using a transvitreal cryoprobe technique.

Workers at Washington University have been injecting liquid *silicone* material to push the retina back in place.

IX. RETROLENTAL FIBROPLASIA

Retrolental fibroplasia is a disease of premature infants which is not clinically detectable at birth but which develops during the first few months of life. It was first described by T. L. Terry in 1942. The earliest sign is an almost angiomatous dilatation of retinal veins and arteries, with great tortuosity. This is followed by the appearance at the periphery of some yellowish solid-looking nodules with pigment changes at their bases. Next there appears an engorgement of retinal veins and a generalized retinal oedema and the appearance of other scattered nodules over the fundus. These proliferate and invade the retrolental space, forming a membranous structure. This membrane is thought to be the anterior portion of the swollen retina. Finally (according to William Councilman Owens and Ella Uhler Owens, of Baltimore) a complete retrolental membrane is formed by extension of peripheral folds of the retina, with proliferative changes and the formation of fibrous bands in the vitreous. Some eyes later develop secondary glaucoma owing to the pushing forward of the lens and iris. The disease is bilateral, but occasionally the course is arrested at some intermediate stage and complete and absolute blindness does not always necessarily result.

The cause is now known to have been due to excessive oxygen given to the infant during early life in the oxygen tent. Hyperoxygenation causes swelling of the retinal tissues which obstructs the normal circulation. Since the oxygen concentration is now never allowed to exceed 40 per cent, the disease has practically disappeared.

Chapter VII

DISEASES OF THE SCLERA

Anatomy: The sclera is the toughest of the coats of the eye, being composed of dense fibrous tissue. It varies considerably in thickness, being thickest at the posterior pole (1 mm) and thinnest at the equator (0·4–0·5 mm). The scleral coat possesses two foramina:

ANTERIOR SCLERAL FORAMEN is situated at the junction of the cornea and sclera and measures approximately 10·6 × 11·6 mm, its greater diameter being transverse. Into this foramen fits the cornea, with the sclera slightly overlapping, like the rim over a watch-glass.

POSTERIOR SCLERAL FORAMEN has a retinal diameter of 1·5–2 mm and an orbital one of 3–3·5 mm. Its function is to provide an exit for the optic nerve. The posterior layers of the sclera in this region are continued backwards along the optic nerve and become fused with its dural sheath.

The anterior scleral layers bridge across the posterior foramen to form the lamina cribrosa, a perforated structure through which pass the fibres of the optic nerve.

In addition to these foramina, the sclera is perforated by various canals through which nerves and vessels enter or leave the eye.

It may be stated at the outset that inflammatory diseases of the sclera are uncommon, a fact which is rather curious in view of the frequency of inflammation of the conjunctiva, the sclera's overlying membrane. There are two distinct varieties found in scleral inflammations, which are totally different clinically: (1) Episcleritis; and (2) Scleritis.

EPISCLERITIS

Episcleritis is really an inflammation of the subconjunctival tissue in which the superficial scleral layers share. The first sign is the appearance of a red inflamed nodule a few millimetres from the limbus. This nodule is the size of a split pea and is hard and tender, with the conjunctiva freely movable over it. The overlying conjunctiva is red and hyperaemic (as it shares in the inflammation), but this redness is definitely localized. The condition is most persistent and is sometimes bilateral and causes a generalized ocular discomfort. The absorption of the nodule may take weeks or even months. Recurrences are frequent.

PATHOLOGY: The nodule consists of aggregations of lymphocytes in episcleral tissue.

AETIOLOGY: Duke-Elder considers that episcleritis is either an allergic reaction to an endogenous toxin or a collagenous disease.

None the less, such a large number of patients with episcleritis suffer from some form of rheumatism or arthritis that it would seem that there must be some connection between these conditions and such superficial ocular inflammations as episcleritis, scleritis, chronic conjunctivitis, etc. It is also found in some cases of rheumatic heart disease, erythema nodosum, rosacea, gonococcal infections, ileitis, diabetes and tuberculosis.

TREATMENT:
1. Local corticosteroids often give great relief and should be tried in all cases.
2. Salicylates can be tried in intransigent cases.
3. Short-wave diathermy on alternate days is helpful in severe and painful cases.
4. Cases that do not respond to the above should be put on general steroid therapy.

SCLERITIS

In this very uncommon condition a diffuse brawny swelling appears on the sclera, which on subsiding leaves the affected area very thin and with a porcelain-blue appearance. It is one of the most painful, prolonged, and eventually the most serious of all eye diseases. Ectasia of the sclerotic in the affected area is not uncommon. Since the deeper scleral layers are affected, an associated iritis or anterior uveitis frequently develops and occasionally sclerosing keratitis supervenes. This is a rare manifestation, where the cornea develops some scattered triangular opacities which, in the course of time, become almost pure white and exactly resemble islands of sclerotic in corneal tissue. Deep scleritis is a very chronic condition and is usually bilateral. It occasionally completely surrounds the cornea, when it is known as 'annular' scleritis. There is a very marked ocular discomfort and the eye is specially sensitive to cold and wind. Ciliary staphyloma and secondary glaucoma are frequent complications.

PATHOLOGY: The seriousness of this disease is due to the accompanying uveitis. The headquarters of the complaint lie in the deep scleral fibres, many of which necrose and giant cells are to be found. Hyaline degeneration supervenes. The disease often affects the corneosclerotic junction, hence the tendency for the inflammation to spread by the ciliary vessels to the anterior part of the uveal tract. Tuberculosis and syphilis sometimes produce a similar condition, hence the appropriate investigations should always be made. Occasionally the thinned-out sclera becomes ectatic in the ciliary region and a staphyloma and secondary glaucoma result.

AETIOLOGY is unknown. Rheumatism is by no means invariably present and young persons are sometimes affected. It can occur in rheumatoid arthritis, polyarteritis nodosa, syphilis, tuberculosis, lupus erythematosus and herpes zoster.

DISEASES OF THE SCLERA

TREATMENT:
1. Careful search for, and treatment of, any possible causative factor.
2. Treatment as for uveitis in general.
3. Frequently the eyes require some protection. Dark glasses or even goggles may be necessary, especially in cold and windy weather.
4. Steroid therapy, both systemic and local, should be given a prolonged trial.

SCLEROMALACIA PERFORANS

This is a rare disease affecting elderly women. Parts of the sclera degenerate exposing bulges of uveal tissue. These changes are accompanied by a severe and progressive iritis which often leads to blindness. Local and general steroid treatment is the only hope in this serious condition.

SCLERAL STAPHYLOMA

The name given to an ectasia or bulging of the sclera. The bulge consists of thinned-out sclera lined with uveal tissue. It occurs as the result of either or both of two factors: (1) Increased intra-ocular tension; (2) Thinning of the sclera.

The commonest conditions which produce these factors are: (1) scleritis, (2) trauma, (3) new growth, (4) tuberculosis, (5) syphilis, (6) severe and prolonged increased tension.

Staphylomata are classified according to their situation:
1. CILIARY, when the bulge occurs in the region of the ciliary body so that this structure lines the staphyloma.
2. INTERCALARY, when the ectasia lies between the iris and the ciliary body, the base of the iris lining the bulge.
3. EQUATORIAL, where the sclera is unsupported by the extraocular muscles. It should be remembered that the normal sclera is thinnest at the equator, hence this naturally weak spot.
4. POSTERIOR, the name given to any ectasia behind the equator. In this form, any of the above aetiological factors may apply, but high myopia is the commonest cause.

BLUE SCLEROTICS

This is a congenital defect where the sclera is so thin that the uveal tissue shines through, giving it a porcelain-blue appearance. The condition is frequently associated with fragilitas ossium and otosclerosis. Both sexes may be affected, but only those suffering from the disease can transmit it.

Chapter VIII

DISEASES OF THE OPTIC NERVE

Anatomy: The optic nerve extends from the chiasma to the optic disc, but for the purpose of this chapter only the part between the optic foramen and the lamina cribrosa will be considered. This portion of the nerve can conveniently be divided into two parts: (1) the orbital portion; and (2) the intra-ocular portion.
  1. ORBITAL PORTION: This part of the nerve is about 25 mm long and extends from the optic foramen to the posterior pole of the globe. It lies very loosely in order to permit free range of movement of the globe. It is surrounded by the recti muscles but is separated from them by fat, in which the ciliary vessels and nerves lie. About 12 mm behind the globe the nerve is pierced by the central retinal vessels. The orbital portion of the nerve is 3–4 mm in diameter and contains both pupillary and visual afferent fibres. The optic nerve should be regarded as a prolongation of the brain. This fact is well known embryologically and can be proved anatomically by the structure of the nerve and its sheaths. It is surrounded by three sheaths continuous with the coverings of the brain:
     a. DURA MATER, which lines the optic canal, divides, part of it being continuous with the periosteum of the orbit and the other portion forming the dural sheath of the nerve.
     b. ARACHNOID, which comes in contact with the optic nerve as it leaves the cisterna basalis, and forms the arachnoid sheath of the nerve.
     c. PIA, attached to the nerve as its pial sheath and forms its interfascicular septa.
       It should be noted that the subdural space is very small but the subarachnoid space is very easily distensible. These two spaces are together called the intervaginal space. These facts are of great importance in considering the pathology of papilloedema.
  2. INTRA-OCULAR PORTION: This portion, the head of the optic nerve, is 1 mm long and traverses the posterior scleral foramen to merge through the lamina cribrosa at the papilla, the spot where the retinal fibres join the optic nerve. At this site the retinal vessels emerge. The head of the optic nerve is visible from the retinal side and is called the optic disc.

Diseases of the optic nerve can conveniently be studied under five headings: (1) Inflammations; (2) Oedema; (3) Atrophies; (4) Congenital abnormalities; (5) Injuries.

I. INFLAMMATIONS

Papillitis is the name given to a true inflammation of the optic papilla and when this occurs it is almost invariably part of a so-called 'neuroretinitis', i.e. an inflammation affecting jointly the retina and the optic papilla. It should be noted that in the early stages of papill-oedema due to a space-occupying lesion in the brain, the ophthalmoscopic appearance of the optic disc almost exactly resembles that of papillitis, but, of course, the pathology of the two conditions is completely different.

SIGNS AND SYMPTOMS: It may be stated at once that a positive diagnosis from the appearance of the optic disc alone is unreliable. Hyperaemia and blurred edges, although textbook signs, are not invariably seen owing to the numerous variations of normal discs. More confidence can be placed in these signs if they are present in the one eye and absent from the other in the same patient, but even this is not entirely infallible, owing to variations between the two eyes of the same individual. Some dilatation of the veins on the disc are visible, and when the disease is at all pronounced, the disc certainly looks pink and the edges are blurred. Some haemorrhages may be present on or near the disc. There is, however, very rarely any marked degree of swelling. At this stage signs of retinitis (exudates, etc.) will be obvious. The symptoms are visual only and often vague. The pupils will be equal and regular, the visual acuity is somewhat impaired, and the vessels show some contraction. The condition is usually bilateral.

AETIOLOGY, PATHOLOGY, PROGNOSIS AND TREATMENT are those of the disease causing the retinitis.

Retrobulbar Neuritis: As its name implies, this is an inflammatory lesion of the *orbital* portion of the optic nerve between the optic foramen and the posterior scleral foramen.

CAUSES: Should be classified as local and general:

LOCAL:
1. Spread of inflammation from surrounding structures, e.g. periostitis, sphenoidal or ethmoidal sinusitis, etc.
2. Haemorrhage into the orbit or optic nerve sheath.
3. Injuries involving fractures of the optic foramen.

GENERAL:
1. Multiple sclerosis frequently causes retrobulbar neuritis and its presence should be suspected especially when occurring in young people.
2. Acute febrile illnesses, especially encephalitis and poliomyelitis.
3. Diabetes.
4. Devic's disease.
5. Leber's disease.
6. Herpes zoster.

98   A SYNOPSIS OF OPHTHALMOLOGY

SIGNS AND SYMPTOMS: This disease is sudden in onset and is usually unilateral. The patient complains of dimness of vision of one eye, associated with pain on movement of the eyeball, especially when looking laterally. The eyeball is tender on pressure and headache may be present. The pupils react to light but show a phenomenon that is almost diagnostic: the contraction of the pupil on the affected side is not sustained but the pupil slowly dilates again even while the light is still fixed on the eye. The fields show a central scotoma, especially for colours, with some peripheral loss also. In a severe case the patient's vision may be so bad that field examination is impossible. More often than not there are no ophthalmoscopic changes, but in severe cases papillitis (q.v.) may be present, and in the worst cases the inflammation may cause degeneration of nerve fibres with partial optic atrophy as the result. This, when present, usually affects the temporal side, causing pallor of the disc in that area. There is one pitfall to be looked for in the diagnosis of retrobulbar neuritis, i.e. an amblyopic eye. Every patient should always be questioned as to the history of an old squint or 'lazy' eye.

PROGNOSIS: Depends upon the cause, but is usually good. In cases of multiple sclerosis relapses are common, bilateral attacks occur occasionally, and there is very slow but progressive loss of vision, the visual acuity following an attack rarely being as good as it was previously. Fortunately, permanent blindness scarcely ever occurs.

TREATMENT: That of the underlying cause, but in every case smoking should be forbidden since tobacco is in itself a potential ganglion-cell toxin and a tobacco amblyopia complicating retrobulbar neuritis might be disastrous. Iodides or salicylates have helped when the cause of the trouble has been uncertain.

Leber's Disease (*Hereditary Optic Neuritis*) is a familial form of optic neuritis occurring in males and commencing in the early twenties or thereabouts. It is bilateral and causes gross visual failure but very rarely complete blindness. A central scotoma and fairly full peripheral fields are the rule, but occasionally total colour blindness occurs. In early stages there are no ophthalmoscopic changes, but later on atrophy supervenes, and temporal or complete pallor of the optic disc is seen. No treatment is of any avail.

PATHOLOGY: It has been suggested that changes in the pituitary gland associated with adolescence and causing pressure on the chiasma have been responsible for this condition. This is very doubtful and in any case does not explain the familial incidence of the disease.

II. OEDEMA

Papilloedema: As has already been mentioned, papilloedema is a totally different pathological entity from papillitis and the only thing they

DISEASES OF THE OPTIC NERVE

have in common is superficial ophthalmoscopic resemblance when the papilloedema is in an early stage. Papillitis is part of a neuroretinitis and is an *inflammation*, whereas papilloedema is an *oedema* due to pressure, a hydrostatic phenomenon, the mechanism of which is discussed under PATHOLOGY, *below*.

CAUSES OF PAPILLOEDEMA:
1. Any condition causing a raised intracranial pressure, e.g. tumour, abscess, aneurysm, subarachnoid haemorrhage.
2. Syphilis.
3. Malignant hypertension.
4. Lead poisoning.
5. Gross nutritional defects (as experienced by prisoners of war, etc.).
6. Some febrile illnesses, especially meningitis.
7. Sudden and severe anaemia, e.g. due to uterine or gastric haemorrhage, etc.
8. Leukaemia.

SIGNS AND SYMPTOMS: Ophthalmoscopically the characteristics of papilloedema are a hugely swollen ('choked') disc, sometimes to the extent of 8 dioptres. Dilated and tortuous veins are present and gross scattered haemorrhages. There is often so much oedema that the disc margins are almost impossible to find. In a later stage exudates also are present and even a macular 'fan'. The visual symptoms are slight in early cases—in fact the vision is sometimes quite normal, but there is usually some constriction of the fields and a careful inquiry may reveal a history of occasional bouts of blurred sight. On the other hand the sight may fail in a matter of a few days to almost complete blindness, with dilated non-reacting pupils, and a visual acuity of hand movements or perception of light only. The curious and unexplained feature of papilloedema is that the visual acuity gives no indication of the amount of oedema present. Sometimes a severe case of 'choked disc' has almost normal sight, whereas another case with comparatively slight oedema may be completely blind. Field changes are present according to the nature and site of the lesion. Central scotomata, especially to colours, are frequently found. In nearly all cases, headache, vomiting, and drowsiness are present. The disease is usually, not invariably, bilateral, and is not necessarily equally advanced in each eye, and the relative degree of oedema present is of very doubtful value in localizing the lesion. The Foster Kennedy syndrome is sometimes found in prefrontal tumours affecting the olfactory nerve. This consists of an optic atrophy on the affected side due to local pressure and papilloedema of the opposite side due to general intracranial pressure. Unilateral papilloedema suggests some local orbital condition, e.g. cellulitis, tumour of optic nerve, haemorrhage into nerve sheath, etc.

PROGNOSIS: In untreated cases the disease runs a chronic course and the prognosis is definitely bad. If the pressure on the nerve is maintained, irremediable damage is done to it and post-neuritic optic atrophy results. When the increased intracranial pressure is relieved by a decompression operation reasonably early, recovery of sight (but usually with some degree of residual visual impairment) can be expected. Likewise syphilitic cases may respond to proper treatment.

PATHOLOGY: In 1869 Schwalbe discovered the continuity between the subarachnoid space of the brain and the optic nerve, and modern views on the pathology of papilloedema are based upon this discovery. In cases of cerebral tumour, a considerably increased pressure is transmitted to the intervaginal space around the optic nerve. The eye nerve fibres are seen to be grossly swollen and cytoid bodies are visible. Neuroglial proliferation occurs and mesoblastic tissue surrounding the vessels is markedly thickened. It will be remembered that the retinal vessels cross this space about 1 cm behind the globe. Most observers now believe that the primary cause of papilloedema is pressure on the central vein as it crosses this very vulnerable space. The theory that papilloedema is an inflammatory lesion has been disproved histologically.

TREATMENT: This is obviously that of the condition causing the trouble, but the most urgent necessity is the prompt relief of pressure by decompression. This should be done as early as possible if the sight is to be saved and should be regarded as an interim measure pending more drastic surgery.

III. OPTIC ATROPHY

'She was blind, but in the orbs themselves there was no visible defect.' LYTTON, *Last Days of Pompeii*

Causes: The first point to remember in considering this condition is the fact that a degeneration of the optic nerve behaves quite differently from a degeneration in a peripheral nerve. If the optic nerve is injured in any part of its course, there is a *descending* as well as an *ascending* degeneration, and the final result is an atrophy extending from the retina to the lateral geniculate body, an atrophy that is complete and final without hope of regeneration. It follows, therefore, that optic atrophy may be caused by a lesion in any one of the following places: (1) in the retina; (2) at the optic disc; (3) anywhere in the optic nerve between the globe and the lateral geniculate body.

RETINAL LESIONS: Every one of these causes atrophy by destroying the ganglion cells.
  1. Pigmentary retinopathy (formerly retinitis pigmentosa).
  2. Any excessive choroidoretinitis.
  3. Any ganglion-cell toxin (tobacco, quinine, etc.).

DISEASES OF THE OPTIC NERVE

4. Retinal vascular lesions such as blockage of central artery, ischaemic amaurosis, etc.
5. Nutritional deficiencies.

OPTIC DISC LESIONS:
1. Papilloedema, where atrophy is due to pressure on the optic nerve behind the disc, a pressure assisted by the mechanical constriction of the disc at the lamina cribrosa.
2. Glaucoma, where the raised intra-ocular pressure causes atrophy and cupping of the disc by pressure from inside the globe.

LESIONS BETWEEN THE GLOBE AND LATERAL GENICULATE BODY:
1. Tabes, retrobulbar neuritis, multiple sclerosis, etc.
2. Pressure by tumours, aneurysms of internal carotid, etc.
3. Inflammatory involvement of the nerve secondary to meningitis, orbital cellulitis, etc.
4. Trauma, e.g. haemorrhage into nerve sheath, damage by fractures, etc.

Although the above classification has accuracy to commend it, the former classification of primary or secondary atrophy possesses at least the merit of simplicity.

PRIMARY OPTIC ATROPHY may be defined as that occurring in the absence of any visible local disease. These cases are generally due to disease of the central nervous system, but in some cases no cause can be found in spite of extensive investigations.

SECONDARY OPTIC ATROPHY is that which follows papilloedema ('post-neuritic'), pigmentary retinopathy and other local diseases which lead to degenerative changes in the optic nerve.

Signs and Symptoms: Ophthalmoscopically, optic atrophy is characterized by a very striking pallor of the disc, which varies from a waxy white to a porcelain-blue colour. The stippling of the lamina cribrosa is very noticeable and the disc edges are so clearly defined. as to give it a punched-out appearance. Shallow cupping (not due to increased tension) may be visible. These variations from the normal appearance are due to the diminished blood-supply. Certain types of optic atrophy have a definite clinical appearance.

1. PIGMENTARY RETINOPATHY (RETINITIS PIGMENTOSA): In optic atrophy secondary to this condition the disc is of a waxy yellow appearance.
2. POST-NEURITIC OPTIC ATROPHY: In these cases fibrous tissue is formed at the disc, and this fills in the physiological cup and overlaps the disc, sometimes extending along the vessels which are constricted by it.

In cases of complete optic atrophy the pupils are dilated and fixed and the patient is quite blind. In unilateral cases a strong consensual reaction is present. When the atrophy is only partial the pupil reactions are sluggish, vision is subnormal, fields generally contracted, and varying degrees of scotomata are present.

Prognosis: It should be noted that the appearance of the optic disc gives no clue as to the visual acuity, some apparently strikingly typical cases of optic atrophy retaining a fair degree of vision. In nearly all cases of primary optic atrophy there is very slow but progressive deterioration of vision leading in the course of years to complete blindness. The prognosis is particularly bad in tabetic cases.

Diagnosis: From the foregoing list of causes of this condition it will be obvious that the diagnosis is not easy. The following investigation should be made:
1. Tabes being the commonest cause, the Wassermann reaction is of prime importance.
2. Complete examination of the central nervous system for multiple sclerosis or other nervous disease. This should include X-ray investigation of the pituitary fossa.
3. The possibility of poisoning should be eliminated, e.g. lead, methyl alcohol, etc.
4. Avitaminosis must be excluded as a cause, especially in those who have been prisoners of war in the East.
5. The possibility of haemorrhages from any source such as uterus, bleeding piles, gastric ulcers and even epistaxis.

Treatment: Entirely limited to that of the condition causing the atrophy.

IV. CONGENITAL ABNORMALITIES

Opaque Nerve Fibres: Normally myelination of the optic nerve fibres ends at the lamina cribrosa, but in some cases medullation (although always lost at the lamina cribrosa) begins again and continues beyond the disc margin. When this happens, the appearance is characteristic, a white leash of wavy fibres being visible and bearing a faint resemblance to the tail of a white horse. The retinal vessels dip in and out of these fibres. They are entirely without significance and no treatment is required. It is of interest to note that in cases of optic atrophy these white fibres disappear.

Colobomata of the Disc: Occur in two forms, the commonest being:
 THE INFERIOR CRESCENT at the lower margin of the disc. This crescent is paler than the disc itself and is often somewhat ectatic. It is due to partial failure of closure of the foetal fissure.
 TRUE COLOBOMA is much rarer and is also due to partial failure of closure of the embryonic fissure. The disc appears to be greatly enlarged and the vessels to have 'gone haywire'. What is taken for the disc is really the sclera and the inner surface of the optic nerve sheath, the nerve itself appearing as a band near the upper part of the coloboma. The coloboma is ectatic and there is usually

grossly defective vision. The cause, again, is defective closure of the foetal fissure.

Congenital Holes: Occur from time to time in the optic disc. They are usually in the temporal portion and appear a dark grey colour owing to the shadow cast by the light from the ophthalmoscope.

V. INJURIES OF THE OPTIC NERVE

The optic nerve may be ruptured in cases of fractured skull or it may be avulsed from the posterior scleral foramen. Very rarely is it injured by penetrating orbital injuries (arrows, knives, etc.), the length of the nerve and the laxity of the tissue in which it is embedded allowing it to be pushed aside. Haemorrhages into the optic nerve sheath are not uncommon. Since the optic nerve does not possess the power of regeneration, any treatment for trauma is useless.

Chapter IX

DISEASES OF THE VITREOUS

Anatomy: The vitreous differs from any other structure of the human body in that it contains no blood vessels, no nerves, no lymphatics, and very few cells of any kind. It is a clear, colourless, translucent, semifluid gel, filling about two-thirds of the volume of the globe, and lying in the space behind the lens, firmly attached at the ora and the optic disc but elsewhere extremely loosely. It is believed to be entirely structureless and the so-called 'framework' which was once thought to 'support' the fluid is now considered to be an artefact. Being semifluid and structureless, it assumes the shape of the globe which contains it.

Pathology: Since the vitreous is completely avascular, it is incapable of inflammation and is unaffected by trauma. In fact it is true to say that any changes that may occur in the vitreous are due to changes in its surrounding structures, the vitreous itself being entirely inert.

Opacities (Muscae Volitantes): Floating specks are very frequently seen by normal people with perfectly healthy eyes. These are usually entoptic images of blood corpuscles, for any non-transparent body that is anterior to the rod-and-cone layer of the retina is capable of producing an image. Often minute cellular specks invisible to the ophthalmoscope can produce muscae. In a variety of pathological conditions these floating bodies may be greatly increased and may prove a serious impediment to vision and become readily visible by the ophthalmoscope. In emmetropic patients they are best seen with the +8 ophthalmoscope lens. Such opacities may be caused by: (1) Fibrinous coagula from the ciliary body or choroid: (2) Collections of leucocytes from the ciliary body; (3) Blood; (4) Crystals; (5) Senile degenerative changes, with increased fluidity of vitreous.

From this list it will be obvious that such conditions as iridocyclitis, choroiditis and myopia all produce vitreous opacities. In fact, it would be true to say that any eye that has had any sort of disease of any part of the uveal tract or retina has vitreous opacities to a greater or lesser degree. One form of vitreous opacity is worth special mention:

SYNCHESIS SCINTILLANS: This is due to a degeneration of the vitreous resulting in increased fluidity and the deposition of cholesterol crystals. These can be seen with the ophthalmoscope (usually best with a +8 lens) as a shower of silver or golden rain when the patient moves his eye. It does not usually affect vision.

DISEASES OF THE VITREOUS

Symptoms: Visual only. The patient complains that a 'speck', a 'spider's web' or a 'tadpole' is floating about in the field of vision, and some intelligent patients can make an accurate drawing of their floating body, which can be verified by the ophthalmoscope.

Treatment: That of the underlying cause, but in the great majority of cases the opacity is 'a visitor who has come to stay'. With the lapse of time, patients become so used to the condition that they regard it as part and parcel of their lives and it ceases to inconvenience them. Patients can safely be reassured.

'Fluid' Vitreous: This is very common in moderate or high myopes. It can also occur as a result of cyclitis or other disease which adversely affects its nutrition. It is accompanied by the presence of gross opacities or synchesis scintillans; sometimes increased fluidity may be the result of senile degeneration of the vitreous and it is not always possible to diagnose it. Its presence adds greatly to the hazards of any intra-ocular operation and especially that of cataract extraction. The tension of the eye gives no indication as to the fluidity or otherwise of the vitreous.

Vitreous Haemorrhage: May occur in any of the following conditions:
(1) Trauma; (2) Arteriosclerosis; (3) Retinopathy; (4) Diabetes; (5) Pernicious or other anaemias; (6) Eales's disease; (7) Undetermined causes.

SIGNS AND SYMPTOMS: A vitreous haemorrhage causes sudden failure of vision in the affected eye, with disappearance of the normal reflex. A red mass can sometimes be seen on oblique illumination and blood cells are visible with the slit-lamp. In every case of vitreous haemorrhage the blood enters the vitreous from one of the retinal vessels.

PROGNOSIS: Recovery from an individual haemorrhage is good, absorption without organization being the rule. 'Never despair of a vitreous haemorrhage' is a sound dictum. The prognosis is far worse in repeated attacks since there is a tendency to organization and the formation of fibrous tissue in the vitreous (*see* RETINITIS PROLIFERANS, p. 77). The presence of some general disease, e.g. diabetes, syphilis, nephritis, etc., also worsens the prognosis.

TREATMENT:
1. Absolute rest in bed is essential for every case until the haemorrhage clears.
2. Vitamin-K therapy is sound and worth a trial.
3. During convalescence, strenuous exercise and stooping and straining should be avoided.
4. In a few cases where the eye has become blind owing to dense vitreous opacities some bold surgeons have tried the drastic measure of aspirating the opaque vitreous and replacing it with

a vitreous implant from a corpse. This is a highly risky procedure and has little to commend it, since a vitreous so full of opaque material probably indicates the presence of iridocyclitis or some other disease of the affected eye.

Pseudoglioma: Certain pathological conditions in the vitreous may give a white or grey pupillary reflex, and when these conditions occur in young children great care must be taken to exclude retinoblastoma. These pseudogliomata can be caused by the following vitreous disorders:
  1. CYCLITIC MEMBRANE behind the lens in plastic iridocyclitis. In this group of cases, however, the membrane is not usually seen clinically since the lens is often cataractous.
  2. SUBACUTE ENDOPHTHALMITIS may occur occasionally without the known presence of ocular inflammation. Meningitis, otitis media or any other serious specific fever can cause it. It is this group that is commonest in early childhood and easily mistaken for glioma.
  3. PERSISTENT VASCULAR SHEATH OF LENS: In these cases there is a gap in the posterior lens capsule with some degree of cataract and a complete hyaloid artery together with its vascular sheath. The artery may contain blood and the blood vessels may be visible on the back of the lens, the general appearance resembling a glioma.

  Other conditions producing pseudoglioma which cannot be classified as diseases of the vitreous (Coats's disease, conglomerate tuberculosis of the choroid, retrolental fibroplasia, etc.) are discussed under their respective headings. For the differential diagnosis between pseudo- and true glioma *see* INTRA-OCULAR NEOPLASMS, p. 159.

Pus in the Vitreous: This occurs in metastatic panophthalmitis, or as the result of perforating injury. The eye is intensely inflamed and the diagnosis is usually obvious. No reflex is present and examination with oblique illumination shows a yellow purulent mass behind the lens.

  TREATMENT: If penicillin treatment has failed, evisceration of the eyeball is indicated.

Persistent Hyaloid Artery: Normally this artery is functionless after the sixth month of fetal life and has disappeared before birth. Remnants are not uncommonly seen in the following forms:
  1. The anterior portion of the artery appears as a tiny threadlike strand attached to the posterior capsule of the lens with its loose end floating about in the vitreous.
  2. Similarly, the posterior portion of the artery may persist. This appears as a grey cord attached to the disc, with its free end moving in the vitreous with every movement of the eye.

3. As a posterior polar cataract, a rounded dot on the back of the lens. This is not, of course, a cataract but the remnant of the artery.
4. Persistent vascular sheath, as mentioned under PSEUDOGLIOMA, *above*.

Usually little or no visual disability results, and it is found in the course of a routine examination. In the case, however, of persistent vascular sheath there is gross visual impairment. No treatment is, of course, possible.

Injuries involving the Vitreous:
'Out, vile jelly.' W. SHAKESPEARE, *King Lear*

1. VITREOUS LOSS: May occur either during the course of an intra-ocular operation or by severe trauma involving a tear of the sclerotic anywhere posterior to the corneoscleral junction. The latter is a very serious condition and usually causes complete destruction of the eye. Occasionally the wound can be sutured, but a good result in these cases is rare.
2. INTRA-OCULAR FOREIGN BODY: May be lodged anywhere within the globe, but it is frequently in contact with the vitreous, hence it will be dealt with in this section. These foreign bodies are of the utmost importance because a retained intra-ocular body is very liable to cause sympathetic ophthalmia. An infinite variety of foreign bodies are found, including minute pieces of steel, air-gun pellets, glass, flint and even wood. The accident is usually caused by hammering or chipping, which results in a tiny piece of sharp metal hitting the cornea with considerable velocity. Occasionally an encapsulated intra-ocular foreign body is found on a routine examination many years after the injury.

    SIGNS AND SYMPTOMS: The patient is conscious of a sudden (but not necessarily severe) and momentary pain in the eye. This may be followed by 'some tears running down the cheek', which is really the escape of the intra-ocular fluid. Soon after the accident there may be no symptoms at all, a fact that sometimes causes patients to neglect seeking advice. A careful examination usually reveals a track from the surface of the cornea leading down to the anterior chamber. Occasionally this is visible to the naked eye, but more often than not a careful search with the loupe or slit-lamp is necessary before it is discovered. If the site of entry is in the sclerotic, it is very unlikely that it will be discovered at all. In the vast majority of cases, however, the foreign body enters through the cornea. The iris may or may not be damaged. The authors have seen cases which show a clearly punched-out hole like a tiny accessory pupil. The lens is usually injured, but if the foreign body was taking an oblique course it sometimes escapes damage. The degree of visual acuity will depend largely upon whether or not the lens has been injured.

It is of vital importance that every case where there is the least possibility of intra-ocular foreign body should be X-rayed. In only a very few cases is it visible to the ophthalmoscope and even radiography has its limitations since a number of these bodies are made of substances that do not produce a shadow. Fortunately, the foreign bodies most commonly found in practice, e.g. steel, lead, etc., show up well. Very accurate localization is essential, for upon this will depend the nature of the operation for its removal.

PATHOLOGY: The nature of the foreign body very largely determines the pathological changes that result from its presence in the eye.

Copper causes a very severe reaction with pus formation and occasionally the extrusion of the foreign body, followed eventually by a shrunken globe.

Iron foreign bodies, after a latent period varying from weeks to years, set up a condition known as 'siderosis'. Part of the iron is dissolved, staining the surrounding tissues, combining with the cellular proteins, and making its way into the vitreous or aqueous. The first clinical sign is the presence of iron as a rusty stain in the cells of the lens capsule where the deposits tend to become arranged in a circular fashion in an area roughly corresponding to the pupil. Rusty stains then appear in the iris and eventually brown granulations appear in the ciliary body, lens, angle of the anterior chamber, cornea, retina and choroid, and even the vitreous may be stained brown. In short: any part of the eye that is in contact with the vitreous or the intra-ocular fluid is liable to become affected and it is probable that these fluids play an important part in the spread of siderosis. The final result is a degenerated eye, with an opaque lens and detached retina.

Other Metals, such as lead, silver, zinc, etc., are more or less inert, and usually remain quiescent, sometimes becoming encapsulated. There is none the less a real risk of sympathetic ophthalmia developing in any of these cases.

Flint or *Stone* is relatively inert, the chief risk being the development of a purulent panophthalmitis.

China or *Glass* produces little reaction, but again there is a risk of sympathetic trouble.

PROGNOSIS: Always bad, and is worst of all in cases where there is injury to the lens. In addition to traumatic cataract, secondary glaucoma may result from the swelling of the injured lens, anterior synechiae narrowing the angle of the chamber, etc. Finally there is the ever-present risk of sympathetic ophthalmia, which is especially true in the case of children.

TREATMENT:
1. *Foreign Bodies in the Anterior Chamber*:
    a. *The Foreign Body is Non-magnetic*: These foreign bodies present difficult problems. They are usually enmeshed in the iris and should be removed if necessary together with a portion of the iris with forceps through a keratome incision.
    b. *The Foreign Body is Magnetic*: Foreign bodies in this situation can usually be removed by a hand magnet through a keratome incision.
2. *Foreign Bodies in the Vitreous*:
    a. *The Foreign Body is Non-magnetic*: It is impossible for a foreign body to remain in the vitreous without gross damage to the sight, and it is almost impossible to remove a non-magnetic foreign body from this situation without severe loss of vitreous. In these circumstances, it is better to remove the eye in good time rather than to wait for serious complications to occur, including the possibility of sympathetic ophthalmia. If the eye is virtually blind it is far safer to remove it.
    b. *The Foreign Body is Magnetic*: It is best to attempt immediate removal with the giant magnet without waiting for X-ray localization. The longer the substance is left in the eye the more difficult is the magnet removal since it becomes embedded in fibrous tissue. If, however, some time has elapsed since the injury, the foreign body should be accurately located and removed by the anterior or posterior route whichever is the easier and less likely to damage the sight. Discussion on the respective merits of these routes is beyond the scope of this work and should be studied in a detailed book on eye surgery. If all efforts with the magnet fail, the eye should be excised forthwith.

It will be obvious from the foregoing that no case of a retained intra-ocular foreign body can be regarded with complacency while such risks as panophthalmitis, siderosis and sympathetic ophthalmia remain.

Chapter X

DISEASES OF THE LENS

Anatomy: The lens is a biconvex structure of highly differentiated epithelium and is composed of three distinct parts: (1) An elastic capsule; (2) The epithelium from which the lens fibres take their origin; (3) The lens substance, which is plastic, and capable (at any rate in youth) of altering its shape according to the tension of the capsule.

The average equatorial diameter of the lens is 9 mm and it has a greater radius of convexity of its posterior than its anterior surface. The lens is supported by the suspensory ligament and lies between the back of the iris and the anterior face of the vitreous. The tiny space between the iris and the lens is called the posterior chamber. The lens consists of fibres in regular layers, the arrangement being similar to the layered structure of an onion. The innermost fibres are the oldest, and, as the epithelium is constantly adding new fibres, the cortex increases with age. Similarly, the nucleus in its turn is being continually augmented by cortex and because the old fibres cannot be cast off, they undergo sclerosis, being massed together in the centre as the nucleus, hence showing increased stratification as growth increases. Layers of optical discontinuity and potential clefts between the ends of systems of fibres are visible with the slit-lamp. These clefts are known as sutures, which resemble a Y (Y) anteriorly and an inverted Y (λ) posteriorly. These sutures run through the whole thickness of the fetal nucleus and form a valuable landmark when examining the lens with a slit-lamp.

Biochemistry of the Lens: A very elaborate subject which in a condensed way can be expressed as follows: In addition to various proteins the lens contains some mineral salts, the most important of which are sodium, potassium, and calcium. The calcium content of the normal lens is fairly constant whereas the potassium content diminishes as age advances, but in a cataractous lens the calcium is definitely increased. As the lens has no blood supply, its nutrition is effected by means of an auto-oxidation system. This is a reversible reaction carried out by glutathionone and for which vitamin C is essential.

Sugar + oxidized glutathionone $\rightleftarrows$ ascorbic acid + reduced glutathionone.

In cases of mature cataract glutathionone and ascorbic acid are both absent.

CATARACT

Pathogenesis: As the lens, like the vitreous, has no blood supply, it is incapable of inflammation but can easily be affected by metabolic changes. Any pathological change in the lens results in the formation of opacities or cataract. Biochemically the essential change in a cataractous lens is the breakdown of lens proteins and subsequent increase in osmotic pressure resulting in an increase in the water content. Many differing factors such as radiant energy, metabolic changes, certain drugs, uveal diseases, senility, etc., all produce the same result in different ways. Taking a senile cataract as a typical example, the following stages can be seen:
1. INTUMESCENCE, when the lens swells and contains excess water. This swollen lens may cause pressure on the iris, shallowness of the anterior chamber leading to glaucoma.
2. MATURITY, when the lens, including the cortex, is opaque and has become dehydrated.
3. HYPERMATURITY, when the lens is flat, yellow, and even more dehydrated, containing calcium and cholesterol. Later the cortex degenerates into a milky fluid, while the nucleus lies loose within the capsule (Morgagnian cataract).

These changes have been tersely summed up by Duke-Elder: 'It may be said that the essential chemical changes causing a cataract involve a hydration followed by a dehydration, an acidification followed by an alkalosis, a replacement of soluble by insoluble proteins, an increase in the calcium and lipoids and an arranging of the concentration of the salts to correspond with that of the blood.

'Metabolically the most important features in the development of cataract are a diminished metabolism, a decrease in permeability and a loss of the substances active in oxidation, cystinine, gluta-thionine and ascorbic acid: whether the relation is causal or consequential a cataractous lens is an asphyxiated lens.'

Signs and Symptoms: The first symptom complained of is that of general mistiness of vision and sometimes of a 'speck' before the eye which remains in the same position and does not move about as is the case with vitreous opacities. Uniocular diplopia is occasionally noted. With an increase in the lens opacities is a diminution of visual acuity and almost every patient complains of a distressing dazzling in bright light owing to the irregular refraction of its rays. A cataract patient walks with his head down, wears dark glasses, hand shading the eye, etc., in contrast to the optic atrophy patient, who looks upward trying to avail himself to the utmost of all the light that is present. A cataract patient, therefore, sees better on dull days. Eventually, as the opacities increase, the vision deteriorates progressively until in the end perception of light alone remains.

Ophthalmoscopically, the earliest changes are usually in the periphery of the lens and the opacities encroach on the pupillary area as maturity progresses. It is of utmost importance to examine the fundi of every cataract case early in the disease, for once it is fairly advanced an adequate view of the fundus is impossible and the success of cataract extraction depends very largely on a healthy fundus. Examination should be made with a +12 lens in the ophthalmoscope which (in an emmetropic eye) brings the details of opacities into focus. The lens system is gradually rotated until fundus details are visible. The progress of a cataract varies enormously, some cases increasing greatly within a few months and others showing little change after many years. Those cases that advance quickly suggest some complication, e.g. diabetes, etc. Cataract is usually bilateral, but one eye is more affected than the other. It often shows quite a remarkable familial incidence.

Varieties: Cataracts can broadly be divided into two headings: (1) Congenital or developmental and (2) Acquired, and the clinical varieties can be listed as follows:

Congenital or Developmental Cataracts
1. Anterior capsular
2. Coronary
3. Fusiform
4. Lamellar (sometimes called discoid or zonular)
5. Nuclear
6. Posterior capsular
7. Punctate (or 'blue dot')
8. Maternal virus infection (e.g. rubella)
9. Suture

Acquired Cataracts
1. Anterior capsular
2. Atopic
3. Metabolic
   Diabetic
   Mongolian
   Myotonic
   Parathyroid
4. Radiation
5. Secondary
6. Senile
7. Toxic
8. Traumatic
9. 'After'

I. CONGENITAL OR DEVELOPMENTAL CATARACT

Is seen in varying forms.

1. **Anterior Capsular Cataract** can be congenital in origin and is due to the delayed formation of the anterior chamber with consequent prolonged contact between the capsule and the primitive cornea. These cases are always bilateral. Generally speaking, the opacity caused by this form of cataract is small and the visual acuity is reasonably good, hence treatment is not required.

2. **Coronary Cataract:** This resembles a lamellar cataract but occurs at puberty. It affects the deep cortical and superficial nuclear layers. Spindle-shaped opacities occur near the periphery while the extreme

periphery, when seen with a dilated pupil, remains clear. Many of these cases remain stationary.
3. **Fusiform Cataract** is an anteroposterior, spindle-shaped opacity which sometimes develops branches resembling coral (coralliform cataract). This is of familial origin.
4. **Lamellar Cataract** (sometimes called discoid or zonular): Occurs usually in the deep cortical periphery of the lens, the nucleus being reasonably clear as also are the superficial layers of the cortex. When seen under a mydriatic it is a discoid opacity surrounded by a clear periphery and enclosing a comparatively clear centre. At regular intervals along the outer edge of the disc jut out projecting opacities that resemble the cogs of a wheel. This type of cataract is usually bilateral and non-progressive until middle age or later, when senile changes may supervene. The visual acuity is frequently surprisingly good. Lamellar cataract is often associated with myopia. It is probably caused by some form of intra-uterine malnutrition, and it occurs most commonly of all in children whose mothers suffered from rubella in the very early stages of pregnancy. This form of cataract is usually associated with hypoplasia of the enamel of some of the permanent teeth, especially the incisors and canines, which have a 'worn' appearance and show transverse striations.

TREATMENT: Entirely depends upon the amount of visual disability.
 1. If the opacity is not dense a careful estimation of the refractive error and the prescribing of appropriate glasses may be all that is necessary. If a visual acuity of 6/18 or more is obtained in the better eye in this way operation is contra-indicated.
 2. If the visual acuity is less than 6/18 in the better eye, the patient will be unable to see to read and his education will be adversely affected. Operative interference is, therefore, indicated. Since the lens fibres of young persons are not sclerosed they will be absorbed if the intra-ocular fluid enters them. Therefore, discission (or needling) is the operation of choice.

   In considering the treatment it must be remembered that operation not only involves the permanent wearing of a thick convex lens (or a contact lens) but it makes accommodation impossible, hence the patient (usually a child) has the drawback of having to wear bifocals or to change his glasses every time he wants to read. Likewise if he plays the piano, draws or paints, a third pair is necessary for occupational use. It would seem, therefore, that a vision of 6/12 or even 6/18 with retained accommodation would be preferable to a vision of 6/6 in an aphakic eye. The treatment, therefore, of lamellar cataracts can be summed up in seven words: *Never operate if it can be avoided.*
5. **Nuclear Cataract** results when the development of the lens is inhibited very early. The nucleus remains opaque but the lens is clear.

6. **Posterior Capsular Cataract:** It is the name given to the posterior vascular sheath of the lens. It does not normally affect vision, but in rare cases the lens becomes involved in fibrous tissue and a complete cataract results.
7. **Punctate (or 'Blue Dot') Cataract:** A common variety where scattered throughout the lens are punctate dots of varying size and showing blue coloration when seen with the slit-lamp. These are non-progressive and cause little or no visual disability and no treatment is required.
8. **Rubella Cataract:** This is a progressive cataract occurring in infants whose mothers developed rubella very early in pregnancy. It is due to the invasion of the infantile lens by the rubella virus. It commences in the nucleus but spreads through the entire lens and is occasionally associated with other congenital abnormalities, e.g. microphthalmos, mental deficiency, congenital heart disease, deafness, abnormal teeth, etc.
9. **Suture Cataract** is without significance. It consists of aggregation by 'blue dots' crowded into the Y-sutures of the lens.

II. ACQUIRED CATARACTS

1. **Anterior Capsular Cataract:** This is sometimes called 'anterior polar cataract'. It is not really a cataract at all inasmuch as there is no opacity in the lens itself. It is formed by proliferation of the cuboidal cells which lie in the capsular epithelium and affects the central pupillary area. The cause of the proliferation is the contact of the lens capsule with the cornea (usually an inflamed cornea), and it is therefore usually due to a perforating ulcer and less frequently to a penetrating wound in early childhood. Only a very short time of contact is necessary to produce this condition. Fortunately, this liability decreases with age, otherwise most intra-ocular operations would be impossible.
2. **Atopic Cataract** is associated with severe dermatoses such as scleroderma, chronic eczema, etc. It is a rapidly increasing form of cataract but the results of operation are good.
3. **Metabolic Cataracts:** Under this heading is a group of cataracts due to the dysfunction of endocrine glands.
    DIABETIC CATARACT: Although not one of the commonest complications of diabetes, in those cases where it does occur it usually affects young adults. It is bilateral and affects the subcapsular cortex and rapidly spreads throughout the entire substance of the lens. The pathogenesis of diabetic cataract is uncertain, but is probably due to osmotic changes causing accumulation of fluid beneath the capsule. Although occurring in patients with sugar in the urine, it is definitely not caused by sugar in the intra-ocular fluid, which is never found in quantities sufficient to produce cataract.

DISEASES OF THE LENS

TREATMENT: As for senile cataract. It is most important that every case should be stabilized before operation. There is definitely more risk in extracting a diabetic cataract than a senile one owing to the frequency of the following complications:

1. *Haemorrhage*: The iris often bleeds very freely, hence the advisability of simple extraction without iridectomy. The possibility of vitreous or choroidal haemorrhage must be remembered also.
2. *Iritis*: The necessary handling of the iris may set up a traumatic iritis. This is an additional reason for avoiding an iridectomy.

However, in spite of all these risks, diabetic patients often do very well and the prognosis is reasonably good. In young people under 25, needling is usually all that is necessary.

MONGOLIAN CATARACT: Really a congenital defect but is usually discovered about puberty. Two kinds of opacities are seen in the lens, an iridescent 'blue dot' type intermingled with dusty crystalline specks resembling those found in myotonia atrophica. The patient's mental condition is such that operation is contra-indicated.

MYOTONIC CATARACT: This is a hereditary disease manifesting itself in early adult life, commencing in the hand and affecting various muscles of the body. It is thought to be due to a pluriglandular deficiency. The opacities consist of cholesterol crystals in the cortex. The patient's general condition may contra-indicate any treatment.

PARATHYROID CATARACT: This is usually seen after removal of the parathyroid gland in the course of a thyroid operation, but it is occasionally idiopathic. As in the case with most metabolic cataracts, the opacities occur in the subcapsular cortex and are of the fine dusty variety. In tetany cataract there is a deficiency of calcium in the blood and an excess of it in the lens.

TREATMENT is for senile cataract.

4. **Radiation Cataract:** Any form of radiant energy can cause cataract, including heat, light (visible, infrared or ultraviolet), radium and X-rays, but far the commonest seen are the 'heat-ray' cataracts. These occur in chain-makers, glass-blowers and other workers who are exposed to heat from furnaces. Chain-makers' and similar cataracts were very commonly seen in the industrial areas of the Midlands until the end of the Second World War. After this, modern furnaces appeared which were fired by oil and stoked by pressing buttons. No flames are visible and often the stokers feel chilly so they have electric fires to keep them warm! As the result of this, 'heat-ray' cataract has largely disappeared. The first person to discover chain-makers' cataract was St. Clair Roberts, surgeon at the Worcester Eye Hospital, as long ago as 1921. It was recognized as an industrial disease in 1927 and much research and detailed

drawings of the condition were made by Lloyd Johnstone, also of the Worcester Eye Hospital, and published in 1944 in *Trans. ophthal. Soc. U.K.*, **64**, 249. A characteristic of this cataract is a small opacity in the posterior cortex. It is shallow and clear-cut in the early stages, but later it cannot be distinguished from a senile cataract. It is commonest in the left eye (the eye which in a right-handed worker is nearer the furnace), but it may be bilateral, in which case the left cataract is the more advanced. Similar cataracts may follow exposure to X-rays and radium, often after a lengthy latent period.

5. **Secondary Cataract:** Results from malnutrition of the lens due to local ocular disease. It will be remembered that the lens receives its nutrition from the intra-ocular fluid which is secreted by the ciliary body; thus in certain inflammatory conditions involving this organ the lens suffers and opacities occur. These usually commence in the posterior cortex, but progress until the whole of the lens is opaque. The opacities are dust-like and increase in number and density with the lapse of time. Secondary cataracts are 'soft', but in late stages the fluid is absorbed and the hard shrunken lens is unable to support the iris, which is tremulous in consequence. This type of cataract is seen in cyclitis, absolute glaucoma, retinitis pigmentosa, choroidoretinitis, high myopia and detachment cases.

   TREATMENT: That of the cause of the condition. Many do not benefit by operation and a careful examination for projection of light should be undertaken in every case, and if not accurate an extremely guarded prognosis should be given, if indeed operation is undertaken at all. A sound rule in complicated cataracts is: do not operate unless you are obliged to do so.

6. **Senile Cataract:** The signs and symptoms of this, probably the commonest of pathological eye conditions, have been described on p. 111 and should be stated again here. It rarely occurs before the age of 50 and the few cases that are seen at an earlier age are usually due to changes occurring in a pre-existing congenital or infantile cataract. It must be emphasized that the diagnosis of senile cataract should only be based upon an ophthalmoscopic examination, for frequently in elderly patients the pupil appears to the naked eye to be of a uniform grey colour. This greyness is physiological in old people and is due to sclerosis of the lens fibres and consequent increase in its refractive index.

   During the growth of a senile cataract the lens goes through the changes described under PATHOGENESIS (p. 111). During these changes a watch should be kept for maturity, the ideal time for operation. When this point is reached oblique illumination throws no visible iris shadow on the lens, for if its cortex is opaque then the pupil is touching the opacity, being separated only by the capsule, hence a shadow is impossible. If, however, there is an area of clear

DISEASES OF THE LENS

cortex surrounding an opaque nucleus (i.e. if the cataract is immature), oblique light throws a distinct shadow on to the opaque lens.

TREATMENT: It may be stated at once that the only treatment is operative. Probably no disease has been more exploited by quacks throughout the ages than senile cataract. No amount of exercises, drops, staring at coloured lights, etc., have ever influenced the course of a senile cataract. The unfortunate patient who is losing his sight and is afraid of an operation often provides a willing and credulous victim for unscrupulous rogues to fleece.

In the early stages, the use of the word 'cataract' should be avoided. It causes needless anxiety and conjures up pictures of operations, blindness, etc., in the mind of a nervous patient. It is far better to say 'slight spots in the lens due to advancing years', etc.

1. In the early stages, vision can often be improved by attending to refractive errors. Owing to an increase in the refractive index of the lens a slight myopia is sometimes produced and correcting this may improve vision greatly. Crookes B lenses should be ordered for sunshine. A weak mydriatic sometimes helps.
2. In unilateral cases with good vision in the unaffected eye, operation is usually contra-indicated, unless the patient is prepared to wear a contact lens or the surgeon to insert an intra-ocular implant, for the difference in refraction between an aphakic and a normal eye is so great that the patient never sees comfortably when using both eyes together. The following exceptions can be made to this rule:
   a. Where a field of vision is necessary for a patient's safety in his occupation;
   b. For cosmetic reasons, to give a black pupil instead of a white one;
   c. To prevent hypermaturity, when operation is much more difficult.
3. In bilateral cases operation is best postponed until the vision in the *better* eye is 6/18 or less. When this occurs and the patient begins to have difficulty in reading, recognizing people, etc., it is time to consider operation on the *worse* eye. The old practice of waiting for maturity and leaving the patient blind in the meantime has been discarded. By far the hardest type of case to advise about operation is the one where the opacities are immature but equally advanced in each eye and the patient cannot see to read, to do his work or to drive his car. In these cases operation is justified even though the cataract is immature. Recently the introduction of alphachymotrypsin, a zonulytic fluid, makes the extraction of immature cataracts a safer procedure. By its use during operation the zonule is dissolved and

the lens can be removed intracapsularly with less risk of breaking the capsule than was previously possible.
4. In every case before extracting a dense cataract the examination for projection of light should be carefully made. The patient should look straight ahead and black out his good eye with his handkerchief. The light from the retinoscope should be shone on to the cataractous eye from varying directions and the patient is instructed to point with his free hand to the source of light. He should be able to locate this without hesitation every time. If he fails in this test it is strong presumptive evidence of an unhealthy retina and if operation is indicated at all, a very guarded prognosis should be given. For the various varieties of operation for cataract *see Chapter XXIII*, OPHTHALMIC OPERATIONS.
5. The question as to whether one or both eyes should be operated upon is a debatable one. The following points should help to influence the decision:
   a. In very old patients or in those that are infirm it is unwise to tempt Providence twice if the result of operation upon one eye is satisfactory.
   b. In younger or very active patients, bilateral extraction is well worth while. There is an increasing tendency at the present time to operate upon both eyes at one sitting. This is a risk the authors are not prepared to take owing to the possibility of tragic results in event of squeezing, vomiting, coughing or even postoperative infection.
7. **Toxic Cataracts:** Certain poisons seem to have a selective action on the lens and can produce cataractous changes which sometimes increase with great rapidity. Their mode of action is unknown. The following are the commonest: (1) Ergot poisoning (usually from eating rye bread); (2) Naphthalene; (3) Thallium; (4) Dinitrophenol, which is sometimes taken for slimming; (5) Steroid therapy sometimes causes cataracts.
8. **Traumatic Cataract:** This is caused by any wound of the lens, whether of a perforating nature or by a ruptured capsule resulting from a blow. When the capsule is injured the intra-ocular fluid enters the substance of the lens, which becomes swollen and cloudy. Traumatic opacities occur most frequently in the posterior cortex and often appear somewhat like a flower with six or seven petals. These usually increase in density until the entire lens becomes opaque. Often white masses of lens matter protrude through the injured capsule and enter the anterior chamber. These masses may be absorbed by the intra-ocular fluid and pass out of the eye through the angle. Rarely very small wounds may cause a local opacity which does not spread Occasionally the escape of lens matter into the anterior chamber

after accidental injury or cataract extraction causes a lens-induced endophthalmitis. This occurs between the 2nd and 14th days after the injury, producing a severe reaction with oedema and vascularization of the iris, KP, occasionally hypopyon and pupillary adhesions which may lead to secondary glaucoma. Secondary glaucoma can also occur without any uveal inflammation. This can be caused by:
1. Swelling of the lens causing a shallow anterior chamber with consequent obstruction of the angle.
2. Blockage of the trabecular network due to macrophages engorged with lens matter.

TREATMENT:
1. Complete rest in bed until the eye is white. Atropine is essential to prevent the iris adhering to the lens capsule. In young persons the entire lens may be absorbed naturally and this may be the only treatment required.
2. Curette evacuation should be undertaken if there is any sign of secondary glaucoma developing. The removal of loose lens matter in this way usually gives prompt relief.

It should be noted that in the operation of 'needling' for congenital cataract, a traumatic cataract is intentionally produced and in the vast majority of cases the lens is entirely absorbed in the course of time.

The following condition is termed 'cataract', but is not genuine cataract at all:

9. **'After' Cataract:** The name given to the slight opacity that follows extraction of the lens or needling of a cataract. The opacity is due to the persistence of the capsule which unlike lens matter is not absorbed by the intra-ocular fluid. Frequently this capsule is almost diaphanous and does not hinder vision, but if it is badly wrinkled or if soft lens matter is adherent to it serious visual impairment may result. Sometimes a postoperative iritis makes this worse by covering the capsule with fibrinous exudate. The capsule is best seen either with the loupe and oblique illumination or with the ophthalmoscope with a +10 lens.

TREATMENT: By 'needling' with a Ziegler's knife, when a hole is cut in the capsule. The improvement in vision after this simple operation is often dramatic.

CONGENITAL ABNORMALITIES OF THE LENS

1. **Coloboma** occurs as a gap, resembling a 'bite' out of the lens at its margin in any meridian. It is caused by a developmental defect in the suspensory ligament.
2. **Subluxation** is a congenital dislocation. It is often associated with Marfan's syndrome (q.v.).

3. Posterior Lenticonus: This is a congenital posterior conical deformity of the lens which causes a gross uncorrectable refractive error.

INJURIES TO LENS

Can result in:

1. Cataract: This can be caused by a concussion injury, due to a direct blow causing rupture of the lens capsule and the entry of intraocular fluid into the lens. A perforating injury, sometimes a comparatively minor one, such as a prick with a thorn when hedge-cutting, can produce the same result (p. 118).

2. Dislocation: This results when the suspensory ligament is ruptured by a concussion injury. The lens may be partly or completely dislocated. It may even lie in the anterior chamber or the vitreous. When visible, the edge of the lens appears as a crescentic grey line. Iridodonesis is present, i.e. tremulous iris owing to lack of support by the absent lens. Iridocyclitis and secondary glaucoma are very liable to supervene. Operative treatment in such cases is often difficult and should only be attempted when the eye has become 'quiet'. Vitreous loss in these cases is frequent so extraction is best done with the vectis.

Chapter XI

GLAUCOMA

'Poor Glaucus! He is as blind as Fortune herself.' LYTTON, *Last Days of Pompeii*

GLAUCOMA is not a disease in itself but a symptom-complex occurring in a variety of pathological conditions with the characteristic sign of raised intra-ocular pressure common to them all. This increased tension can be caused in one of three ways:
1. An increased pressure in the intra-ocular capillaries causing congestion and increased secretion of fluid. There is increasing evidence that local corticosteroids tend to decrease the outflow of intraocular fluid.
2. A normal secretion of intra-ocular fluid with diminished drainage at angle of anterior chamber or obstructed circulation at the pupil.
3. A less important factor is biochemical changes in the intra-ocular fluid resulting in increased protein or cell content.

Of these three factors, the first two are of major significance. Since the uveal tract is spongy in structure, when congested it can easily become sufficiently engorged to impede or even obstruct the canal of Schlemm, the normal drainage channel of the eye. In addition, any engorgement is aggravated by the liberation from the uveal tract of histamine-like substances which cause further uveal vasodilatation with increased capillary permeability, thus causing a vicious circle. Of course, even when the canal of Schlemm is obstructed, some drainage can occur through efferent capillaries of the iris and ciliary body, but this is an inefficient route and is certain to result in increasing intra-ocular pressure.

Glaucoma is classified under two headings:
1. PRIMARY: Where the cause of the condition is still uncertain, dependent upon one or more of the three factors mentioned above.
2. SECONDARY: Where the cause is known.

PRIMARY GLAUCOMA

The gonioscope has thrown much light on the pathology and causation of primary glaucoma. It occurs in two forms: (1) Narrow angle glaucoma; (2) Glaucoma simplex or open angle glaucoma. These must be regarded as completely differing diseases having one sign in common—the raised intra-ocular pressure.

Narrow Angle Glaucoma: The characteristic of this type of glaucoma is periodic attacks of raised intra-ocular tension associated with corneal oedema resulting in visual impairment and the sensation of 'haloes'. These attacks tend to recur and result eventually in a marked increase in ocular tension which can become permanent and lead to complete blindness. It usually occurs in people well over middle age and is most common in hypermetropes. The anterior chamber in these cases is noticeably shallow, the iris is well forward, and the angle of the chamber is unduly narrow. The actual seat of the obstruction is at the trabecular network which becomes fibrotic and compresses or obliterates Schlemm's canal (Greer's *Ocular Pathology*, 1972). This narrow angle can be accounted for in three different ways:

1. Hypermetropes have small eyes with relatively large lenses which tend to obstruct the angle mechanically.
2. In the fifth decade of life and later, the lens tends to increase in size which in its turn can obstruct filtration by mechanical pressure.
3. In quite a number of cases there is a hereditary factor. From the foregoing, it is clear that anything that tends to dilate the pupil in a patient with small eyes or a narrow angle will be liable to precipitate an acute attack. When the iris is fully dilated in a patient with a shallow anterior chamber, the folds at its base can easily cause severe obstruction. Hence, any mydriatic is dangerous in a patient with a shallow anterior chamber. A variety of other causes may help in producing an attack. These include worry, emotional stress, exhaustion, vasomotor instability and not infrequently an attack follows a severe 'cold' or other virus infection.

SIGNS AND SYMPTOMS: The patient has periodic attacks of dim vision associated with a sensation of 'haloes' around lights, but in the early stages there is no pain and the eye remains white. Occasionally the condition is bilateral. These attacks often occur in the dark evenings, especially at cinemas, watching television, etc. The tension may be raised to 35–60 mm Hg. The attacks usually pass off spontaneously and the patient takes little notice of them. Eventually, however, a characteristic acute attack is sure to occur when the already narrow angle becomes closed. There is a sudden onset of very acute pain in the eye and over the entire area supplied by the fifth nerve. The pain is usually severe and is often accompanied by vomiting. The tension is very greatly raised, the vision severely impaired and the patient may be quite ill. Examination reveals an acutely congested conjunctiva with ciliary flush, the cornea is 'steamy'-looking, the pupil ovoid about three-quarters dilated and does not react. The tension is very high, occasionally readings of 60–80 mm Hg have been registered. In untreated cases, the fields contract, the vision is lost and the root of the iris becomes adherent to the posterior corneal surface (peripheral anterior synechiae). In such cases the tension remains permanently high, the eye feeling as hard as a

GLAUCOMA 123

golf ball. In addition, the eye remains red and irritable, the disc becomes cupped and chronic congestive narrow angle glaucoma supervenes.

The final phase in untreated cases is *absolute glaucoma* when the eye is totally blind, the cornea appears like ground glass and occasional vesicles or bullae are present. The anterior chamber is all but absent, and the iris is atrophied with a broad pigment zone visibly surrounding the pupil (ectropion uveae). The pupil assumes a peculiar greyish hue. Staphylomata of the sclerotic (due to greatly increased tension) are sometimes observed. The eye is frequently very painful.

DIAGNOSIS: For the diagnosis of acute attack and its differentiation from acute iritis, *see* p. 59.

It is most important to bear in mind that early diagnosis, long before an acute attack occurs, is of fundamental importance. Too much stress cannot be placed upon the symptom of 'haloes' and attacks of dimness of vision, especially when they are associated with a shallow anterior chamber. A patient with the above symptoms should be thoroughly investigated as follows:

1. SLIT-LAMP EXAMINATION: Gives a rough idea of the shallowness or otherwise of the anterior chamber.
2. GONIOSCOPY (*see* p. 253): Will establish for certain the narrowness or otherwise of the angle.
3. TONOMETRY: May be helpful but it must be remembered that the tension is often normal between attacks so no reliance can be placed upon a single normal measurement. The patient should be admitted to hospital and 4-hourly tensions taken over 24 hours. If all these are normal, 'provocative' tests should be undertaken. The most reliable tests used at the present time are:
    a. Mydriatic Test: Mydrilate or similar drops should be administered, and the tension taken after half an hour's interval. From earlier remarks, it will be remembered that this test is not without its dangers and the patient must be kept under observation until full miosis occurs. A rise of tension after a mydriatic test is suggestive.
    b. Dark-room Test: The patient is left in a completely darkened room from $\frac{1}{2}$ to 1 hour until the pupils are fully dilated. The tensions should then be taken and compared with those found under normal conditions. A difference in tension of 8 mm Hg or more is certainly pathological. This test is reliable in 70 per cent of cases.
    c. Water-drinking Test: The patient is given 2 pints of water to drink immediately on waking in order to lower the osmotic pressure of the blood. The tensions should be taken later and

if there is a difference of 6 mm Hg or more over normal conditions, it should be regarded with suspicion.

d. Priscol Test: A subconjunctival injection of 10 mg of priscol is given. If the tension rises more than 14 mm in 1 hour the test is certainly positive.

e. Prone Position Test: A significant rise in tension is found in many patients with narrow angle glaucoma after lying for 1 hour in the prone position. This is as reliable as the dark-room test and safer than the mydriatic one.

It must be stressed that negative results in all these tests cannot exclude glaucoma, but a positive test in any one of them is very suggestive. At this stage, before studying the treatment of glaucoma, the reader is advised to refresh his memory on the pharmacology of drugs which act on the intra-ocular muscles (p. 43).

TREATMENT OF THE EARLY CASE:
1. If the patient is seen early (i.e. complaining of 'haloes', but without raised tension) miotic drugs such as pilocarpine 1 per cent or eserine ½ per cent should be used regularly. This should be continued *ad infinitum* if operation is refused.
2. Peripheral iridectomy should be performed to restore communication between the anterior and posterior chambers. Early operation in these cases carries a very good prognosis. It should be carried out as soon as the diagnosis is established. Operation on both eyes is advisable.

TREATMENT OF ACUTE CONGESTIVE CASES:
1. Eserine 1 per cent should be instilled every 5 minutes for half an hour in the hope of drawing the iris away from the angle. This should be continued at hourly intervals until the pupil is small and the pain has ceased. Short-wave diathermy sometimes relieves the pain. Morphine should be given if need be.
2. In cases that have responded to this, subsequent instillation of eserine ½ per cent three times a day usually suffices. This should be continued until the eye is white. Cases that do not respond should be tried on 1 per cent DFP drops. This is a very powerful miotic.
3. Dehydration treatment sometimes helps. This is achieved by oral glycerin (1·5 g to each kg of body-weight). This acts through diminishing the formation of intra-ocular fluid.
4. The amount of intra-ocular fluid formed can be reduced by carbonic anhydrase inhibiting drugs such as acetazolamide or dichlorphenamide, and the use of these tablets or injections in conjunction with other methods is always recommended for a few days.
5. When there is no response to the above treatments, a broad iridectomy under general anaesthesia is indicated within 24 hours

A retrobulbar injection of procaine and adrenaline is effective in lowering the tension before operation.
6. Pilocarpine 1 per cent should be instilled into the unaffected eye twice a day as a precautionary measure.
7. In cases that have responded to conservative treatment, an iridencleisis or filtering operation should be undertaken, if possible before the patient is discharged from hospital. Also a prophylactic iridectomy on the unaffected eye is indicated. Patients frequently decline to return once they have gone home free from pain, and such cases run a serious risk of recurrence and their subsequent attacks may not always end so happily.

TREATMENT OF ABSOLUTE GLAUCOMA:
1. Excision is the only certain method of relieving the patient from this painful condition.
2. If for any reason this is refused, a retrobulbar injection of 3 ml of 2 per cent novocain and 90 per cent alcohol in equal parts is always worth a trial and gives relief which often lasts for many months.

Glaucoma Simplex (Open Angle or Chronic Glaucoma): Differs completely from narrow angle glaucoma in aetiology, pathology, symptoms, treatment and prognosis. It occurs in middle life or later, is most commonly found in arteriosclerotic patients, and is by no means associated with a shallow anterior chamber. Both sexes are affected and the condition is usually bilateral, one eye being more advanced than its fellow.

SIGNS AND SYMPTOMS: These are often conspicuous by their absence. There are no premonitory 'haloes', no pain or discomfort, and the first thing noticed by many patients is that the vision of one eye has become seriously impaired. This is frequently discovered accidentally, or it may be found during a routine refraction. In some patients, presbyopia increases at an undue rate, the patient having to have much stronger lenses than is usual at his age. Indeed, when this is found during a refraction, glaucoma simplex must be excluded. Good central vision is often retained until very late in the disease. Therefore, good visual acuity on a test chart is not inconsistent with advanced glaucoma simplex. The following are the fundamentally important signs:

FIELDS: The earliest changes are to be seen on a 'Bjerrum' screen. These vary from a 'baring' of the blind spot in a very early case to Seidel's sign—a sickle-shaped scotoma involving the blind spot later in the disease. Peripheral fields are sometimes affected early, the most consistent change being the loss of part of the nasal field (Rönne's step) in the form of a quadrantic notch which, as the disease progresses, gradually increases until it reaches the fixation point. This nasal loss is accompanied by a general peripheral constriction. In very late stages only a small patch of temporal vision remains, the central vision being lost, and 'tunnel' vision of a few degrees only remains through a tiny paracentral area on the temporal side of the disc.

DISCS: Unlike narrow angle glaucoma, cupping is often an early sign and two factors combine to bring this about:
   a. *Mechanical*: The optic nerve is the first structure to be affected by an increase of intra-ocular tension. The posterior scleral foramen is a weak spot and the nerve tends to be depressed backwards, the depression forming the 'cup'.
   b. *Vascular*: Duke-Elder (*Diseases of the Eye*, 1970, 15th ed., p. 302) considers that vascular sclerosis and subsequent ischaemic atrophy of the optic nerve with degeneration of its supporting tissues is the major factor. He stresses that this sclerosis is present in almost every case of glaucoma simplex. This view would explain the occurrence of cupped discs in those cases where the tension is comparatively low.

TENSIONS: The intra-ocular tensions present considerable problems in these cases. Taken casually in the outpatient department they may often be found to be low. Thus admission for periodic tensions over 24 hours is essential in any suspected case. Physiologically there is a normal diurnal variation of tension of 2 or 3 mm Hg rising slightly in the morning or afternoon, or both (biphasic), but usually falling in the evening. In glaucoma simplex the difference in intra-ocular tensions tends to level out in favour of the higher reading, in time leading to a permanently raised tension. A diurnal variation of more than 5 mm Hg should be regarded with suspicion even though the highest peak it reaches is considered to be within normal limits. This frequent variation in intra-ocular pressure spread over a period of time produces an insidious change in fields, discs and eventually in visual acuity.

PATHOLOGY: The changes noted in these eyes are the result of a combination of pressure and vascular sclerosis causing the cupping and optic atrophy already described. In advanced cases much of the uveal tract becomes atrophied. The angle of the anterior chamber is not usually narrow but there is evidence of increased trabecular resistance and endothelial proliferation of the canal of Schlemm which interferes with the normal drainage mechanism in spite of a sometimes wide angle.

DIAGNOSIS: As there are no prodromal symptoms, the diagnosis depends upon thorough investigation of the three signs described above, supplemented by the results of the five provocative tests on p. 123.

GLAUCOMA

TREATMENT: Recent opinion undoubtedly regards open angle glaucoma as a disease that is best treated medically, especially since the introduction of the more powerful miotics. For their mode of action *see* p. 43.

1. Miotic treatment at the earliest stages in both eyes is essential. Pilocarpine 1–2 per cent is the first choice as it is less irritating than eserine. It should be given whether the anterior chamber is deep or shallow and should be continued after operation. It is of value for its vasodilatory effects even in open angle cases.
2. If the tension is not controlled by pilocarpine, the stronger cholinergic drugs, such as Eppy, DFP and phospholine iodide, should be used. DFP is a most powerful miotic and when used in 0·25 per cent solution produces extreme miosis. Sussman of New York recommends its use in carefully selected chronic narrow angle cases and in aphakic glaucoma as well as in simple glaucoma.
3. Carbonic anhydrase inhibitors, such as diamox, should be used orally. It is now possible to get 'sustained release' diamox capsules which release their contents gradually over a period of 8 hours, thus ensuring a more steady action of the drug.
4. Leopold of Pennsylvania suggests that the combination of acetazolamide and digoxin reduces the formation of intra-ocular fluid.
5. Adrenergic agents combined with anticholinesterase drugs have recently been popular in the treatment of open angle glaucoma. One of these, guanethidine (Ismelin), is a systemic antihypertensive drug that also lowers the intra-ocular pressure. Recent work shows that when used as a 5 per cent solution, the drug has a beneficial effect in lowering ocular tension.
6. Epinephrine and similar sympatheticomimetic drugs can be tried in wide angle glaucoma but on no account in narrow angle cases owing to their mydriatic effect. They can be used in conjunction with pilocarpine if necessary.
7. A variety of operations has been devised with the idea of establishing drainage between the anterior chamber and the subconjunctival tissues. These are briefly discussed in the chapter on OPHTHALMIC OPERATIONS (p. 225) but for fuller details reference to a textbook on ophthalmic surgery is essential.

PROGNOSIS: The only cases that carry a good prognosis are those diagnosed and treated early. In later cases the outlook is far from good whether operation is performed or not. Operations themselves are by no means free from danger. If, however, the tension is not controlled by miotics and if the fields are narrowing, something must be done. The results of operation are uncertain and variable. The best that can be hoped for is some arrest of the progress of the disease. In low tension glaucoma (vascular type)

PROPRIETARY DROPS USED FOR GLAUCOMA

PROPRIETARY NAME	MAKER	THERAPEUTIC INGREDIENT(S)
Eppy	Smith & Nephew	Stable adrenaline 1 per cent
Ismelin, 5 per cent	Ciba	Guanethedine sulphate
Lyophrin	Alcon	Adrenaline hydrogen tartrate 2 per cent
Phospholine iodide: 0·06 per cent, 0·125 per cent, 0·25 per cent	Farillon	Ecothiopate iodide
Prostigmin	Roche	Neostigmine
Tosmilen	Astra	Demacarium bromide 0·25 per cent

the prognosis is worse; the visual acuity tends to drop and the fields tend to become increasingly constricted whether operation is undertaken or not.

SECONDARY GLAUCOMA

This is almost invariably due to either or both of two factors: (1) Mechanical obstruction of the angle; (2) Increased viscosity of the intra-ocular fluid.

It will be obvious that either of these may seriously embarrass the drainage of fluid and a combination of the two may well be disastrous. These two factors can be brought about by a variety of causes:

1. *Iridocyclitis* resulting in a highly albuminous intra-ocular fluid containing leucocytes, pigment granules and exudates which tend to block the filtration angle. Furthermore, iris bombé may occur, which effectively stops the intra-ocular circulation.
2. *Perforated cornea.* This condition may cut off the angle of the anterior chamber by adhesions between the iris and the cornea (anterior synechiae).
3. *Lens changes.* Intumescent lens in rapidly progressive cataract cases can cause secondary glaucoma by mechanical obstruction of the angle. Similarly, traumatic rupture can also block the angle.
4. *Dislocation of lens,* when the angle may be blocked by the lens pushing the iris forwards, or even by the lens itself entering the anterior chamber and causing obstruction.
5. *Intra-ocular haemorrhage* whereby a sudden increase in pressure is caused and the normal methods of drainage are quite incapable of coping with the excess. Furthermore, the accumulation of blood corpuscles tends to block the filtration angle.
6. *Thrombosis of the central retinal vein.* The actual cause of the glaucoma which follows this condition is uncertain. Some authorities believe that the venae vorticosae are affected by thrombosis as well, others believe that this form of glaucoma is due to albuminous exudate in the vitreous. The modern view is that it is due to new

vessel formation in the region of the trabeculae of the anterior chamber. (*See* THROMBOTIC GLAUCOMA, p. 70.)
7. *Intra-ocular tumours*, either by the growth itself or by an associated retinal detachment pushing the lens forwards. Sometimes glaucoma may result from the growth involving a vortex vein.

SIGNS AND SYMPTOMS: Those of acute glaucoma. The diagnosis is obvious from the disease causing it.

TREATMENT:
1. The golden rule is: *Always treat the disease causing the secondary glaucoma*, e.g. if due to iritis, push atropine. Never be tempted to treat it with eserine as for acute primary glaucoma.
2. In addition to treating the cause, relief of the tension must be given urgently if the sight is to be saved. This is best done by posterior sclerotomy, iridotomy or similar simple operation that can be repeated if necessary.
3. The use of phospholine iodide drops and diamox has undoubtedly relieved some cases of secondary glaucoma and is always worth a trial, particularly where the condition does not respond to atropine.

Glaucoma Capsulare is an obstructive form of glaucoma due to deposits of debris on the iris, ciliary body and lens. They are particularly noticeable on the anterior capsule where they are rubbed off by movements of the iris and they accumulate in the angle, thus obstructing drainage. These deposits are now considered to be an indication of degenerative changes in the uveal tract and not due to exfoliation of the capsule.

INFANTILE GLAUCOMA (BUPHTHALMOS)

Buphthalmos is totally different clinically from the adult form of glaucoma. The child has an obviously large eye. The earliest symptoms are photophobia, lacrimation and general ocular discomfort. These may lead an unwary observer into diagnosing an ocular infection. It is caused by a congenital defect in or blockage of the angle, with consequent impairment of drainage and rise of tension. Occasionally the canal of Schlemm is absent from birth. Infantile glaucoma is sometimes associated with von Recklinghausen's disease and Sturge–Weber syndrome. It is nearly always bilateral and is far commoner in boys than in girls. Since it is a disease of childhood, the greater elasticity of the sclerotic allows the eye to enlarge under the increased tension and the sclera becomes thinned and appears of a bluish shade owing to uveal pigment showing through this thinned-out membrane. The cornea, for the same reason, is forced forwards and becomes globular, causing an apparent anomaly: a glaucomatous eye with a very deep anterior chamber. Splits appear in Descemet's membrane and the lens is forced somewhat backwards, thus depriving the iris of its support and causing iridodonesis. The elongation

130 A SYNOPSIS OF OPHTHALMOLOGY

	NARROW ANGLE GLAUCOMA	GLAUCOMA SIMPLEX (OPEN ANGLE)	BUPHTHALMOS
AGE OF ONSET	Fifth decade or later. Sometimes earlier	Sixth decade or later. Sometimes earlier	Early childhood
TYPE OF PATIENT	High strung. Nervous. Emotional. Vasomotor instability	No specific pyschological type. May be phlegmatic. Sometimes arteriosclerotic	Boys more commonly than girls
ANTERIOR CHAMBER	Shallow	Usually normal	Abnormally deep
ANGLE OF CHAMBER	Narrow	Variable. Often wide	Closed by embryonic tissue
'HALOES'	Present periodically	Absent	Absent
DISCS	Late cupping	Cupping early	Very deep cupping
TENSIONS	*Early*. Raised slightly on provocative tests only *Late*. High	Not high in early stage. Exaggeration of normal diurnal variations	High
FIELDS	Involvement a late sign	Peripheral fields involved early (nasal step). Central involvement a very late sign	Early involvement
OTHER CHARACTERISTICS	Attacks of blurred vision noticed at same time as the 'haloes'	Sometimes accommodative failure	Iridodonesis axial myopia. Thinning of sclera
MIOTIC TREATMENT	Essential. Earlier the better	Indicated for their vasodilatory effects. Pilocarpine for preference	Useless
OPERATIVE TREATMENT	*Early*. Peripheral iridectomy *Congestive attack*. Broad iridectomy *Late*. Filtration operation	Defer unless fields or tensions not controlled. Filtration operation best or cyclodialysis	Goniotomy for preference. Filtration operations often not satisfactory
PROGNOSIS	Good if diagnosed early	Fair if diagnosed very early. Otherwise bad	Bad

of the eye from pressure results in some axial myopia. Deep cupping of the disc is the rule. This condition must not be confused with congenital megalocornea (q.v.), a harmless condition which is never associated with glaucoma.

Prognosis: Definitely bad, except in cases treated really early.

Treatment: Miotics are useless. The usual glaucoma operations (trephining, iridencleisis, etc.) are variable in their results, usually inclining to the bad! The best modern operation is goniotomy, where the trabeculae of the angle are severed by a special knife, thus opening up drainage when the buphthalmos is due to obstruction of the angle by embryonic remains. A filtering operation is required when the corneal diameter is less than 14 mm as the canal of Schlemm is often absent in such cases. Even with most modern surgery the eventual results are not good and many pupils at Schools for the Blind are there on account of infantile glaucoma.

The student may find that the table given opposite helps to clarify the symptomatology and treatment of the three main types of glaucoma; narrow angle glaucoma, glaucoma simplex and buphthalmos.

Chapter XII
DISEASES OF THE ORBIT

'Its ruddy orbit.' JAMES PAYN, *To the Unknown Eros*

Anatomy: A detailed account of the anatomy of the orbit would be beyond the limited scope of this volume and the student is referred to textbooks on the subject. Very briefly, the orbital cavity is pear-shaped and bounded by a bony roof, floor and walls. In the adult its total capacity is 29 ml and it contains the following structures, all of which are of fundamental importance to the ophthalmologist:

OPTIC FORAMEN: Situated at the apex of the orbit. It is 4–6 mm wide and transmits the following structures:
  1. Optic nerve with its sheaths.
  2. Ophthalmic artery.
  3. Sympathetic nerves.

SUPERIOR ORBITAL (SPHENOIDAL) FISSURE leads from the orbit to the middle cranial fossa and transmits:
  1. The three cranial nerves that supply the extrinsic muscles of the eye—the third, fourth and sixth nerves.
  2. The three branches of the ophthalmic division of the fifth nerve.
  3. The ophthalmic vein.
  4. The orbital branch of the medial meningeal artery.
  5. Sympathetic fibres supplying the ciliary ganglion.

INFRA-ORBITAL (SPHENOMAXILLARY) FISSURE: Lies between the lateral wall and the floor of the orbit and thus communicating with the pterygopalatine fossa, the only important structure transmitted being the second division of the fifth nerve.

FOSSA FOR THE LACRIMAL GLAND: A depression situated at the anterolateral aspect of the roof.

TROCHLEAR FOSSA: On the anteromedial aspect of the orbit and provides attachment for the pulley of the superior oblique muscle.

LACRIMAL FOSSA: Situated on the anteromedial aspect of the medial wall of the orbit and contains the lacrimal sac.

RELATIONS OF BONY ORBIT: By far the most important facts to be borne in mind by the practising ophthalmologist are the relations of the bony orbit, which are as follows:
  SUPERIOR: The anterior cranial fossa, the frontal sinus and the supra-orbital sinus (when present).
  INFERIOR: The maxillary antrum, the palatine air cell
  LATERAL: The medial cranial fossa, the temporal fossa and the pterygopalatine fossa.

DISEASES OF THE ORBIT

MEDIAL: The ethmoidal air cells, the nasal cavity and, posteriorly, the sphenoidal sinus.

It will, therefore, be seen how the orbit, in all its aspects except laterally, is intimately related to the various nasal sinuses. These points should be borne in mind in considering possible spread of sinus infection.

EXOPHTHALMOS

Exophthalmos (or proptosis) is the name given to abnormal protrusion of the globe. Seeing that the orbit is, with the exception of the anterior foramen, completely encased in bone, the only direction in which its contents can expand is anteriorly. It therefore follows that in the event of an orbital inflammation, space-occupying lesions, etc., the eye will be pushed forwards and exophthalmos will result, the only limit to protrusion of the globe being its attachment to muscles and the optic nerve, all of which can become stretched to the utmost limits of their elasticity.

Causes:
1. BILATERAL EXOPHTHALMOS: High myopia; Graves' disease; Exophthalmic ophthalmoplegia.
2. UNILATERAL EXOPHTHALMOS: Orbital cellulitis; Thrombosis of cavernous sinus; Arteriovenous aneurysm; Tumours of the orbit; Orbital periostitis; Haemorrhage into the orbit; Emphysema of the orbit; Empyema of one of the nasal sinuses; Lymphosarcoma; Burkitt's lymphoma (in Africans); Hodgkin's disease.

These various causes of exophthalmos are dealt with individually under their appropriate headings.

ENOPHTHALMOS

Enophthalmos or abnormal retraction of the globe is a comparatively uncommon condition and is caused by:
1. Injuries involving fractures of the bony wall of the orbit.
2. Fibrous tissue formation following severe orbital cellulitis.

CELLULITIS

An acute purulent inflammation of the cellular tissues.

Causes:
1. Sepsis following penetrating injuries.
2. Spread of inflammation from neighbouring structures, e.g. nasal sinuses, etc.
3. Facial erysipelas.
4. Metastatic spread of pyaemia.
5. Sepsis following operations (e.g. enucleations, etc.).

Signs and Symptoms: The patient is acutely ill, with a raised temperature and often rigors. There is marked exophthalmos of the affected side, with gross brawny oedema of the lids. Pain is severe and is increased by movements of the eye, which are greatly restricted. The vision is not usually affected and the fundus (if the lids can be opened sufficiently for it to be seen) is usually normal. An abscess may form and may point either in the skin of the eyelids or it may discharge through the conjunctival fornix. There is considerable risk of panophthalmitis, meningitis and cavernous sinus thrombosis. The condition is usually unilateral.

Treatment:
1. The fullest doses of systemic antibiotics are indicated with or without chemotherapy by mouth. This should be administered at the earliest possible moment. This treatment is very successful in the vast majority of cases.
2. If there is not a prompt response to these measures, while the treatment is being continued, an incision should be made and the orbit explored for pus. Even if this is not found the tension is relieved and improvement may result.

CAVERNOUS SINUS THROMBOSIS

The reader is advised at this stage to refresh his memory of the anatomy of this important structure and its emissaries. He will then be reminded that this very grave condition can be caused by spread of infection from any of the following regions: the face, nose, orbit, the globe, the meninges, the pterygoid fossa and even from the mastoid region, as well as a metastatic manifestation of septic conditions elsewhere.

Signs and Symptoms: In the early stages the signs and symptoms resemble those of orbital cellulitis with one important exception: 50 per cent of cavernous sinus thrombosis cases are bilateral. The pain is most severe owing to involvement of the ophthalmic division of the fifth nerve and marked ocular palsies occur. The pupil is usually dilated and fails to react and the cornea is anaesthetic. Some degree of papilloedema is often present. Cerebral symptoms, rigors and vomiting are the rule.

Treatment: Fullest doses of systemic antibiotics should be tried, but the chances of success are very slender unless treatment is started early in the disease. In late cases the prognosis is very grave.

ORBITAL PERIOSTITIS

May occur anywhere, but is most commonly found at the margins.

Causes:
1. Trauma.
2. Extension of inflammation from neighbouring structures.
3. Tuberculosis (in children).
4. Syphilis (in adults).

DISEASES OF THE ORBIT

Signs and Symptoms: Differ with the situation of the lesion.
1. When the margin is involved there is obvious swelling, which is tender and related to the bone. Some displacement of the lid occurs, but exophthalmos is not present.
2. When the lesion is deeper in the orbital cavity the signs and symptoms are more vague. There is exophthalmos, deep-seated orbital pain and some ocular palsies may occur. Frequently there is severe supra-orbital neuralgia. These cases may greatly resemble orbital cellulitis.

Treatment:
1. This depends upon the aetiology and the results of investigations undertaken to exclude the causes listed.
2. Treatment as for orbital cellulitis should be commenced forthwith and an exploratory incision if necessary should not be delayed for too long.

NASAL SINUSITIS AND OCULAR DISEASE

From the relations of the nasal sinuses to the orbit briefly summarized at the start of this chapter, it is not very surprising that a purulent infection of any of them can give ocular symptoms. This fact is even less surprising in view of the thinness of the bony wall that separates them from the orbit. In the case of the ethmoidal air cells the thickness is only that of parchment. The sinuses that most commonly cause orbital involvement are the ethmoids, the frontals and the sphenoids.

Ethmoiditis may cause exophthalmos and oedema of the upper lid accompanied by pain, tenderness, severe headaches and unilateral nasal discharge. Fluid from these air cells enters the orbit and may even cause orbital cellulitis.

Frontal Sinusitis usually manifests itself (so far as ocular diseases are concerned) as a dense swelling at the upper and inner margin of the orbit. This is sometimes associated with slight exophthalmos and a downward displacement of the globe. Frontal headaches and tenderness are always present.

Sphenoidal Sinusitis is much more insidious and the usual ocular sign is retrobulbar neuritis owing to the close relationship between the optic nerve and the sphenoidal cells.

In addition to *direct* spread of infection to the orbit, it must be remembered that sepsis in any of the nasal sinuses can act as a focus for causing metastatic mischief elsewhere in the eye (e.g. iridocyclitis, endophthalmitis, etc.).

Treatment of Nasal Sinusitis: This lies entirely within the province of the nasal surgeon, but consultation between the ophthalmologist and nasal surgeon is often advisable in obscure cases. Occasionally the nasal surgeon may require his ophthalmic colleague's opinion on the advisability of exploration of the orbit. In these cases, collaboration is essential and the oculist must be prepared to undertake the orbital exploration if deemed necessary.

EXOPHTHALMIC GOITRE

Exophthalmic goitre is the commonest cause of exophthalmos. It is a disease of metabolism and the general signs and symptoms include enlargement of the thyroid gland, tachycardia, tremors of hands, sweating and great nervousness. Apart from exophthalmos, the following eye signs are seen: (1) Defective convergence (Möbius's sign), (2) lagging of the upper lid (von Graefe's sign), (3) retraction of the upper lid (Dalrymple's sign), (4) imperfect lid closure when blinking (Stellwag's sign).

Pathology: This disease is said to be due to a combination of overactivity of the thyroid and of the anterior lobe of the pituitary. It is this latter factor that is believed to be the actual cause of the exophthalmos.

Treatment is the concern of the general physician. The exophthalmos itself rarely requires the services of an oculist.

PULSATING EXOPHTHALMOS

This condition results from a communication between the cavernous sinuses and the internal carotid artery. It is nearly always an aftermath of trauma, but isolated cases have been reported when syphilis or arterial degeneration has been responsible.

Signs and Symptoms: There is marked exophthalmos accompanied by great congestion of the retinal, conjunctival and angular veins. The latter vein pulsates synchronously with the facial artery. Exophthalmos in these cases can be reduced temporarily by pressure on the eyeball or by compressing the common carotid artery. A loud rushing noise (bruit) is audible on auscultation over the globe and this is most distressing to the patient, who is conscious of it all the time. Much neuralgic pain is present owing to involvement of the upper division of the fifth nerve. Untreated cases tend to progress and to lead to death from haemorrhage.

Treatment:

1. Ligature of the carotid artery is indicated and often gives great relief.
2. If this is only partially successful the second carotid artery should be ligated after a few weeks have elapsed to allow a collateral circulation to be formed.

EXOPHTHALMIC OPHTHALMOPLEGIA

This condition is one of exophthalmos associated with immobility of the external ocular muscles and gross oedema of the conjunctiva. This oedema may be so great as to cause a complete eversion of the conjunctiva, with ulceration and necrosis. It is most commonly found in patients who have had thyroid operations, and is believed to be due to excess of the anterior lobe pituitary secretion.

Causes: Professor Mann has classified these cases into three groups:
1. PRIMARY DEFICIENCY OF THYROXINE with compensatory excess of thyrotrophic hormone. These cases not only show no sign of overactive thyroid, but their basal metabolic rate is diminished and there may even be slight myxoedema.
2. PRIMARY EXCESS OF THYROXINE: These cases are usually those of Graves' disease which have undergone removal of the thyroid gland, and a compensating excess of thyrotrophic hormone results. In this group the basal metabolic rate is very variable.
3. PRIMARY EXCESS OF THYROXINE AND THYROTROPHIC HORMONE occurring at the same time, i.e. cases of toxic goitre which develop ophthalmoplegia during the course of the disease and without any thyroid operation. All this group have high metabolic rates and the patients may be acutely ill.

Pathology: Gross oedema and infiltration of all the extra-ocular muscles are present. The swelling is so great that the normal muscular movements are quite impossible and the oedematous muscles within the orbit produce exophthalmos in exactly the same way as a space-occupying lesion will displace the eye.

Prognosis: This is a serious disease from the point of view of the eye and often involves its loss from exposure. The disease tends to regress spontaneously and very slowly, but the eyes seldom return completely to normal.

Treatment:
1. If at all severe, prompt tarsorrhaphy (if necessary bilateral) is called for. If that is not done many eyes will be lost. This is the only local treatment of any use.
2. A medical colleague should be called in to advise on general treatment, since it is necessary to give thyroid treatment to all cases in the first group, to some cases in the second group, but never to those in the third.
3. X-ray treatment to the orbits and/or the pituitary fossa has been undertaken in many cases but the results are uncertain.
4. In severe cases orbital decompression may be required.

ORBITAL TUMOURS

Tumours of the orbit and the optic nerve, although very distinct entities, give rise to identical signs and symptoms. Orbital tumours are by no means common in spite of the somewhat formidable list of their varieties.

Cystic Tumours:
MICROPHTHALMOS WITH CYSTS: The eye in these cases cannot usually be discovered clinically. Instead a fluctuating cystic tumour

is present, which is connected with the shrunken globe. The cyst contains retinal tissues. This condition is due to imperfect closure of the embryonic fissure.

DERMOIDS are usually found at the upper and outer angle of the orbit.

MENINGOCELES AND ENCEPHALOCELES occur most frequently at the upper and inner angle of the orbit, but are occasionally found posteriorly. These swellings often pulsate and can be compressed. They become tense on straining and cerebrospinal fluid can be removed by aspiration.

PARASITIC CYSTS: Extremely rare.

Simple Tumours:
1. BONY TUMOURS: Exostoses and osteomata may develop either from the bony orbit or from one of the sinuses related to it.
2. ANGIOMA: This is usually congenital and grows very slowly. It increases in size on stooping, straining, etc., since it is usually connected with an orbital vein.
3. CAVERNOUS LYMPHANGIOMA (OR CYSTIC HYGROMA): Non-encapsulated and is liable to attacks of recurrent inflammation, with tenderness, pyrexia, etc.
4. LYMPHOMA OR CHLOROMA: May occur in leukaemic diseases.
5. LIPOMA, CHONDROMA, FIBROMA, NEUROFIBROMA: All occur, but are very uncommon.

Malignant Tumours:
1. ROUND-CELL SARCOMA: Usually occurs in childhood or late in life and varies greatly in malignancy.
2. MELANOTIC SARCOMA: Usually arises from pigmented cells in the sclera or it may invade the orbit from the choroid.
3. CARCINOMA: Usually secondary to a growth in the breast. Sometimes it arises from the lacrimal gland, lids, or nasal sinuses. In infants it may be secondary to neuroblastoma of the suprarenal gland.

Pseudo-tumours: Very rarely, a patient is seen who presents all the signs and symptoms of an orbital tumour and at operation nothing but a mass of chronic inflammatory tissue is found. The pathology is unknown. Probably any case of suspected orbital tumour which regresses spontaneously is an inflammatory pseudo-tumour.

Treatment: Treatment of orbital tumours is identical with those of optic-nerve tumours (*see below*).

TUMOURS OF THE OPTIC NERVE

These are usually described as intradural or extradural according to their site of origin. The former are the more common. Secondary malignant tumours can occur in the optic nerve.

Glioma: An intradural growth arising from the neuroglial tissue of the optic nerve. It commences as a fusiform enlargement of the nerve

DISEASES OF THE ORBIT

resembling a 'wiped joint' on a pipe and increases in size until it becomes as large as a pullet's egg. It occurs chiefly in children, is non-malignant and does not cause secondary deposits, spreading only by direct extension. It is not to be confused with the very malignant 'glioma' of the retina (retinoblastoma).

Endothelioma (Meningioma): This tumour resembles a glioma in every respect but it originates from the cells lining the arachnoid sheath of the optic nerve. It is, therefore, extradural. This, too, is a relatively innocent growth which spreads locally only.

Signs and Symptoms: The cardinal sign common to every case is unilateral and progressive exophthalmos. This exophthalmos is rarely directly forwards; there being nearly always some lateral or downward displacement of the globe. Ocular movements are impaired with resulting diplopia, and in late stages atrophy of the optic nerve results from compression.

Diagnosis may be difficult. One of the first points to be determined is whether the tumour is a primary orbital one or whether it has spread from a neighbouring structure. Radiographs of sinuses, Wassermann reaction and a white blood count are indicated, and a complete overhaul is advisable to exclude the possibility of metastases from a primary growth elsewhere.

Treatment:
1. Exploration of the orbit by Krönlein's operation is the method of choice; a portion of the tumour should be removed for section.
2. In cases where this has proved to be non-malignant, local removal can be attempted. It is sometimes possible to do this without injury to the globe or the optic nerve.
3. In very malignant tumours the entire contents of the orbit should be removed (exenteration of the orbit), followed by deep X-ray or radium treatment.

INJURIES OF THE ORBIT

May involve both the bone and the soft structures that lie within its walls. Fractures of the orbital margin are usually obvious from irregularity of outline, tenderness, crepitus and emphysema of the subcutaneous tissues. Fractures of the deeper parts of the orbit result from penetrating injuries, fractured skull, etc., and can only be diagnosed for certain by X-rays. Any of these fractures may involve one or other of the nasal sinuses. A deep fracture is often complicated by injury to other structures within the orbit, e.g. optic nerve, muscles, etc. Occasionally a 'blow-out' injury occurs, i.e. a direct blow on the eye ruptures the orbital floor and some of the orbital contents are blown out into the antrum or palatine nasal sinus. An orbital haematoma may cause exophthalmos. Finally it should be remembered that orbital injuries of this type may be caused at childbirth by a forceps delivery.

140 A SYNOPSIS OF OPHTHALMOLOGY

Treatment: According to the condition found.
1. Wounds should be cleaned, trimmed, dusted with sulphonilamide powder and sutured. Antitetanus serum should be given when necessary.
2. The more conservative the surgery the better, e.g. orbital foreign bodies are better left in situ rather than run the risk of removing them with probable damage to important structures. In these cases, the surgeon is likely to do more harm than the foreign body.
3. Even involvement of nasal sinuses can be treated expectantly unless orbital cellulitis supervenes.
4. 'Blow-out' injuries require early surgery to release the blown-out inferior rectus muscle and to keep it in place with a terylene implant.

Chapter XIII

DISEASES OF THE EYELIDS

Anatomy: The eyelids are highly specialized folds of skin which cover the anterior orbital foramen and protect the cornea. The gap between the upper and lower lids is known as the palpebral fissure. Each lid is divided by a sulcus on its anterior surface into orbital and tarsal parts. The extremities of the palpebral fissure are the canthi, the lateral canthus forming an acute angle whereas the medial is somewhat rounded. The drainage arrangements of the conjunctiva are situated near the inner canthus, which also encloses a semilunar fold of mucous membrane known as the plica, at the base of which lies the caruncle. Section of an eyelid reveals four layers: (1) Cutaneous; (2) Muscular; (3) Fibrous (tarsal plate); (4) Conjunctiva.

EYELID MUSCLES:
  THE ORBICULARIS MUSCLE completely encircles the anterior orbital foramen and acts as a sphincter on forced closure of the lids. This important muscle is supplied by the seventh nerve.
  THE LEVATOR INSERTION, which is supplied by the third nerve and the function of which is to lift the upper lid.

GLANDS: The following glands are present in the eyelids:
  TARSAL GLANDS: A single row of 30–40 glands in the upper lid and 20–30 in the lower. These are almost straight sebaceous tubules lying in the substance of the tarsal plate, closed at their upper ends and opening at the lid margin.
  ZEIS'S GLANDS, which are the sebaceous glands at the roots of the eyelashes.
  MOLL'S GLANDS: These are sweat glands.
Both eyelids are rich in blood vessels and their supply is derived from both the facial and ophthalmic arterial systems. In the case of the lower lid the internal maxillary artery contributes as well through its infra-orbital branch.

LID MARGINS: About 5 mm from the inner canthus of each lid is situated the lacrimal papilla, a slightly raised eminence on the summit of which is the punctum. The lid margins are lined with the ciliae at their outer boundaries and their inner ones are marked by the openings of the tarsal glands. Between these two landmarks is the 'grey line'. This is of great importance, for along this line the lid can easily be split for surgical purposes. The lid margin is cutaneous up to the gland openings but conjunctival posterior to them.

142 A SYNOPSIS OF OPHTHALMOLOGY

Diseases of the eyelids will be considered under the following headings: (1) Inflammatory diseases; (2) Diseases due to malpositions; (3) Tumours of the eyelids; (4) Congenital abnormalities; (5) Injuries of the eyelids.

I. INFLAMMATORY DISEASES

'With eyelids heavy and red.' THOMAS HOOD, *Song of the Shirt*

Blepharitis is one of the commonest eye diseases, especially in children. It occurs in two clearly defined clinical forms:

ACUTE BLEPHARITIS: Usually occurs concurrently with some other local skin or ocular conditions, e.g. phlyctenular conjunctivitis, acne keratitis, facial eczema, etc. This should be regarded and treated as a spread of infection to the lids from the inflamed surrounding tissues. When these tissues return to normal the blepharitis usually subsides.

CHRONIC BLEPHARITIS: Many of these cases are symptomless, but some get a mild irritagion, soreness of the eyes and photophobia. Both the lid margins are red and hyperaemic, the cilia become encrusted and in some cases adhere, especially when waking in the mornings. In very severe cases the margins become thickened and slightly indurated, and many of the cilia drop out. Ulceration is sometimes present. The aetiology is very uncertain in any given case, but the following factors may contribute:

1. Seborrhoea of scalp.
2. General debility, malnutrition, etc.
3. Uncorrected refractive errors.
4. Unhealthy occupations, especially those involving exposure to heat, dust, wind, smoke, etc.

BACTERIOLOGY: Smears and cultures from chronic blepharitis cases show a variety of flora; staphylococci and Morax–Axenfeld bacilli are found, but in a surprising number of cases the culture shows saprophytic organisms only and a number are even sterile.

TREATMENT:
1. Try to remove any aetiological factor as suggested above.
2. Before undertaking any local treatment, the lids should be thoroughly cleaned with cotton-wool, soaked in warm water, and all adherent scales or discharge removed.
3. Local antibiotics such as chloramphenicol often act like a charm and are best used in ointment form, applied to the lid margins three times a day. This should be used regularly for 3–6 weeks according to the severity of the case, and should be persisted in even though apparent clinical cure results earlier.
4. In resistant cases some other wide-spectrum antibiotic ointment should be used. The choice would depend upon the nature and sensitivity of the causative organism.

5. If an allergic factor is suspected, steroid therapy should be tried in addition to antibiotics, if necessary. Alternatively, gutt. antazol co. is sometimes helpful.
6. If seborrhoea is present in the scalp or there is an excess of dandruff, it must be energetically treated.
7. The old-fashioned treatment of regular painting of the lids with gentian violet or similar dyes is worth trying in resistant cases.

It must be realized that chronic blepharitis may be very resistant to treatment and liable to relapse. If one form of treatment does not give improvement within a month, the changes should be rung and something else tried. When the condition responds, treatment should be left off. It is useless to prolong it indefinitely in the hope of preventing relapses. The patient should be told frankly that *control* rather than *cure* must be expected.

Hordeolum or 'Stye' is an abscess of Zeis's glands. There is a localized hard tender swelling often with gross oedema of the lid and much pain. The abscess usually discharges through the ciliary margin, with great relief to the patient. Epilation of the offending lash is often helpful. The causative organism is nearly always *Staph. aureus*, and the infection is liable to spread along the lid margin causing acute blepharitis and involvements of other Zeis's glands. Hence successive outbreaks of styes are common.

TREATMENT:
1. Hot bathing is indicated. This is best done by means of a wooden spoon covered with cotton-wool. The spoon should be dipped in a bowl of hot water and held at first near the closed eyelid and later in contact with it. Incision (which is excessively painful) is scarcely ever necessary, nearly all cases discharge spontaneously on this treatment.
2. Oc. chloramphenicol 0·5 per cent should be applied three times a day to the eyelids after they have cooled down from the hot bathing.

Chalazion (Meibomian or Tarsal Cyst): This condition is usually symptomless and the patient is concerned on account of cosmetic reasons only. The only sign is a rounded swelling present in the upper or lower lid.

PATHOLOGY: This is not a true cyst, but a granuloma of the tarsal gland. Section shows lymphocytic infiltration and epithelial proliferation, with giant-cell formation. The inner portion of the chalazion degenerates and liquefies, hence the jelly-like substance that is removed on curetting. Occasionally the chalazion will fibrose leaving a hard nodule which is permanent but smaller than the original cyst.

TREATMENT:
1. Very small chalazia are best left alone, for when the eyelid is injected with local anaesthetic they are often difficult to locate and incise.
2. Medium or large chalazia should always be dealt with from the tarsal aspect. The lids should be injected with novutox or other local anaesthetic and a drop of 2 per cent cocaine instilled in the conjunctiva. A vertical or cruciform incision is made in the chalazion, the contents are evacuated, and the walls of the gland thoroughly curetted with a spoon.

Cellulitis of the Eyelids: The eyelids are liable to any form of infection that may attack the skin anywhere, and owing to their laxity of structure, gross oedema may occur on comparatively little provocation. Gnat bits, styes, dacryocystitis and even a very acute conjunctivitis can produce oedema. A similar condition can result from allergic conditions (e.g. exposure to *Primula obconica*, *Rhus toxicodendron*, etc.), sensitivity to drugs (e.g. atropine, boracic, etc.). If the oedema is due to any septic infection cellulitis may result. In such cases there is in addition to oedema, redness, tenderness, brawny induration and much pain in the affected lid. In untreated cases an abscess may follow. Any unexplained cellulitis of an upper lid may be due to a frontal sinus infection.

TREATMENT: Oedema itself in the absence of infection requires no special treatment. It always subsides, usually rapidly. The only treatment should be directed towards the cause of the condition, and when this happens to be allergic the response to antihistamine treatment can be very dramatic. Cellulitis is a different matter and needs prompt attention.
1. Hot spoon bathing 3-hourly.
2. Full doses of chemotherapy according to age of patient.
3. In the few cases that progress to abscess formation the lids should be incised if necessary.

Syphilis of the Eyelid may occur in two forms:
1. PRIMARY SORE: This usually affects the conjunctiva of the lid margin and appears as an indurated ulcer associated with an enlarged pre-auricular or submaxillary gland. Indeed the presence of this sign should always put the ophthalmologist on his guard, for it nearly always indicates a serious infection, e.g. tuberculosis, syphilis, etc.

   TREATMENT: If recognized early and the diagnosis is confirmed by examination of scrapings, local excision may be undertaken, due regard being paid to its situation and possible resulting deformity.
   PROGNOSIS in treated cases is good.

2. GUMMATA (SYPHILITIC TARSITIS): These bear a superficial resemblance to a chalazion but they are usually multiple and the

DISEASES OF THE EYELIDS

whole tarsal plate is grossly enlarged and indurated. The preauricular or submaxillary glands are involved. Pain is uncommon.
TREATMENT: Energetic antisyphilitic remedies are indicated, followed by a course of iodides by mouth. Improvement is usually rapid.

II. DISORDERS DUE TO MALPOSITION OF LIDS

Trichiasis is a condition where the cilia instead of growing forwards are pointing backwards and coming into contact with the conjunctiva or cornea, with resulting irritation.

CAUSES: Congenital distichiasis, spastic entropion, severe blepharitis, trachoma, scarring from injuries, burns, etc.

SIGNS AND SYMPTOMS: The patient complains of a feeling of irritation in the eye and often thinks that a foreign body is present. Recurrent corneal ulceration occurs, and, as these areas heal, vascularization and corneal opacities result. In the course of time vision deteriorates greatly owing to these corneal irregularities.

TREATMENT:
1. In slight cases epilation or the destruction of the hair follicles by electrolysis may be all that is required.
2. In severe cases operations similar to those for entropion are indicated. Operative details are outside the scope of this volume and the reader is referred to textbooks on eye surgery.
3. Contact lenses play a valuable part in the treatment of very obstinate cases. Not only do they prevent the cilia from coming into contact with the cornea, but in many cases they result in much better sight since they abolish the unevenness of the corneal surface which reflects irregularly the light rays as they enter the eye.

Entropion: Turning inwards of the lid (almost always the lower one) is due to one of two causes: spasm or scarring.

SPASTIC ENTROPION is a disease of advancing years and is caused by a spasm of the orbicularis muscle. It is commonest in persons with sunken and recessed eyes, which for this reason are unable to give adequate support against the sphincter action of the orbicularis.

TREATMENT:
1. In slight cases temporary relief can be given by strapping the skin of the lower lid in an everted position by adhesive plaster. Temporary improvement can also be obtained by injecting the lid with local anaesthetic and alcohol.
2. Cautery treatment may give great relief, which may last for months or even years and can always be repeated. The technique is as follows: The lid is injected with novutox and a double row of deep punctures is made with the cautery in

the skin immediately below the ciliary margin. These punctures are made along its entire length at a distance of about 2 mm from each other and about 2 mm from the row above. The rows of punctures should not be opposite each other but should be arranged in a 'mocked' fashion as gardeners plant flowers in a bed.

In very severe cases a triple row can be made but this is rarely necessary. This treatment breaks the spasm and the resulting scarring usually pulls the cilia forwards, with great relief to the patient.
3. Operation, such as Weis's or Wheeler's operations, may be undertaken in severe cases.

CICATRICIAL ENTROPION results either from trachoma or trauma and is a natural mechanical result due to scar tissue distorting the lids, conjunctiva or tarsal plate.

TREATMENT: If the case is one of any degree of severity either operation or contact lenses may be indicated.

Ectropion: The sagging and partial eversion of the lower lid. The condition is an extremely ugly one from the aesthetic point of view since the lid appears to have a rim of red, velvety, raw-looking flesh. Apart from the disfigurement, there are other highly disagreeable symptoms. The patient has a troublesome epiphora, because the punctum is no longer in contact with the conjunctiva, and an irritable conjunctivitis, and in severe cases keratitis results from exposure. This condition can be due to the following causes:
1. Paralysis of the orbicularis muscle from any cause.
2. Senility, when general laxity of the subcutaneous tissues combined with loss of tone of the orbicularis muscle causes sagging of the eyelid.
3. Scarring of the lids or the skin in the neighbourhood of the lids from any cause, e.g. trauma, burns, operations, severe blepharitis, etc.

TREATMENT:
1. Cautery puncture as described under ENTROPION is indicated and is a very successful treatment in milder cases. In ectropion the punctures are made in the exposed mucous membrane, the first row being immediately posterior to the ciliary margin. Special care must be taken to avoid injury to the punctum or canaliculus. The punctures must be deep, and quite frequently three rows are required. The resulting scarring often improves the position of the lid greatly and the treatment can be repeated when necessary.
2. For more severe cases a variety of operations varying from simple procedures such as Snellen's sutures or the 'VY' operation to Kuhnt's or Blaskowicz's operations, with various modifications,

DISEASES OF THE EYELIDS 147

have been devised. Details of these appear in books on operative surgery.

Ptosis: This is a drooping of the upper lid and is due to the following causes:

1. Increase in the weight of the lid due to infiltration, cysts, chronic blepharitis, etc.
2. Far more commonly it is due to paralysis (partial or complete) of the levator muscle. Ptosis may be congenital or acquired, unilateral or bilateral and partial or complete. In the latter case the pupil is completely covered by the lid and vision is only possible by looking upwards and bringing the frontalis muscle into action.

   In partial cases the pupil is usually about half covered and the patient has to tilt his head upwards to see clearly in front of him. Cases of bilateral partial ptosis give the patient a very 'sleepy' and stupid appearance. Congenital cases are bilateral, although both lids are not necessarily affected to the same extent, and these cases are often accompanied by a limitation of upward ocular movement. Acquired ptosis is usually unilateral and is most commonly due to a partial or complete third-nerve paralysis, often the result of cerebral causes of trauma involving injury to the muscle or its nerve supply. It must be remembered that bilateral ptosis in young persons is the first sign of myasthenia gravis. If this disease is suspected 1 ml of prostigmin should be injected; if this results in the disappearance of, or marked improvement in, the ptosis, which returns again later, the diagnosis is certain.

TREATMENT: Must when possible be aimed at the cause. It is frequently a manifestation of cerebral syphilis, and these cases often respond to the appropriate treatment. In congenital or undetermined causes the following may be tried:

1. A ptosis bar can be fitted to the rim of spectacles if worn. This bar is made to project backwards and to take the weight of the lid. An exact fit is necessary and a careful adjustment must be made every time the glasses are put on. This cannot be regarded as a very satisfactory method of treatment.
2. A contact lens with a specially made 'ptosis ledge' has the same effect.
3. Various operations including Hess's, Motais's, Greeves's and Blaskowicz's have been successful. The student is referred to larger textbooks for details of these and other ptosis operations.

Lagophthalmos: The inability to cover the eyes when the lids are shut. It may be due to many conditions: (1) Exophthalmos; (2) Paralysis of orbicularis; (3) Ectropion; (4) Scarring due to burns, trauma, trachoma, etc.

The signs, symptoms, and treatment are dealt with under EXPOSURE KERATITIS (q.v.).

III. TUMOURS
Innocent Tumours:
DERMOID CYSTS: Occasionally occur as cystic swellings under the skin of the upper lid. These have already been described under TUMOURS OF THE ORBIT (p. 138).

NAEVI: These are usually in the form of pigmented moles on the mucocutaneous margin of the lids. They scarcely ever become malignant.

HAEMANGIOMATA: Another variety of naevus can occur in two forms:
1. TELANGIECTASIS or port-wine coloured aggregations of dilated capillaries which often resemble a spider's web.
2. CAVERNOUS HAEMANGIOMA, which are dilated subcutaneous venous spaces and appear as a bluish swelling which becomes dense on straining, holding the breath, etc. This condition may be present in Sturge–Weber's syndrome and buphthalmos.

XANTHELASMA: The name given to the small, yellow, plate-like spots that occur in the skin of both lids in the region of the inner canthus. They are of no significance and only occasionally require treatment for cosmetic reasons. Their pathology is uncertain, but they are believed to be due to cholesteraemia, and their presence always in the same situation is attributed to the vascular anastomoses between the blood supplies from the internal and external carotid arterial systems.

PAPILLOMATA: Occur from the lid margins and if untreated tend to become pedunculated owing to the movements of blinking.

HORNS: May be formed by the massing of the epidermic cells which cover a papilloma. They may become very hard, of considerable length and most disfiguring. Occasionally a horn can be of sebaceous origin, i.e. formed from the hardened sebum from a gland.

NEUROFIBROMATOSIS (PLEXIFORM NEUROMA): May involve the lids. Grossly enlarged nerves are palpable, running subcutaneously like a series of hard beads. Similar swellings may occur in the temporal region, and other nerves such as the ciliary, optic, etc., may be affected as well.

MOLLUSCUM FIBROSUM: A pedunculated tumour of lobular structure. It is covered by skin and contains fibrous and connective tissue. These tumours are often multiple and may be one of the ocular manifestations of von Recklinghausen's disease.

TREATMENT OF INNOCENT TUMOURS:
1. The aim should be to remove the tumour with the minimum damage to the lid. This is of great importance, for resulting

DISEASES OF THE EYELIDS

scarring or loss of tissue might cause epiphora, imperfect closure of the lids, etc.
2. Owing to extreme vascularity of the lids, electrolysis, diathermy or the electric cautery is the method of choice for the removal of small lid tumours. Papillomata, horns, etc., can be conveniently and permanently removed by grasping the tumour with toothed forceps and burning around its base. In all such cases it is very important to burn down deep, to ensure that the tumour base is completely destroyed.
3. Some tumours (e.g. naevi, telangiectasis) may be removed with carbon dioxide snow. Others (dermoids, cavernous haemangiomata) should be dissected out. An alternative treatment is the injection of some sclerosing agent. No treatment is required until the age of 3 years as sometimes there is a spontaneous improvement.

Malignant Tumours:

RODENT ULCER: A basal-cell carcinoma; is the commonest malignant growth of the eyelid. It is a disease of late middle or old age, and starts as a wart on the skin (not on the mucocutaneous margin) which has often been quiescent for years but the surface of which has recently 'become raw and formed a scab'. This scab comes off on little provocation such as rubbing the face with a towel. The ulcerated area remains quite painless and spreads very slowly indeed, but in all directions, in depth as well as extent. In grossly neglected cases it may invade the orbit, the nose and even the cranium. It never gives rise to secondary deposits.

TREATMENT: If seen reasonably early, the treatment of choice is excision, but if this procedure is likely to endanger the eye subsequently from exposure, radium or X-rays may be tried provided a careful watch is kept on the case afterwards.

CARCINOMA AND SARCOMA:

CARCINOMA: Carcinoma of the squamous-cell type occurs most commonly at the mucocutaneous junction of the lids. It commences as a wart-like growth which ulcerates, leaving everted and indurated edges, and slowly progresses. It rarely causes secondary deposits in spite of glandular involvement.

SARCOMA is very rare in the eyelid. It may be of the spindle- or round-cell variety or it may occur as a malignant change in a pigmented naevus. Growth is slow but sure, and the eye is lost from exposure. Glandular involvement and secondary deposits are more common in sarcoma than in any other growth of the eyelid.

TREATMENT: These require more drastic measures. Complete removal and even exenteration of the orbit if necessary should be undertaken as soon as possible.

IV. CONGENITAL ABNORMALITIES OF THE EYELIDS

Coloboma: Occurs as a wedge-shaped gap in the margin of one of the lids (usually the upper one). It is frequently associated with other congenital defects both in the eye and elsewhere, e.g. coloboma of iris, hare-lip, cleft palate, etc.

Epicanthus: A semilunar skin fold which joins the upper and lower lids at their inner angle, and may overlap the caruncle and puncta. It is usually associated with a broad nasal bridge and wide pupillary distance. This fold is bilateral and hides from view part of the sclerotic at the inner angle of each eye. This frequently gives the appearance of an internal squint to anyone untrained in ophthalmology, hence many children with epicanthus are referred to the outpatients' department or school clinic for 'a squint'. A negative cover test will clinch this diagnosis.

TREATMENT is very rarely required. Usually the deformity becomes less noticeable with the lapse of time, but in exceptional cases plastic surgery may be justifiable, the operation of choice being that of Spaeth. For details see textbooks on eye surgery.

Distichiasis: A rare condition where two parallel rows of eyelashes are present, the second row being posterior to the normal one and causing irritation by contact with the cornea. This condition is usually bilateral and both upper and lower lids may be affected.

TREATMENT: Electrolysis of each cilium of the posterior row.

Very rarely, other gross lid abnormalities are seen: cryptophthalmia, where the palpebral fissure is absent, the eye being hidden by skin; ablepharon, where the lids are absent, and microblepharon, where they are abnormally small. All these conditions are often associated with other gross abnormalities in the eye, usually due to failure of closure of the fetal fissure. Sometimes congenital defects are present in other parts of the body, e.g. syndactyly. Finally it should be remembered that plexiform neuroma (q.v.) is considered by some authorities to be a congenital condition.

V. INJURIES OF THE EYELIDS

Wounds: Wounds of eyelids are a very common occurrence. Those that are only skin deep normally heal well and rapidly, with a minimum of scarring and no distortion. Wounds requiring the greatest care are those that split the eyelid throughout its entire thickness. These require the most careful suturing and every effort must be made to ensure that the margins are in exact opposition, otherwise the resulting irregularity may be unsightly and epiphora and even exposure of the cornea may result. Care taken over these wounds is amply repaid by good results. The finest nylon sutures on eyeless needles are the best for this type of work.

Burns of the Eyelids: If of any appreciable depth these must be regarded as major injuries since the resulting scarring may cause serious distortions which may tax the ingenuity of the plastic surgeon to repair. Any coagulant treatment must be avoided and either a Thiersch graft applied or dressings with tulle gras, ung. penicillin, or other bland treatment that does not adhere to the burnt area.

Haematoma ('Black Eye'): Always results from a direct blow and may cause so much swelling that the eye cannot be opened. This usually absorbs well and requires no special treatment. Cold bathing helps to reduce the swelling and to ease the discomfort.

Symblepharon: The name given to an adhesion between the eyelid and the globe. Any form of trauma which causes loss of conjunctiva from both tarsal and bulbar surfaces will result in this condition if the two denuded areas remain in apposition. It is a common sequel to lime and other caustic burns and it may occur as the result of diphtheria, tuberculous ulceration, etc. Symblepharon always impairs the ocular movement, hence the commonest symptom is diplopia. In severe cases closure of the eyelids may be impossible, and exposure of the cornea with all its attendant dangers may result.

TREATMENT:

1. PREVENTIVE: In every injury or disease likely to result in symblepharon both fornices should be explored daily with a glass rod with ung. chloramphenicol or petroleum jelly, as much of the ointment as possible being pushed into the fornix. This may break down adhesions which tend to form while the process of healing is taking place.
2. CURATIVE: Treatment is operative only. The symblepharon must be broken down and some form of graft applied to cover the raw surfaces. One of the authors (C. M.-D.) has devised a simple method which has succeeded in a number of cases—a graft consisting of egg and prepared amniotic membrane. A piece of membrane from a hard-boiled duck's egg (this membrane being tougher than that of a hen's egg) is removed and folded on itself with the smooth sides outwards. This is trimmed to the approximate size of the area to be covered. The egg membrane is then surrounded with a double layer of prepared amniotic membrane and the whole stitched in position with fine silk sutures. The eyelids should be stitched together. On the seventh day the eyelid stitches are removed, likewise the egg membrane, by which time the amniotic graft has usually 'taken'. It will be found that amniotic membrane is very much easier to manipulate and to place in position when thus backed with egg membrane, and the whole graft can be sutured in position comparatively easily. Other grafts possible for use in symblepharon operations can be taken from conjunctiva or

mucous membrane. The normal routine at most hospitals is to take a graft from the patient's buccal mucous membrane. This is highly successful but it takes a long time to perform.

Ankyloblepharon: Ankyloblepharon means the adhesion between the lid margins. It is usually due to the same causes as symblepharon, but in very rare cases it is congenital. The adhesions may be extensive even throughout the entire length of the lid margins or they may be partial, as is artificially produced in a median tarsorrhaphy.

TREATMENT is surgical only. If the condition is associated with extensive symblepharon, it is very doubtful whether operation will benefit the patient. In cases without symblepharon the lids should be separated by snipping with scissors, and during the process of healing the lid margins must be kept apart as far as possible. An egg and amniotic membrane graft (as described under SYMBLEPHARON) may be applied to the lid margins in these cases, especially if the ankyloblepharon is extensive.

Chapter XIV

DISEASES OF THE LACRIMAL APPARATUS

DISEASES OF THE LACRIMAL GLAND

Anatomy: The lacrimal gland is a serous tubulo-racemose gland made up of very small lobules and is situated at the upper and outer corner of the orbit beneath the septum orbitale and the orbicularis muscle. It shows considerable variation in form, but its anterior aspect is always closely related to the expansion of the levator tendon which cuts deeply into this substance, dividing it into upper and lower lobes, which are, however, connected by a narrow isthmus of gland tissue. The upper lobe, which is the size of an almond, runs parallel to the orbital margin; the lower lobe, which is half the size of the upper, lies under the levator and is adherent to the palpebral conjunctiva, into which its twelve ducts open at the upper fornix.

Surgically the lower lobe is the more important, for its removal severs these ducts (which carry the secretion of both lobes) and is the equivalent of extirpating the entire gland.

In addition to the lacrimal gland, some microscopic accessory glands (Krause) are present, which open into the conjunctiva at the fornices. These, together with the goblet cells present in the conjunctiva, are sufficient to moisten that structure reasonably adequately even when the main gland is extirpated.

Diseases of the lacrimal gland are very uncommon.

Dacryo-adenitis may occur and may lead to abscess formation and lacrimal fistula. Occasionally tubercle bacillus attacks this gland.

Sjögren's Syndrome (Keratoconjunctivitis Sicca): This is thought to be due to primary dysfunction of the lacrimal gland. (*See* p. 19.)

Mikulicz's Syndrome: Consists of a bilateral enlargement of the lacrimal and parotid glands. Its aetiology is uncertain and may be due to such varied factors as syphilis, tuberculosis or leukaemia. Sections of these glands show lymphocytic infiltration and giant cells; in later stages this is followed by fibrosis.

Heerfordt's Disease (Uveoparotid Fever): Enlargement of the lacrimal as well as the parotid glands may occur in the course of this disease, which is referred to under DISEASES OF THE UVEAL TRACT, p. 45.

'Mixed' Tumour: Mixed tumour of the lacrimal gland may occur, but this is much less frequent than the mixed tumour found in the parotid gland. It is endotheliomatous in nature and soft and non-malignant. Very occasionally sarcomatous changes supervene.

Carcinoma: May occur in this gland but it is very rare.

154 A SYNOPSIS OF OPHTHALMOLOGY

Retention Cysts (Dacryops): May result from the blockage of one or more of the ducts. This causes a cystic swelling in the upper fornix.

It must be borne in mind that any disease which causes enlargement of the lacrimal gland may result in proptosis and displacement of the globe, with consequent limitation of ocular movements and diplopia.

DISEASES OF THE LACRIMAL PASSAGES

Anatomy: The lacrimal passages conduct the tears from the eye to the nose. They commence at the puncta and are situated at the summit of the lacrimal papillae of both upper and lower lids, and they lead through the upper and lower canaliculi to the lacrimal sac, thence to the nasolacrimal duct which opens into the nose.

PUNCTUM: Each punctum lies about 5–6 mm from the inner canthus on the posterior edge of the lid margin. It is normally in apposition with the conjunctiva and is, therefore, invisible except when the lid is everted.

CANALICULUS extends vertically upwards in the case of the upper (downwards in the case of the lower) for 2 mm. It then turns at a right-angle, to run horizontally for about 6 mm before it opens into the lateral aspect of the lacrimal sac.

LACRIMAL SAC: Lies in the fossa of the lacrimal bone at the lower part of the medial wall of the orbit. It is approximately 14 mm long by 5 mm wide and is completely enclosed by the periosteum, which splits in this region—the superficial layer (the lacrimal fascia) covering the sac and the deeper layer lining the bone. The posterior surface of the sac is adherent to the deeper periosteal layer. Important relations which the ophthalmologist should remember are the angular vessels which lie superficially and just medially to the sac.

NASOLACRIMAL DUCT: The downward continuation of the sac to the inferior meatus of the nose. It is in two parts: (1) the interosseous part lying in the bony nasolacrimal canal; and (2) the intermeatal part lying in the mucous membrane of the nose.

These two parts vary considerably in length, but the average is 12 mm and 5 mm respectively. The meatal portion opens at the ostium lacrimale in the inferior nasal meatus 30 mm behind the nares and 16 mm above the floor of the nose.

Diseases of the lacrimal passages can be considered under two headings— inflammations and obstructions. Before considering these in detail it would be well to consider one symptom common to all diseases of the lacrimal passages:

Epiphora: Tears are an alkaline fluid containing appreciable quantities of sodium chloride and an antibacterial enzyme, called lysozyme which is potent enough to inhibit most air-borne bacteria before they have time to infect the cornea or the conjunctiva. Under norma

DISEASES OF THE LACRIMAL APPARATUS

circumstances the amount of tears secreted is just sufficient to moisten the eye, any surplus being evaporated. When an excess of tears is produced the lacrimal passages come into play to drain the overflow, but if the secretion of tears is so great that these passages cannot cope with them, or if, for any cause, any part of these passages is obstructed, then epiphora results. It is obvious, therefore, that epiphora can be produced in one of two ways: (1) by an increased secretion of tears; (2) by an obstructed drainage system.

INCREASED SECRETION is due to a reflex stimulation of the endings of the fifth nerve, e.g. cold winds, smoke, corneal foreign bodies, pungent fumes, etc. In this category can also be included ocular inflammations, excessive sunlight, bathing in chlorinated water, etc.

OBSTRUCTED DRAINAGE may occur anywhere in the passages due to absence, occlusion or obstruction of any part of them. Spaeth reported that prolonged use of local epinephrine causes casts of the nasolacrimal ducts to form. These cause obstruction with epiphora and can sometimes be expelled into the nasopharynx by syringeing. A punctum which is not in contact with the conjunctiva also prevents drainage as effectively as would an obstruction.

Apart from being an unpleasant and irritating symptom, epiphora results in a diminution of the lysozyme content, with consequent lowering of the resistance of the affected eye to invading bacteria. This fact should be borne in mind by the surgeon before undertaking any intra-ocular operation on a patient with this symptom.

INFLAMMATIONS AFFECTING THE LACRIMAL PASSAGES

Dacryocystitis commonly occurs as a chronic infection. The signs and symptoms are epiphora with a swelling in the region of the tear duct which, on pressure, discharges a mucopurulent fluid through the canaliculus. Occasionally dacryocystitis occurs in an acute form accompanied by great pain, redness and swelling of the skin over the sac, often extending into the eyelids. The whole area is acutely tender. If abscess formation does not take place the condition slowly settles down to that of chronic dacryocystitis. This condition sometimes occurs in newborn infants. It may be stated categorically that untreated chronic dacryocystitis never cures itself. Nothing but extirpation of the sac can get rid of this troublesome and potentially dangerous condition.

AETIOLOGY: The cause of dacryocystitis may be either an obstructed tear passage or an upward spread of infection from the nasal mucosa.

156 A SYNOPSIS OF OPHTHALMOLOGY

PATHOLOGY: Cultures taken from the fluid expressed from the sac in these cases may show a variety of virulent pyogenic bacteria including *Staph. pyogenes* and pneumococci. There is no doubt that these bacteria which have such ready access to the eye constitute an ever-present threat like the 'sword of Damocles'. Corneal ulceration and hypopyon may result on little provocation and an intra-ocular operation undertaken without first removing the sac (or sealing off the punctum with the cautery) would run a grave risk of panophthalmitis.

TREATMENT:
1. In early stages periodic syringeing of the lacrimal passages may relieve the obstruction and ease the epiphora. At first the syringed fluid returns to the eye via the upper canaliculus, but, if repeated, communication with the nose may be re-established. Penicillin and other antibiotics have been introduced in this manner, but are probably useless. It is very doubtful whether this treatment really cures the condition, since most cases recur sooner or later.
2. If the above fails, and especially if there are nasal symptoms, the advice of a laryngologist should be sought as to whether any pathological condition (e.g. polypi, deviated septum, etc.) is present in the nose which might be causing an upward spread of infection or obstructing the ostium. Treatment of such conditions may cure the patient in a small proportion of cases. In those cases that do not respond, extirpation of the sac may be undertaken. After operation the epiphora slowly improves and the discharge is 'clean water' (tears) instead of 'dirty water' (infected mucopus) liable to infect the eye. These tears evaporate normally, but in cold weather, etc., the epiphora may again become somewhat troublesome. For this reason surgeons prefer a dacryocystorhinostomy operation (*see below*) whenever possible.
3. In every case of recent lacrimal obstruction the operation of dacryocystorhinostomy may be advised, since, if successful, a drainage channel from the eye to the nose is restored. The student is advised to consult textbooks for details of this operation.
4. Most surgeons regard probing in these cases as tending to do more harm than good; when a probe is forced through to the nose damage cannot fail to be done to the inflamed mucous membrane lining the duct, and after withdrawal of the probe fibrous stricture is liable to result.

Lacrimal Abscess: This condition frequently complicates acute dacryocystitis. The abscess usually points at the level of the lower end of the sac and occasionally a fistula remains.

TREATMENT:
1. Immediate injection of long-acting penicillin and full doses of chemotherapy in an early stage may prevent abscess formation.

DISEASES OF THE LACRIMAL APPARATUS

2. In infants drain the abscess by probing.
3. Frequent hot spoon bathing is indicated and incision if the abscess points.
4. In cases of fistula, the whole area should be opened up and every trace of epithelial lining of the sac should be curetted away.

OBSTRUCTIONS OF THE LACRIMAL PASSAGES

These may be congenital or acquired and may occur at any point between the punctum and the ostium. The symptom common to all is epiphora.

Blockage of the Punctum: Very rarely this occurs as a congenital condition (imperforate punctum), but it is frequently seen as a result of scarring following trauma. In these cases the punctum may be very difficult to locate even with a careful examination with a loupe. It should be remembered here that if, owing to slight ectropion, the lower punctum is not in contact with the conjunctiva the effect is just the same as if an obstruction was present.

TREATMENT:
1. If the punctum can be found it should be slit open and a probe inserted daily.
2. If no trace is to be found and it is impossible to get the probe into the canaliculus, Stallard's operation may be performed. This is a comparatively simple and ingenious procedure whereby the fundus of the sac is sutured to the conjunctiva near the inner canthus, thus enabling the tears to drain away, short-circuiting the punctum and canaliculus.

Blockage of the Canaliculus: This may be caused by three factors:
1. CONGENITAL ABNORMALITIES are sometimes found. There may be atresia of the canaliculus or it may be present as a groove instead of a tunnel.

   TREATMENT: Stallard's operation as described above is the simplest and best treatment.
2. CONCRETIONS AND MECHANICAL OBSTRUCTIONS are not uncommon. These may be caused by a fungus infection such as streptothrix or actinomycosis, or even by mechanical blockages such as an eyelash.

   TREATMENT: The canaliculus should be slit up and the concretion or obstruction removed and the canaliculus curetted.
3. TRAUMA: The canaliculus may be obstructed by scarring or by direct injury. If a troublesome epiphora results, Stallard's operation offers the best prospect of relief.

Blockage of the Nasolacrimal Duct: This may be due to:

DELAYED CANALIZATION: Very frequently infants of a few weeks or months old are brought to the oculist because of unilateral (or sometimes bilateral) epiphora. There has been no question of any infection and the discharge is watery and not mucopurulent. Very many of these cases cure themselves spontaneously, and Foster-Moore considered that these are due to delayed canalization. As the child grows there comes a time when suddenly almost dramatically the watering ceases. This means that the duct has opened up. This may happen at any time from a few months up to 2 years of age.

TREATMENT:
1. If the case is a mild one and the discharge is clear expectant treatment should be carried out until the patient is at least 6 months old in the hope that canalization may be completed by a normal if delayed process. Mucopus will be expressed.
2. Ung. chloramphenicol or other antibiotics three times a day for 2–4 weeks seems to improve these cases and is always worth a trial, even if only to relieve the added infection.
3. In more severe and intractable cases, particularly if the discharge is mucopurulent, the punctum should be dilated and probe passed through to the nose.

TRAUMA: The commonest traumatic cause of blockage of the duct is injudicious and energetic probing either in infancy or in vain efforts to treat lacrimal obstruction in adults. It cannot be too strongly emphasized: (1) that probing should rarely if ever be undertaken in an adult—syringeing may or may not do good but it cannot do harm; probing can and does. (2) In infants probing, if undertaken, should be gentle and without force. A solitary probing is sufficient. Repeated probings are harmful and likely to cause stricture of the nasolacrimal duct. Apart from injudicious probings, a fractured maxilla is the commonest cause of traumatic occlusion of this duct.

TREATMENT is unsatisfactory, dacryocystorhinostomy offering the only hope of cure.

Chapter XV

INTRA-OCULAR NEOPLASMS

CARCINOMA, sarcoma and retinoblastoma (formerly called 'glioma') all occur intra-ocularly, but the first is always secondary to a primary growth elsewhere. None of them is of common occurrence and all of them are definitely malignant. The first two occur in the uveal tract and the last is a growth of the retina itself.

Pathology: There are four stages in the progress of all the primary intra-ocular neoplasms:
1. THE QUIESCENT STAGE: Early in the disease when the growth remains localized and is causing little interference with either the vision or the drainage of the eye.
2. THE STAGE OF GLAUCOMA: The onset of this symptom depends upon whether the growth has invaded a vortex vein, or has pushed the lens and iris forward, thus blocking the filtration angle.
3. THE STAGE OF EXTRA-OCULAR EXTENSION: Occurs when the growth has penetrated some of the scleral canals that contain the ciliary vessels and nerves, and hence has entered the orbit. Alternatively, it may have affected the nerve head and extended for some distance along the optic nerve.
4. STAGE OF METASTASIS: Secondary growths occur—common in the liver, but may affect other organs. In some intra-ocular neoplasms this stage occurs quite late, often a number of years after the eye has been removed.

CARCINOMA OF THE CHOROID

Carcinoma of the choroid is always secondary to a primary growth elsewhere in the body, and it most commonly follows a carcinoma of the breast. It is usually bilateral and its presence in the eye is a sure sign that other secondary growths are occurring in different organs of the body. These tumours sometimes fluoresce (p. 257).

MELANOMA OF THE IRIS

This is one of the rarest of the intra-ocular neoplasms. It commences as a pigmented nodule anywhere on the surface of the iris, sometimes occurring as a proliferation of a pre-existing pigmentary naevus. Growth at first is slow, but later it goes rapidly through the four stages described. Diagnosis when the nodule is solitary is very difficult, but it is obvious when satellites make their appearance and gradually enlarge. If slit-lamp examination shows the vessels over the nodule the diagnosis of sarcoma is very probable.

Differential Diagnosis: The following conditions may cause nodules on the iris: congenital melanomata, tuberculosis, syphilis, sarcoiditis, leukaemic conditions and leprosy. The appropriate measures to exclude these must be taken before the diagnosis is established.

Treatment:
1. A short period of observation is justifiable during which slit-lamp examination and photographs should be undertaken regularly.
2. If the tumour grows, a nodule should be removed by iridectomy or iridocyclectomy and submitted to histological examination.

Prognosis: Good in cases when local removal is undertaken early.

MELANOMA OF THE CHOROID

Malignant melanoma of the choroid may occur at any age, but it is commonest in the fifth decade of life. It is always unilateral, and although it may occur anywhere in the choroid it is commonest at the posterior pole. It commences as a lens-shaped growth which pushes the retina before it as it enlarges. Bruch's membrane offers some resistance to its progress, but it eventually bursts through and forms a sort of head through the opening. The constriction by the opening through Bruch's membrane produces a neck which is connected to the main mass of growth which lies in the choroid behind. Thus on section it somewhat resembles a collar stud. As it grows, the head pushes the retina forwards, which soon becomes detached, and albuminous fluid accumulates behind it. If the fluid is excessive and if the head of the growth is not attached to the retina, diagnosis from a simple detachment may not be easy. As

	SIMPLE DETACHMENT	MALIGNANT DETACHMENT
AGE	Any age	Commonest in fifth decade
HISTORY	Sometimes follows trauma	No trauma
ONSET	Sudden	Sometimes sudden, often gradual
REFRACTION	Commonest in moderate myopia	Irrespective of refractive errors
TRANS-ILLUMINATION	Clear	May be dull
TENSION	Normal or soft	If tension is raised it is diagnostic
SITE	Commonest in lower half	Anywhere. If small and confined to upper part or posterior pole, it is diagnostic
APPEARANCE	Parallel folds and nodules that may move on ocular movements	May appear rounded and fixed
PIGMENT	If present at all, is usually at periphery	Pigment on summit of detachment is very suggestive
HOLE OR TEAR	Almost always present	Scarcely ever present

the disease progresses glaucomatous changes supervene and secondary cataract may occur. The usual four stages of intra-ocular neoplasms are seen.

Diagnosis: Not infrequently a sudden retinal detachment is the first sign of melanoma of the choroid, thus differential diagnosis between simple and malignant detachments is of vital importance. This can be conveniently studied in tabular form. Sometimes a choroidal naevus can closely resemble an early melanoma. This usually occurs as a rounded, bluish, slightly raised swelling near the posterior pole. It is about one or two discs in diameter. Such a naevus must be watched with utmost care and if there is any doubt about it, it should be destroyed by light coagulation. Recently workers in the University of Munster have devised an ingenious method of diagnosing malignant tumours by retro-illumination. The curved transilluminator is inserted retrobulbarly and the operator watches through the dilated pupil. In malignant cases the shadow of the tumour can be clearly seen. More recently the early diagnosis has been greatly helped by fluorescein angiography (q.v.).

Histology and Prognosis: These growths are usually pigmented but not necessarily so. Spindle-cell variety is the commonest, but cylindrical, endothelial and round-cell varieties occur, as also do angiosarcomata. Staining with silver always reveals the presence of a greater or less amount of reticulin fibres. Observations by Callender, Sorsby and others show that the less reticulation present the greater the liability to metastasis, and hence the worse the prognosis. Likewise these observers believe the lower the pigment content the lower the mortality. Greer considers that the type of cell is the important factor in prognosis, those with epithelioid cells having the worst. When sending eyes that have been excised for histological report the pathologist should always be asked to report on these three important prognostic factors: reticulation, pigment content and cell type. Untreated cases are invariably fatal, as are most of those when excision is delayed until intra-ocular expansion has occurred. Occasionally metastasis is slow and may be delayed for anything up to 30 years.

Treatment:
1. Immediate excision when the diagnosis is established. The optic nerve should be cut off as long as possible in case the growth has invaded it.
2. If any extra-ocular growth is found the orbit should be exenterated and treated with X-rays.
3. In the event of the eye with the growth being the only eye with vision, treatment with radon seed, light coagulation (*see* p. 91) or laser beam is justifiable provided that a very careful watch is

kept on the patient for a prolonged time afterwards, and excision is performed at the first sign of recurrence.
4. In cases of melanomata very near the disc (where the differential diagnosis is always difficult and uncertain) treatment with the laser beam is indicated.

MELANOMA OF THE CILIARY BODY

Differs in no vital respect from melanoma of the choroid except that detachment occurs rarely and glaucoma commonly in these cases. Displacement of the lens occurs and the ciliary circulation is impeded, resulting in a dilatation of the anterior ciliary vessels overlying the tumour. When the growth involves the angle a dark crescentic mass (superficially resembling a dialysis) is visible, upon which vessels may be seen with the loupe or slit-lamp. These growths are dull on transillumination. In all other respects, histology, prognosis, treatment, etc., this condition is identical with sarcoma of the choroid.

RETINOBLASTOMA

Retinoblastoma (formerly called 'glioma of the retina') is a very malignant intra-ocular neoplasm which affects infants and young children usually under 5 years of age. The name 'glioma' was ill chosen, for it is in no way related to glioma (astrocytoma) of the optic nerve, a growth which never gives rise to metastasis. No less than 25 per cent of retinoblastoma cases are bilateral, and when this occurs these two growths are both primary and are not connected with each other by metastasis. Frequently there is a family history of retinoblastoma and sometimes several children in one family are affected. Duke-Elder considers that this condition is a congenital one although it may remain quiescent for some years. There is no preference for either sex.

Signs and Symptoms: Occasionally the presenting sign is a squint of sudden origin but usually advice is first sought on account of one sign which is invariable and of fundamental importance: the child has developed a 'white pupil'. If the case is neglected the disease makes the usual progress of a malignant intra-ocular neoplasm outlined under General Pathology at the beginning of this chapter. The quiescent stage becomes glaucomatous and this is quickly followed by extra-ocular extension and general metastasis. Local extension is along the optic nerve to the brain and secondary deposits may occur in the cranium, liver, and elsewhere. The total duration is usually less than twelve months.

Pathology: Most authorities believe the disease to be congenital but that its manifestations are delayed for a few years. Sections of these growths often show a striking resemblance to embryonic retinal tissues, and some of the 'rosettes' which are a histological characteristic of the disease resemble malformed rods and cones. Very soon

after the disease is discovered, daughter growths appear all around it and in other parts of the eye. As has already been stated, in the 25 per cent of cases where retinoblastoma appears in the second eye, this is another primary growth and not either a metastasis or an extension via the chiasma. From the pathological point of view two forms of retinoblastoma are described according to their manner of growth:
1. GLIOMA EXOPHYTUM, where the growth tends to grow outwards involving the choroid.
2. GLIOMA ENDOPHYTUM, where it tends to grow inwards and invade the vitreous.

The appearances of these two types in their early stages differ. The latter appears as a white cheesy-looking mass involving the vitreous, whereas the former when seen early appears simply as a detached retina.

Differential Diagnosis: Other conditions which resemble glioma are called collectively 'pseudoglioma'. The following should be borne in mind: (1) Tuberculosis of the choroid; (2) Congenital abnormalities, such as fibrovascular sheath of lens; (3) The aftermath of infantile iritis with inflammatory exudates in the vitreous and sometimes detached retina; (4) Retrolental fibroplasia; (5) Coats's disease; (6) *Toxocara canis*, q.v., p. 206.

Treatment:
1. Excision of the eye at the earliest possible moment, cutting the optic nerve as long as possible (this latter precaution should always be taken when dealing with any intra-ocular neoplasm).
2. Exenteration of the orbit if the growth has appeared outside the eye followed by widespread irradiation.
3. In cases of doubt decision should be given in favour of excising the eye, for a pseudogliomatous eye is always virtually blind. All such excised eyes should be sent to the pathologist for a report.
4. In no case should a child's eye be excised without the corroborative opinion of a colleague.
5. When an eye has been removed for retinoblastoma the most careful periodic watch should be kept on its fellow. If any sign of growth is detected in it, it is justifiable to attempt treatment with radioactive application to save the child from complete blindness. Stallard has reported encouraging results from this. This treatment should be reserved for metastatic cases or those where the only 'seeing' eye is involved. More recently, laser treatment has become a useful adjunct to radiotherapy or photocoagulation.

Chapter XVI

OPTICAL ANOMALIES OF THE EYE

The optics of these eyes.' SIR THOMAS BROWNE, from *Religio Medici*

ALL optical errors described in this section are those which prevent the exact focusing of images on the retina and all the symptoms to which these errors give rise are directly or indirectly due to this imperfect focus. A detailed account of the theory and practice of refraction would not only be out of place here, but it would fill a whole volume of equal size. It is intended merely to give a brief description of the commoner refractive errors and their treatment.

HYPERMETROPIA

Occurs when the rays of light entering the eye are brought to focus behind the retina, i.e. when virtually the eye is shorter than normal. This condition is physiological in childhood and since the eye grows with the rest of the body, the condition has a tendency to remedy itself. Occasionally hypermetropia may be pathological, e.g. the retina may be pushed forwards by a growth which has the effect of shortening the axial length of the eye. Axial hypermetropia is by far the commonest variety. Alteration of the refractive index of the lens, partial subluxation, etc., are far less common causes. Hypermetropia of 6 dioptres is the equivalent of 2 mm of shortening of the optic axis.

Symptoms: Vary with the age of the patient. In children and young persons there may be no symptoms at all, since their power of accommodation is such that they can without conscious eyestrain overcome the defect and bring the rays of light to focus on the retina. If the hypermetropia is considerable the effort of accommodation is also considerable and eyestrain or headaches will result. This is particularly noticed on close work. The strained feeling may cause blinking, lacrimation, and in neglected cases may lead to conjunctivitis or blepharitis. In children (especially if one eye is more hypermetropic than the other) convergent squint may result. In older patients the symptoms are twofold:
1. Blurring or mistiness of distance vision. Quite frequently 1 dioptre of hypermetropia may cause the distance vision to drop to 6/24 or less, whereas it may be 6/5 when corrected. This is especially true in patients who have passed the fifth decade of life.
2. Great difficulty may be caused by near work. The near focus recedes, small print appears blurred, headaches and eyestrain occur. In

short, presbyopic symptoms occur before the age at which presbyopia is normally noticed. It should be emphasized, however, that provided adequate glasses are worn constantly a presbyopic addition is very rarely required before the patient is 45.

Finally, it must be remembered that, as mentioned under glaucoma (q.v.), a hypermetropic eye is *ipso facto* predisposed to glaucoma.

Treatment:
1. The golden rule is: no symptoms, no glasses.
2. When symptoms occur, the appropriate glasses should be ordered but the hypermetropia must never be over-corrected.
3. Whether glasses should be worn constantly, or for near work only, depends upon the severity of the symptoms and the visual acuity. If the distance vision is markedly improved with glasses they should be worn constantly.
4. In the case of high hypermetropia glasses should always be ordered for constant wear.

MYOPIA

This is the converse of hypermetropia. In myopia the rays of light entering the eye are brought to focus in front of the retina, i.e. it is virtually a longer eye than normal. Increase in the axial length is the commonest cause of myopia, but it may also be due to alterations in the refractive index of the lens (especially in early cataract cases) and to abnormal curvature of one of the refractive surfaces of the eye, e.g. conical cornea, posterior lenticonus, etc.

Myopia is very rare in infancy but it often occurs in childhood and increases considerably during the years of growth. Once growth is over any marked increase in myopia is unusual. Any severe degree of myopia occurring during childhood or adolescence must be viewed with great concern since these cases are usually rapidly progressive and lead to partial-sightedness or even blindness later in life. This is the so-called 'malignant myopia'.

Examination: Fundus examination is occasionally difficult in myopia, especially by direct ophthalmoscopy. This difficulty largely disappears if the fundus is examined through the patient's own glasses. With the pupil dilated and the ophthalmoscopic lens system set at 'O', a good view can be obtained by this technique in almost every case.

Symptoms: In moderate myopia symptoms are usually visual only. The child cannot see the blackboard and the adult is unable to recognize people or to read the titles on the cinema screen. In cases of high myopia the vision may be bad indeed owing to the pathological changes mentioned below:

In some cases 'floating specks' are seen, and the eye may appear unduly large and prominent. Occasionally a squint appears which is usually divergent, convergent squint being exceptional in myopia. Lastly, it must be remembered that a myopic eye is predisposed to retinal detachment in just the same way as a hypermetropic one is to glaucoma.

Aetiology: Largely unproven, but the following theories are held:
1. Developmental weakness of the sclera, especially in the posterior part and often hereditary. It is commoner in women than men and some races (e.g., the Jewish and Japanese) are particularly liable to myopia. This weakness allows the eye to stretch because of the intra-ocular pressure. This theory is the most generally accepted one by modern ophthalmologists.
2. Excessive close work. This is hard to believe, since it frequently occurs in labourers and others who read little. Also, forbidding reading in moderate cases does not prevent myopia from increasing.
3. Abnormal convergence always present in myopia causes tension in the intra-ocular muscles, which, in turn, raises the intra-ocular pressure, hence causing an axial lengthening of the eye.

Pathology: Unlike hypermetropia, myopia causes a whole train of pathological intra-ocular changes. The commonest of these is the 'myopic crescent' seen on the temporal side of the disc. This is probably a congenital condition aggravated by some dragging on the optic disc due to the formation of a posterior staphyloma. This staphyloma is a bulge at the posterior pole of the eye which causes degeneration of and tears in the underlying choroid and retina. White spots or branching white streaks are visible in the region of the disc and macula, and areas of choroidal atrophy appear which coalesce in severe cases. Much of the retinal pigment disappears, with the result that the choroidal vessels are clearly seen. In addition to these fundus changes, degenerative changes also occur in the media, the vitreous becoming more fluid than normal and gross floaters being visible.

Prognosis: Broadly speaking, the younger the onset of myopia, the worse the prognosis, for it is an error which nearly always increases during growth. If, say, -2 or -3 dioptres of myopia are found in early childhood, in a comparatively few years this may increase to -12 or -14, and later in life the various changes described under pathology are likely to occur. Moderate myopia in adults is of good prognosis (except for the ever-present possibility of detachments of the retina), whereas high myopia is always to be regarded as serious.

Treatment:
1. Appropriate glasses should be ordered, but care must be taken to avoid any over-correction. Full correction is permissible in all except young children, where it is wise to under-correct by at least 1 dioptre.

2. Generally speaking, the practice of ordering a weaker correction for close work than is worn in the distance is to be deprecated in persons under 40 years of age. There is nothing to be gained by anticipating presbyopia and this practice discourages convergence.
3. In myopic children, glasses should be worn all day, otherwise their mental development suffers, since they become indifferent to the things around them just because they cannot see them clearly. This in its turn drives them to close things and they become 'bookworms'.
4. Reading matter must not be held too close to the eyes and excessive close work should be discouraged. Reading in poor illumination is not permissible. In the case of schoolchildren with progressive myopia, reading need not be forbidden for this would irretrievably ruin all their future prospects, but it is wise to forbid excessive non-essential or extraneous reading.
5. Operative treatment (the removal of the lens) is sometimes undertaken for high myopia and occasionally good results are seen. This procedure is, however, fraught with danger since a myopic eye is an unhealthy one. If operation is undertaken it should be needling, and the only suitable cases are patients under 30 years of age with a myopia exceeding -12 dioptres. It also presupposes a healthy fundus.

PRESBYOPIA

'Why has not man a microscopic eye?' ALEXANDER POPE, from *An Essay on Man*

A physiological condition due to the gradual sclerosis of the lens that occurs with the passage of years. In order to understand this, brief mention must be made of the physiology of accommodation.

Physiology of Accommodation: Rays of light entering the eye must be brought to a focus on the retina if the image is to be seen clearly. Hence, some sort of mechanism is necessary that can adjust the focus from distance to near objects and vice versa. Theoretically, there are two possible methods by which this difficulty can be overcome: (1) If the distance between the lens and the retina could be varied, i.e. if the eye was telescopic, it would be able to focus near and distance objects in the same way that most cameras do. This mechanism is, in fact, present in the eyes of certain fishes. (2) If the lens could alter its radius of curvature and become sometimes more and sometimes less convex, this would have the same effect. This is, in fact, the method in use in the eye and the process of varying the lens convexity is known as 'accommodation'. Briefly, this is as follows:

The substance of the lens is of plastic material and is capable of adjusting its shape to that of the capsule which encloses it. This capsule is elastic and its shape depends upon the amount of tension exercised upon it by the ciliary muscle. When the muscle contracts, the suspensory ligament slackens, tension is taken off the capsule and the plastic lens fills the 'slack' by becoming more convex. This enables the lens to bring near objects to focus on the retina. The plasticity of the lens decreases with age owing to sclerosis of its substance, hence it loses its power of accommodating itself to the tension imposed by the capsule. When a patient reaches 65–70 years of age this progressive sclerosis is complete, hence those living to very advanced years need no further correction than they required at 70 years of age.

Presbyopia is not to be regarded as a defect which commences at the age of 45 and goes on progressing until old age. It commences very much earlier, indeed it is present throughout life, but does not manifest itself until the near point of the eye has receded so that it makes reading uncomfortable. In emmetropia this occurs at about the age of 45, earlier in hypermetropia, and in myopia it may be much later.

Treatment is by correcting lenses.

1. Accurate refraction for distance must be carried out whether the patient requires to wear distance glasses or not; and
2. To the distance correction add convex lenses as follows:

Age	Correction
45	+0·75
47	+1·25
50	+1·50
55	+2·00
60	+2·50
65	+2·75
70	+3·00

    The above is an approximate guide only and not a rule-of-thumb correction. Some patients will accept less than these figures and this should be encouraged whenever possible because the smaller the reading correction, the greater the depth of focus. Rarely should +3·00 be exceeded and +3·50 should be regarded as the absolute maximum in normal cases. Occasionally in patients with a low visual acuity due to such pathological conditions as macular degeneration, lens opacities, etc., higher corrections can be prescribed. These are seldom satisfactory, for printed matter has to be held unpleasantly close to the eyes due to the short focal length of the powerful correcting lenses.

3. If a patient's work is held at a greater distance from his eyes than normal reading, e.g. compositors, artists, musicians, carpenters,

etc., then the above correction will be too strong. For such occupations a correction of about 1 dioptre less should be ordered.
4. Other occupations involve work at a closer distance than normal, e.g. ophthalmic operations, watchmaking, fine needlework, engraving, etc. A strong presbyopic correction in these cases will interfere with convergence and will cause great discomfort. Occupational glasses of this type should consist of the appropriate presbyopic correction incorporating prisms (base in) to make convergence possible.

MULTIFOCAL LENSES

At this stage the value of multifocal lenses should be considered. Bifocal lenses have been commonplace for decades and with them a presbyope who has to wear glasses constantly has the great advantage of being able to see in the distance and near objects without having to change his glasses. They have, however, one drawback which begins to be obvious during the fifth decade of life onwards: When the reading segment requires an addition of $+1\cdot50$ or more, the depth of focus for reading is reduced so that when a $+3\cdot0$ addition is reached there is only a focus of 10–13 cm where small print is really clear. With such a reading correction it is quite impossible to see anything clearly that is 60–90 cm away. There are, of course, a lot of patients whose occupation involves such intermediate reading, e.g. clergy who read from a desk or stall, teachers who walk round their class inspecting pupils' work, etc. Such cannot see intermediate distances with their reading correction and if they have a special pair of weak glasses with a long focus these glasses are unsuitable for small print, threading needles, etc. The best answer for these patients is a multifocal lens. Three varieties are obtainable:

Trifocals: In prescribing these the required distance correction is ordered with the presbyopic addition according to age. The intermediate lens is normally half the reading addition, e.g. a patient of 65 wears a $+2\cdot0$ correction for distance in each eye. He requires a $+2\cdot5$ addition for close work. Therefore his intermediate requirement for arm's length work is $+1\cdot25$ (half the reading addition). Trifocals should then give him perfect sight for distance, reading and intermediate work. If the patient is used to bifocals he should have no trouble in coping with trifocals.

Varilux Lenses: This type of lens gives clear vision for distance, near and intermediate vision without a 'jump' in focusing. The lens power is graduated optically so that when the patient lifts his head and looks through the lowest part of the lens he gets the maximum near vision and the focal length recedes as he looks higher up the lens. In theory this sounds ideal but it does involve adjusting the tilt of the head to get the correct focus and in practice many patients prefer trifocals.

Zeiss Gradal Lenses: These are similar in principle to Varilux lenses but they are considered better optically and have technical advantages. At the time of writing they are just being introduced so it is not yet possible to assess their advantages over the Varilux type.

The following points should be borne in mind when considering any form of multifocal lens:
1. They are not required unless a patient has to wear glasses constantly.
2. The necessity for them does not normally arise until the patient is 50 years of age or upwards. Younger presbyopes have sufficient accommodation left to manage with bifocals.
3. The patient must have a modicum of intelligence and be willing to persevere sufficiently to overcome the initial difficulty. The type of person who 'cannot get on with bifocals' will never cope with any form of multifocal lenses.

Given these three conditions and an occupation where good intermediate sight is required, these lenses are ideal.

TINTED LENSES

'I am too much i' the sun.' W. SHAKESPEARE, *Hamlet*

Sensitivity to light varies with the individual and there is no recognized norm hence no test can be applied to determine whether or not darkened glasses should be ordered. If the patient is genuinely sensitive to sunlight to the extent of causing discomfort, lacrimation, screwing-up eyes, etc. nothing but good can come from ordering tinted lenses. These will not only relieve the symptoms but will give the patient increased visibility by cutting out glare. There are many different tinted lenses manufactured under different names but a choice can nearly always be made from one of the following:

1. **Polaroid:** These are of very lightweight plastic material which is easily scratched. They are only available as plano hence cannot be made up to an individual prescription; thus they are of no use to anyone who wears glasses constantly. They can be bought as 'clip-ons' but these are seldom satisfactory.
2. **Crookes Lenses:** These are excellent and a large range is available which can be dispensed to any prescription. Of those available nearly all needs can be met from one of the following:
   a. CROOKES ALPHA OR A 2: This tint is a very light one suitable for patients who work indoors under bright conditions, i.e. fluorescent lighting, on drawing boards, etc. They are of no use as sun glasses.
   b. CROOKES B 1: This is the best tint for outdoor use in this climate. It cuts out ultraviolet light, improves visibility without impairing colour relationships, e.g. geraniums still look red and lobelias blue!

c. CROOKES B 2: This is the tint of choice when a really dark sun glass is required for cruising, mountaineering above the snow line, skiing, etc. but they are too dark for normal wear in this country.
3. **Zeiss Umbramatic:** In recent years these have come to the fore. They are photosensitive and increase in darkness with the intensity of the light. They can be dispensed to any prescription and are an excellent proposition. However, even in dull light a very slight tint remains.

In the absence of eye disease darkened glasses (except for Umbramatic, Crookes Alpha or A 2) should not be worn indoors nor on dull days. If young people suddenly take to wearing dark glasses indoors it might be an indication that they are taking some drug which has a mydriatic sideeffect. Lastly, sun glasses should never be worn when motoring at night to eliminate dazzle from oncoming headlights. This is extremely dangerous as such glasses cut out all visibility except for the small area illuminated by headlights, thus making pedestrians, cyclists, etc., quite invisible if they are at the side of the road.

ASTIGMATISM
'They see not all clear.' HENRY VAUGHAN, from *The Night*

This is another troublesome form of refractive error which differs from hypermetropia and myopia. The corneal radius of curvature (in the case of *corneal* astigmatism) varies in two meridians at right-angles to each other. This is a complicated condition involving the optical considerations of Sturm's conoid, but very simply it may be explained as follows: instead of the cornea resembling a section of a perfect sphere, it is shaped like the back of a spoon, i.e. more curved in one meridian than the other. It, therefore, follows that objects reflected by the meridian of greater curvature are brought to a focus before those reflected by the meridian of lesser curvature. This will result in indistinct vision in some meridians, for instance the letter L may be seen as I, if its horizontal part is not seen clearly, X may resemble K, B is mistaken for the letter R, etc. Astigmatism may be congenital or acquired. If the latter, it is usually due to trauma, such as operation for cataract, etc., or it may even be due to pressure from a cyst. Irregular astigmatism occurs as the result of corneal nebulae, but as this cannot be corrected optically it will not be discussed here.

Signs and Symptoms: Astigmatism is very liable to cause eyestrain, especially on accommodation, owing to the effort of the eye to bring to a focus a circle of least diffusion upon the macula. Print appears blurred, and the eyes tire easily. On the distance test a characteristic of astigmatism is the inability to read the lower lines of test type completely. If a patient reads say, 6/6 *partly*, or 6/9 *partly*, this is very suggestive of astigmatism. The plain hypermetrope or myope can usually read the whole line correctly even though they cannot read very far down the chart. Often comparatively slight astigmatism causes more eyestrain and discomfort than severe astigmatism, but the severe cases result in much more blurring of vision.

Treatment: May not be required unless there is complaint of eyestrain or unless the patient is conscious of indistinct vision. The only treatment possible is the ordering of correcting lenses after a careful refraction. Slight cases, and especially those that are not associated with any hypermetropic error, need wear glasses for close work only, but those of a moderate or marked degree will be more comfortable if they wear them all the time.

APHAKIA

Denotes an eye from which the lens has been removed and has in consequence some very serious optical drawbacks. Assuming that the eye was previously emmetropic, the aphakic eye is a highly hypermetropic one to the extent of about +10 dioptres, and if the cataract was removed by corneal section (as opposed to needling) the resulting scarring produces usually about 2 dioptres of astigmatism in addition. Furthermore, the retinal image in aphakia is one-third larger than that in the normal eye. Hence if one eye is normal and the other aphakic, the two images cannot be fused and binocular vision, except with the aid of a contact lens (q.v.) or intra-ocular implant, is impossible. Lastly the aphakic eye has lost its power of accommodation so any patient, however young, will be dependent upon two pairs of glasses and not infrequently a third pair may be necessary for intermediate distances if any of their work or hobbies is done at arm's length. It will thus be seen that aphakia has many serious drawbacks which must be carefully considered before advising extraction. There is no doubt whatever that 6/12 or even 6/18 vision with accommodation is preferable in some cases to a vision of 6/9 or even 6/6 without it.

ANISOMETROPIA

'It is vain to treat them as if they were equal.' JAMES ANTHONY FROUDE, from *Party Politics*

Indicates a big difference in the refractive state between the two eyes. Minor differences are almost the rule, but when a large difference is present, vision is usually uniocular and there is sometimes amblyopia and divergence in these cases.

Treatment:
1. If one eye is emmetropic it is questionable whether glasses should be ordered even though a correcting lens improves the sight of the anisometropic eye. Each case of this type has to be dealt with on its own merits and a hard-and-fast rule cannot be made.
2. In no case should the difference in power of the lenses between the two eyes exceed 4 dioptres, otherwise the disparity in sizes of retinal images may make fusion impossible.

3. Occasionally a compromise can be effected to diminish the difference in strength between the two lenses, i.e. over-correcting the one eye and under-correcting the other. The golden rule in this difficult problem of prescribing for anisometropia is this: order whatever is most comfortable to the patient whether this is theoretically correct or not.
4. As in the case of aphakia, contact lenses can overcome anisometropia, but not all cases are suitable for them, and of those that are suitable not all will tolerate them.

Chapter XVII
ANOMALIES OF OCULAR MOVEMENTS

'My eyeballs roll.' ALEXANDER POPE, from *Eloisa to Abelard*

ALL eye movements are carried out by synchronized action of the six extra-ocular muscles which are attached to the globe. In addition to these muscles, the levator, though not inserted into the globe, is functionally associated with the superior rectus, and thus should be reckoned as an indirect oculomotor muscle.

Anatomy and Physiology: All these extra-ocular muscles, including the levator, and with the single exception of the inferior oblique, arise from the annulus of Zinn at the apex of the orbit encircling the optic nerve and the lower half of the superior orbital fissure.

INTERNAL RECTUS: The thickest and best developed of all the extrinsic muscles. It runs parallel to the inner orbital wall and is inserted into the sclera 6 mm from the limbus. Its action is adduction and it is the muscle of convergence. Its nerve supply is from the third nerve.

EXTERNAL RECTUS: The antagonist of the internal rectus; it runs close to the lateral orbital wall to its scleral insertion 7 mm from the limbus. It is an abductor and is supplied by the sixth nerve.

SUPERIOR RECTUS: Runs close to the orbital roof and immediately below the levator muscle and is inserted 8 mm from the limbus. It is the chief elevator of the eye, but it also helps in adduction and inward torsion of the globe. It is supplied by the third nerve.

INFERIOR RECTUS: Passes forwards and outwards similarly to the superior rectus but below the globe. It is inserted 6·5 mm from the limbus. Its primary function is to turn the eye downwards (depressor), and in this respect antagonizes the superior rectus. Its subsidiary functions are adduction and outward torsion of the globe. It is also supplied by the third nerve.

SUPERIOR OBLIQUE: Runs in the angle formed by the junction of the roof and the inner wall of the orbit. Just short of the orbital margin its tendon passes through a cartilaginous pulley, the trochlea. By means of this pulley it turns backwards and outwards under the superior rectus, to be inserted into the sclera and the upper and outer aspect of the globe. Its principal action is to depress the eye, especially when adducted, and in a subsidiary capacity it helps in abduction and intorsion. It is supplied by the fourth nerve.

ANOMALIES OF OCULAR MOVEMENTS

INFERIOR OBLIQUE: Is unique among the extra-ocular muscles in that it does not arise from the apex of the orbit. Instead, it takes its origin from the anteromedial aspect of the orbital floor, thence passing outwards and backwards beneath the inferior rectus to be attached to the postero-lateral surface of the globe. Its chief action is that of elevating the eye, especially when adducted. It also helps in abduction and extorsion. Its nerve supply is from the third nerve.

THE LEVATOR: Runs immediately below the orbital roof and above the superior rectus muscle, to which it is adherent by its fascial sheath. It is attached by a tendinous expansion to the skin of the upper lid, the tarsal plate, the conjunctiva at the upper fornix, and by means of two 'horns' to the medial and lateral orbital margins. Its action is to elevate the upper lid and the conjunctival fornix. The superior rectus and the levator are closely associated both anatomically and physiologically, hence on looking upwards not only is the eye elevated but the upper lid and the conjunctival fornix also. Its nerve supply is from the third nerve.

It will be appreciated from a study of the action of the extrinsic muscles that every movement of the eye from the primary position (i.e. looking directly forwards) is a complicated synkinesis in which certain groups of muscles contract and their antagonists not merely relax but are actively inhibited. To make it more complicated, this synkinesis is a binocular one, hence adduction of one eye is synchronous with abduction of the other, yet in convergence this binocular synkinesis is inhibited and both eyes turn inwards. If it is remembered that underaction of any one of the twelve muscles involved in all ocular movements may produce diplopia, it must be admitted that the perfect functioning of these muscles represents a degree of precision which the most exacting engineer will admire.

BINOCULAR VISION AND DIPLOPIA

'Double the vision my eyes do see, and double vision is always with me.' WILLIAM BLAKE, from *To Thomas Butts*

It will be convenient at this stage to consider binocular vision and diplopia because in the event of dysfunction of any one of the twelve extrinsic muscles just described, binocular single vision ceases and diplopia occurs. Normally when the eyes are directed at any object it is seen clearly although the two retinal images are not identical, a fact that can be appreciated by the obvious 'shift' noticed when looking at the relative positions of two distant objects and covering each eye alternately. These two slightly different images are fused psychologically and it is this fusion that gives the impression of depth, solidity, etc., and makes possible accurate visual judgement and co-ordination between eyes and hand which play such a large part in giving man supremacy in the animal creation. This function of binocular vision depends, of course, on frontally placed eyes. In animals with laterally placed eyes binocular vision is either impossible or the binocular field is very small.

Supposing that one extra-ocular muscle ceases to function, the result will be that the visual axes will cease to be parallel in all directions of gaze and the image ceases to fall on the fovea, hence a second and blurred image is seen. This is binocular diplopia and is an extremely distressing and unpleasant symptom causing gross upset of visual judgement and sometimes leading to vertigo and even vomiting. It is, of course, immediately relieved by blacking out either eye.

Unilateral diplopia and polyopia also occur, but these are of totally different causation. They are indicative of a lesion in the refractive media of the eye such as lens opacities, dislocated lens, etc., which diffuses the entering rays of light to different points on the retina. This is, of course, relieved by covering the affected eye only.

Anomalies of ocular movements can be stated under three headings: Paralytic strabismus; Concomitant strabismus; Nystagmus.

PARALYTIC STRABISMUS

As its name implies, paralytic strabismus is due to paralysis or paresis of one or more of the extra-ocular muscles and may be due to any lesion between the cerebral nuclei and the muscles themselves.

Signs and Symptoms:
1. Diplopia on looking in the direction of action of the affected muscle.
2. Limitation of movement of the eye when looking in the direction of action of the affected muscle.
3. The secondary deviation is greater than the primary. The patient in most cases fixes an object with the unaffected eye, and the paralysed eye will show a deviation. This is the primary deviation. If he is made to fix with the affected eye, the deviation of the other eye is the secondary deviation.

    This sign is of considerable importance, for it is diagnostic of paralytic strabismus, especially if it is of recent onset. Where there is extra-ocular muscle paralysis of long standing, secondary muscle changes may take place and the deviation comes to resemble concomitant strabismus, where the two deviations are equal.
4. Vertigo and occasionally vomiting.
5. Inaccurate visual judgement, e.g. past pointing.
6. In an unconscious effort to avoid the symptoms the patient may sometimes adopt a compensatory head posture in order to get the two eyes into some position where fusion of the two images is possible. A head tilt which dates from infancy due to ocular imbalance is known as ocular torticollis. It always compensates for a restriction of a vertically acting muscle.

ANOMALIES OF OCULAR MOVEMENTS

Examples of Paralytic Strabismus: Either one muscle or a group of muscles may be affected according to the aetiology:

IN A COMPLETE THIRD-NERVE PARALYSIS ptosis always occurs which masks the diplopia, and in addition to the external muscles the pupil is also paralysed and does not react to light or accommodation.

IN EXTERNAL RECTUS PARALYSIS the affected eye may be limited in movement outwards beyond the midline. There may be a manifest convergent squint in the primary position of gaze and the head may be turned towards the affected side.

IN SUPERIOR OBLIQUE PARALYSIS there is limitation of movement in the direction of the main action of the affected muscle, i.e. looking downwards and inwards. The chin may be depressed and the head turned. There may also be a definite head tilt to overcome the torsion and reduce the vertical deviation. Negotiating stairs causes much discomfort and giddiness: the patient closes one eye and holds on to the banisters.

Aetiology: The lesion may be anywhere between the nucleus and the muscle and may be due to any of the following causes:

1. CONGENITAL: Absence or mal-insertion of muscle.
2. TRAUMATIC: Either affecting the muscle sheath or the nerve nucleus. A haemorrhage is commonly responsible.
3. INFLAMMATORY: Syphilis, meningitis, encephalitis, etc.
4. TOXIC CONDITIONS: Alcohol, lead poisoning, diphtheria, etc.
5. VASCULAR CONDITIONS: Cerebral haemorrhages or thromboses.
6. SYMPTOMATIC: Indicating general disease such as multiple sclerosis, myasthenia gravis, progressive muscular atrophy, etc.
7. NEOPLASTIC: Pressure from tumour.

It must be emphasized that vascular lesions are responsible for most cases seen. Formerly acquired syphilis was the chief aetiological factor.

Prognosis: Depends upon the aetiological factor. A surprising number of cases tend to improve with the lapse of time and with appropriate treatment.

Treatment: Depends mainly upon the aetiological factor causing the squint, but the following remarks apply to almost all cases:

1. Diplopia calls for either covering the affected eye with a shade or wearing the appropriate prismatic correction.
2. Orthoptic treatment sometimes helps by exercising partially paralysed muscles.
3. Occasionally in old-standing cases operative interference is indicated, e.g. tenotomy or recession of an antagonistic muscle or a tendon transplantation, such as planting a strip of superior and inferior rectus tendon into a paralysed external rectus.

Ocular Torticollis occasionally occurs as a compensatory mechanism for avoiding diplopia and is particularly common in cases of congenital mal-insertions or absence of muscles. In contradistinction from real torticollis the following points should be noted:
1. The sternomastoid muscle is supple and not contracted.
2. The head tilt is less obvious.
3. Paresis of one or more of the vertically acting extra-ocular muscles clinches the diagnosis.

CONCOMITANT STRABISMUS

In concomitant strabismus the neuromuscular mechanism of the eye is intact, the squint being of a functional nature, in this respect differing from a paralytic strabismus which has just been described. A squint of this type may be convergent or divergent and it may be monocular or alternating. It may also be constant or occasional.

In investigating any case of suspected squint the first thing to be done is to be sure whether or not a squint exists. Quite a number are more apparent than real, e.g. epicanthus may stimulate strabismus by hiding part of the sclerotic at the inner canthus. Myopia or hypermetropia may deceive some, since the visual axis of the eye (the line from the fovea to the fixation point) differs from the optic axis (the line on which the cornea, lens and centre of rotation are situated). Proof of the existence of a squint depends upon the *cover test*. The oculist holds a pen 0·7–0·9 m (2½–3 ft) from the patient's eyes. A card is held to cover the patient's right eye, hence he is fixing the pen with his left. If the left eye moves outwards to take up fixation, a manifest left divergent squint is present. If it moves inwards, a manifest convergent squint is demonstrated. If, however, the left eye was already fixing the pen, the cover test should be repeated covering the other (left) eye. If the right eye then moves to take up fixation then a right convergent or divergent squint exists, according to the direction in which the eye moves. No such movement by either eye means that no squint is present. The cover test should then be repeated for distance fixation since a squint may be present when a patient looks into the distance even though none may be found on near fixation. Patients with alternating squint can fix with either eye voluntarily, but none the less they usually have a 'favourite' eye and most of the time they fixate with this. This is a useful fact to bear in mind when considering cosmetic operation. If in doubt as to which eye to straighten it is best to avoid choosing the 'favourite' one.

Amblyopia: In paralytic strabismus it has been mentioned that the most distressing symptom is diplopia. It may well be asked 'How is it that this scarcely ever occurs in concomitant strabismus?' The theory is that in order to avoid diplopia the image of one eye is unconsciously suppressed by a process of cerebral inhibition, just as one image is voluntarily suppressed by students when they use a monocular microscope keeping both eyes open. This psychological suppression is often made easier by a refractive error which is usually greater in the 'suppressed' eye. This suppression if continued for a prolonged time leads ultimately to amblyopia. This theory has some weak points: it does not explain the absence of diplopia in cases of alternating squint where the vision of each eye is often normal and the refraction emmetropic. From the foregoing it is obvious that patients with concomitant squints never have full binocular vision and are usually amblyopic to a greater or lesser extent. The amblyopia may be slight, with a vision of possibly 6/12; or it may be extreme, when hand movements only may be visible. The degree of amblyopia depends upon two factors: (1) The age of onset —the earlier the onset the greater the degree of amblyopia. (2) The length of time that has elapsed before treatment. It should be particularly remembered that a case of squint cannot be treated too early. To tell the mother of a squinting child of, say, a year old that 'He may grow out of it' is about as true as telling the mother of a child that needs circumcision that the foreskin may shrink with growth! Every case of squint needs investigation and the younger the patient the more urgent the need if severe amblyopia is to be avoided. Ten months old is not too young to refract and if need be to order glasses.

Eccentric Fixation: When amblyopia is long-standing the fixation may move in the squinting eye from the fovea, i.e. central fixations, to any area between the fovea and the optic disc. Where this condition exists it is called 'eccentric fixation'.

It is diagnosed by investigation using a visuscope. A circle of light has a black star in its centre; when the light is directed on to the retina the star should settle on the fovea if central fixation is present. If the star falls on any other retinal area between the fovea and the optic disc then eccentric fixation is present. The fixation may be unsteady, wandering, or fixed in nature. The fixing eye should be examined first and then the squinting eye.

Signs, Symptoms and Aetiology: Convergent squint is nearly always a disease of childhood and often of infancy. No attention need be paid to transient squints which occur before 6 months of age and are due to lack of development of the fusion faculty. Again, care must be taken in infants to differentiate between a squint and normal accommodation. If a rattle is dangled about 0·3 m (1 ft) from an infant's nose it will naturally converge to fix it, and this should not be confused with a squint. If, however, the infant turns one eye when fixing a distant object then a pathological condition of squint exists. Sometimes a convergent squint is not only in the horizontal plane; often an upward deviation may be present. This may be due to inferior oblique overaction or to a congenital mal-insertion or other

muscular abnormality which is discoverable only at operation. The angle of squint may vary from 5° (less than this is not clinically discoverable) to 45° or 50°. In a surprising number of cases a squint manifests itself soon after a febrile illness or a psychological upset. It is frequently associated with hypermetropia, a fact which may be explained by the accommodation convergence reflex. Hypermetropes have to accommodate strongly to focus near things and this strong accommodation causes a correspondingly strong convergence. There is, therefore, a very fine dividing line between the excessive convergence of hypermetropia and the onset of concomitant strabismus. The convergence of accommodation in hypermetropes cannot be the only cause of the squint for the following reasons:
   1. Hypermetropia may exist without a squint.
   2. Occasionally squints are present in myopes.
   3. Sometimes hypermetropes have a divergent squint.
   4. Convergent squint may occur in emmetropic eyes.
The visual acuity in a squinting eye is (except in alternators) usually but not always subnormal to a greater or lesser extent. This is discussed under AMBLYOPIA (q.v.).

Treatment: There are four general lines of treatment in any case of squint: optical, occlusive, orthoptic, operative. Any or all of these may be required in a given case, so a brief general view of each of these will first be given before discussing their application to any particular case.

OPTICAL: In every case an accurate refraction must be carried out. In children under 6 years of age, which represents the vast majority of squint cases, Ung. atropine 1 per cent should be used twice daily for 3 days before the day of the test, but *not* on the actual day of testing. In older children instillation of mydrilate 1 per cent or other quick-acting mydriatic is permissible. In young children the normal full correction should be ordered, but as they grow older, and particularly if the squint disappears when they wear glasses, the correction may be reduced. In every case an annual review should be made. In all cases where the squint is associated with a refractive error, correction with appropriate glasses as early as possible may well check the deviation completely and avoid such complications as amblyopia.

OCCLUSIVE: A careful periodic watch should be made in every case of squint and in particular the visual acuity of each eye should be recorded if the patient is old enough. If, as is usually the case, amblyopia is present, an attempt should be made to improve the visual acuity of the squinting eye by occluding it or its fellow, known as the inverse and direct method of occlusion. The following methods of occlusion can be used which should be carried out under orthoptic supervision:

ANOMALIES OF OCULAR MOVEMENTS 181

1. Complete occlusion with Elastoplast or non-allergic adhesive patches are excellent for a severe case and is the only satisfactory way of securing *total* occlusion. It is rather irksome and demands cooperation on the part of both the patient and its mother. The Elastoplast has to be changed daily.
2. Second best to the Elastoplast method is an extension occlusion made to fit the patient's glasses from zinc oxide plaster.
3. Sellotape occlusion consists simply of sticking Sellotape on one lens of the patient's glasses.
4. Atropine occlusion is suitable only for very young children and consists in the nightly application of Ung. atropine 1 per cent to the sound eye in order to paralyse its power of accommodation.

In any severe case of amblyopia a thorough course of occlusion is necessary before orthoptic treatment can be undertaken. It is surprising how the visual acuity in an amblyopic eye can improve with occlusion. It is not uncommon for a vision of 1/60 to improve to 6/24 or more on total occlusion for a month or two.

ORTHOPTIC: When the visual acuity in the amblyopic eye has improved sufficiently, orthoptic exercises should be ordered. These are carried out by trained personnel with special instruments and aim at producing simultaneous macular perception, fusion and stereopsis. It must be admitted that orthoptic treatment is in some cases prolonged and requires cooperation on the part of the child and its parent. It is, however, in many cases abundantly worth while, for it may be rewarded by a *real* cure (with fusion and stereoscopic vision) as opposed to a *cosmetic* cure (a straight but amblyopic eye). This treatment may involve weekly attendances for many months and unless the parents are prepared to go through with it thoroughly no good will result. It must also be admitted that a number of cases, even of those who are cooperative, fail to respond to treatment. Not every case responds to binocular training, but every suitable case should at least be given the opportunity. Cases of eccentric fixation (*see* p. 179) do not respond to usual orthoptic methods and call for the use of pleoptics.

In some cases of convergent squint where excessive convergence persists in near fixation only, in spite of wearing glasses, the temporary use of a miotic may help to control this convergence excess. When combined with binocular exercises and occasionally the use of bifocal glasses the result is often good, but in other cases surgery is required to obtain a lasting and good result.

PLEOPTICS: Professor Bargerter of St. Gall is the pioneer in the treatment of eccentric fixation by these methods. He devised the pleoptophore by means of which the eccentrically fixing part of the retina is dazzled and the use of the fovea is stimulated. In St. Gall and elsewhere the treatment is residential with sessions of pleoptics alternating with school lessons. A 75 per cent or more cure is claimed. Pleoptics are used at Moorfields Hospital after the normal period of occlusion. The simplest method is by 'Haidinger's brushes' which cause polarized light to fall on the macula. The child sees a rotating brush, the centre of which is only visible at the fovea. Looking at this centre encourages normal fixation. This method is suitable for home treatment. The projectorscope is a more elaborate and expensive instrument aimed at attaining the same result by dazzling the extrafoveal area of the retina. A 70 per cent cure rate can be obtained by this method. After the eccentric fixation is cured by pleoptics, normal orthoptic training is necessary to establish binocular vision and fusion.

Finally, it must be remembered that pleoptic treatment is arduous and the instruments expensive. It would be unnecessary if more squints were diagnosed really early and treated before eccentric fixation is established. Prevention is better (and easier!) than cure.

OPERATIVE: Is indicated in the following conditions:
1. When a squint persists in spite of wearing the correct glasses and having orthoptic treatment, operation is required to help the patient obtain binocular single vision. In such cases operation should not be long delayed otherwise amblyopia will result. Orthoptic treatment in suitable cases may be indicated before and after the operation.
2. In squints of long duration where a good cosmetic result is required, even though there is no chance of regaining binocular vision. A late age is no contraindication in this group.

Operation should be undertaken early—probably 4–6 years is the best age, but if the squint is a severe one or if there is reason to believe that amblyopia may occur, operation can be undertaken much earlier. In other words, surgical treatment should not be regarded as a last resort and for cosmetic reasons only, long after everything else has failed and all hopes of binocular vision are lost. It is rather a useful accessory before or after other treatment.

ROUTINE PROCEDURE IN A CASE OF SQUINT: Having discussed the four main lines of treatment in general terms we will endeavour to answer the question 'What is the routine treatment when a child of, say, 5 years of age is brought for advice about a concomitant squint?'
1. Vision should be recorded if possible by means of the 'E' test.
2. The patient should be refracted under atropine and the necessary correction ordered.

ANOMALIES OF OCULAR MOVEMENTS

3. The glasses should be worn all the day without any exception at all.
4. If the squint persists occlusion is advised. If there is any suggestion or definite confirmation of eccentric fixation, then the squinting eye is occluded (inverse method). The fixation is checked on the visuscope at each visit and when the fixation is almost central then the cover is changed to the good eye. If the vision in the squinting eye is less than 6/60 total Elastoplast occlusion is necessary.
5. Orthoptic training should be undertaken as soon as the vision in the amblyopic eye is normal or has reached its limit of improvement.
6. Operation is necessary if the eye still turns in spite of giving the above measures a trial of, say, 6 months. Operation should not be postponed indefinitely or permanent amblyopia will result.
7. After operation, a further course of orthoptic exercises should be tried and the patient should be refracted 12 months after the first test.

Alternating Squint: As mentioned earlier in the chapter, alternating squint is a condition where the patient can fix an object with either eye at will, but the eye that is not fixing turns inwards (or occasionally outwards). These cases frequently have no refractive error, hence glasses will not help them and the visual acuity is usually normal in each eye, but binocular vision does not develop. Orthoptic treatment is useless in alternating squint.

TREATMENT:
1. Refraction and correction of any obvious error even if only for the sake of improving the visual acuity.
2. Cosmetic operation, if necessary, is the only other possible form of treatment. In a true alternator it is immaterial which eye is chosen for operation but the author prefers to operate on the eye that fixes least. Most patients with alternating squint have a marked preference for one eye. An attempt should be made to ascertain their 'favourite' or 'best' eye and operation should be performed on the other one.

Divergent Squint: There are the following varieties:
1. PRIMARY CONCOMITANT DIVERGENT SQUINT: This may be either constant or intermittent and may be due to:
   a. Divergence excess: the deviation being more marked on distance fixation. Good vision is usually present in each eye and emmetropia or a negligible refractive error is the rule in such cases. Good convergence on near vision is generally found.
   b. Convergence weakness, when the deviation is more marked on near vision.

2. SECONDARY DIVERGENCE: This results from myopia, anisometropia, serious visual impairment following eye disease or injury, and similar causes which affect one eye only, the vision in the other being good.
3. CONSECUTIVE DIVERGENCE following surgical treatment of convergent squint.

Divergence is really a natural tendency for the eye to find its most comfortable position and is comparable to the position of semi-flexion which is assumed by an injured limb. A divergent squint is a worse cosmetic disability than a convergent one since it gives the patient a 'crafty' appearance.

TREATMENT:
1. Refraction and correction of any error is the first treatment. It must be remembered that in cases of anisometropia only rarely should there be a difference of more than 4 dioptres between the two correcting lenses.
2. A course of fusion training and convergence exercises by the orthoptist may help.
3. If the above measures fail operation is indicated.
4. Cosmetic operation is not usually very successful in blind or badly amblyopic eyes. If the divergent eye lacks the stimulus of vision, recurrence is probable. Operation is, however, well worth trying.

Latent Squint: It has previously been mentioned that binocular vision depends upon the fusion of two slightly dissimilar retinal images. It sometimes happens that this binocular vision is maintained with difficulty owing to the tendency of one muscle or group of muscles to overact or underact, thus making it easy for the eye to deviate. This tendency to deviation is really a condition of latent squint and is termed 'heterophoria'. The phorias are named as follows:

Tendency to lateral deviation (commonest) = exophoria.
Tendency to medial deviation = esophoria.
Tendency to upward deviation = hyperphoria.
Tendency to downward deviation = hypophoria.

When the muscle balance of the two eyes is normal without any tendency to deviation the eyes are said to be in a state of orthophoria.

The unconscious efforts of a heterophoric eye to maintain fusion may cause a considerable amount of eyestrain and sometimes the effort is too much for the individual and the latent squint becomes an actual one for a short time. This is especially liable to occur with physical exhaustion and after too much close work, such as studying for examinations, etc. Print may look blurred, supra-orbital headaches may occur, and occasionally, when the eye 'wanders', diplopia may result. Generally speaking, cases of exophoria are rarely troublesome. One of the authors has approximately 22° of exophoria and is entirely without symptoms and perfectly comfortable with his normal hypermetropic correction. Esophoria also rarely gives symptoms, but even a slight case of vertical phoria may give much trouble. This difference in symptoms between the horizontal and vertical phorias is capable of a simple explanation: every time the eyes accommodate, synergistic action between the internal and external recti takes place and these movements are part and parcel of our daily life. Horizontal phorias therefore involve no synergistic muscular disturbance. At the most it is an exaggeration of a normal movement. A vertical phoria, however, involves the complex and unusual adjustment between the superior rectus and inferior oblique on the one hand and the inferior rectus and superior oblique on the other. Experience with the RAF during the war has proved that vertical phorias have occasionally been the sole cause of bad landings.

DIAGNOSIS is made by cover test, the Maddox wing test for new fixation and the Maddox rod test for distance fixation. In latent squint it is the eye under cover that must be observed for movement when the cover is removed. A latent squint is revealed if the eye moves to take up fixation and regain binocular single vision. For the Maddox rod test a spotlight is illuminated (or a candle will serve the purpose) at 6 m distance from the patient. A 5-cylinder Maddox rod is placed in the trial frame before one eye with its cylinders horizontal, the other eye remaining uncovered. If the patient is orthophoric a red line appears to go vertically through the light. In the event of exophoria or esophoria the line appears to be to one side of the light. The Maddox rods are then rotated until they lie vertically. Here, in the orthophoric eye the red line appears horizontally through the spotlight, but if hyperphoria or hypophoria is present it appears to be above or below. The amount of phoria is measured by the strength of prism that has to be placed before the Maddox rod to make the line come exactly through the light. This test should also be carried out for near vision at 35 cm.

Many other ingenious tests have been devised to measure muscle imbalance. Space prevents a description of them, but the most commonly used is the Maddox wing test. Less often used are the Bishop Harman's diaphragm and the 'red–green' test.

TREATMENT:
1. Generally speaking in the case of all phorias the rule is 'no symptoms, no treatment'. If discovered in the course of a routine examination it is probably wiser not to mention it to the patient. Any refractive error must, of course, be corrected.
2. Optical treatment consists in incorporating the correct prism with whatever spherical or cylindrical correction may be necessary. The prismatic strength necessary for correction should be

divided between the two eyes. If there is a hyperphoria of, say, 4°, instead of placing a 4° prism before one eye, a 2° prism is placed base up before one eye and a similar prism base down before the other. It is important to remember that prisms are very rarely indicated except for the vertical phorias. If they are ordered for the horizontal ones many patients find them difficult to tolerate. Never order a prism if it can be avoided.
3. Orthoptic exercises play a definite part in the treatment of horizontal phorias and these should always be tried before prisms.
4. If prisms are considered unavoidable they should be first tried out in a 'clip-on' frame, worn over the patient's own glasses. This tests the patient's tolerance and shows whether the symptoms are relieved, thus enabling the surgeon to judge whether it is wise to incorporate them irrevocably in the glasses.
5. Very rarely operative correction may be necessary.

CONVERGENCE INSUFFICIENCY is a form of latent squint and is seen in patients of any age, although young adults are most commonly affected. It may be associated with any refractive error and it not infrequently occurs in patients who are emmetropic. The symptoms are difficulty and discomfort on close work which cease as soon as the patient discards the near work and looks into the distance. Examination with the Maddox wing test reveals exophoria for near objects, whereas in the distance the patient may be orthophoric or even esophoric. These cases of insufficiency of convergence often respond well to orthoptic treatment or even to home exercises. A simple and beneficial exercise is as follows: The patient holds a pencil vertically in his right hand at eye level. He fixes this with both eyes and gradually brings it nearer until his near point is reached and he can no longer see it binocularly. This exercise is repeated 20–30 times a day and after doing it five times consecutively the patient should look into the distance to relax his accommodation. It is of utmost importance in these cases to ascertain that any refractive error is adequately corrected.

NYSTAGMUS

A curious anomaly of ocular movement consisting of quick involuntary oscillations of the eyeball nearly always in the horizontal direction. Both eyes are usually affected, but it may be more pronounced in one than the other. Genuine unilateral nystagmus is exceedingly rare. Nystagmus can be seen at its best by watching passengers in a railway train looking through the windows at objects, e.g. telegraph wires, as they cross their field of vision. This form of nystagmus is, of course, physiological and is due to the eye's efforts to keep a fast-moving object focused on the macula. Nystagmus also occurs in a variety of pathological conditions such as disease of the labyrinth or cerebellum, multiple sclerosis, etc

ANOMALIES OF OCULAR MOVEMENTS

Ophthalmologists, however, are chiefly concerned with two varieties: (1) Congenital nystagmus; (2) Miner's nystagmus.

Congenital Nystagmus: Better described as infantile, for it is very doubtful whether infants are born with it. It usually commences in an infant of a few months old and is often due to some ocular defect interfering with vision, e.g. congenital cataract, corneal opacities, albinism, colobomata, marked refractive errors, etc. Defects of this type seriously impair vision and deprive the infant of the power of fixation. The oscillating movements are due to the efforts on the part of the child to fix some object he wishes to see. They represent the unconscious 'groping' of the maculae.

TREATMENT: Entirely that of the causative condition. The condition of congenital nystagmus is inconsistent with good vision even in those cases without obvious disease and when the refractive error is adequately corrected. The visual acuity is rarely better than 6/18 in either eye, and in those cases associated with ocular disease the vision is proportionately worse.

Miner's Nystagmus: Affects only those miners who have worked underground for a long period and it is claimed that it does not occur in miners who work in well-illuminated pits. The patient looks ill and worried and is emotionally unstable. He complains of insomnia, headaches, giddiness, photophobia, sweating, palpitation and tremors. The nystagmus is of a very fine type and is often difficult to elicit. If suspected but not seen, the following technique may reveal it: ask the patient to stand with his arms above his head and to bend to touch his toes six times in rapid succession. The eyes should be examined immediately after this. If the nystagmus is not found then the patient should be told to look upwards and examination carried out with the head in this position.

AETIOLOGY:
1. Poor illumination as mentioned.
2. The strain of continual looking upwards when working at the coal-face.
3. Uncorrected refractive errors.

PROGNOSIS AND TREATMENT: The disease is primarily a psychogenic one and like all neuroses a prolonged time off work is indicated. Of first importance in treatment is attention to insomnia. Unless this is done the patient may be haggard and ill for months. Furthermore, the miner when recovered must permanently leave off underground work and must be given a surface job. If this is done, the prognosis is very good; if not, recurrences are almost certain.

Chapter XVIII

SUBJECTIVE VISUAL DISTURBANCES

Sundry visual symptoms of an entirely subjective nature occur in a variety of both organic and functional diseases. These symptoms can be classified approximately under two headings: (1) Disturbances of visual sensations, and (2) Disturbances of visual fields.

DISTURBANCES OF VISUAL SENSATIONS
'Is this a dagger that I see before me?' W. SHAKESPEARE, *Macbeth*

These are nearly always due to functional conditions and almost any type of visual sensation may be affected. Disorders of visual acuity are seen in cases of amaurosis and amblyopia. Colour sensation anomalies occur in colour-blindness. Disturbances of form sense are seen in hallucinations, and more complex disturbances of visual sensations are found in such psychological conditions as word-blindness, etc.

Amaurosis Fugax: The name given to transitory blindness. It occurs in uraemia, pregnancy toxaemia and nephritis. The onset is sudden and it is usually bilateral, and may last anything from a few seconds to 48 hours. No fundus changes are present (except occasionally in albuminuric retinopathy) and the pupil reaction is normal, thus proving that the lower centres are not involved. It is probably due to toxins affecting the cells of the cerebral cortex. Amaurosis may occur in non-toxic conditions due to temporary cerebral ischaemia e.g. migraine, arteriosclerosis and Raynaud's disease, and in healthy patients it is not uncommonly caused by vasomotor changes as in sudden rising from the lying to the standing position. Also it may result from a temporary circulatory failure.

Amblyopia: Partial loss of sight has already been discussed (*see* p. 178). When due to old-standing squint or refractive errors it is always unilateral. Unilateral amblyopia (very rarely bilateral) also occurs in retrobulbar neuritis. Bilateral amblyopia occurs in various toxic conditions such as tobacco or quinine poisoning. Hysterical amblyopia is a definite clinical entity which occurs usually in young, intelligent, highly strung patients and is more common in women than in men. It may affect one or both eyes, and has one very constant clinical feature: the fields show spiral contraction. At the commencement of taking the field it is reasonably full, but contracts down with each movement of the arc until finally it is only a few degrees off the fixation point. These fields when plotted on the chart resemble a cochlea or concentric spiral. Many cases are difficult to diagnose and the greatest care must be taken to exclude organic disease. In hysterical amblyopia the pupils are always normal in reaction—a most helpful factor in diagnosis which differentiates it from many organic lesions.

Migraine: Causes very unpleasant visual disturbances. It nearly always occurs in intelligent highly strung patients who lead a 'high-pressure' type of life, and especially where tension is associated with overwork and worry. An attack is usually ushered in by a feeling of general malaise accompanied by a shimmering central scotoma which greatly diminishes visual acuity, but rarely involves the fixation point. Bright geometrical patterns resembling fortifications are seen in different spectral colours and homonymous hemianopia may be present. These visual phenomena are followed by a splitting headache, usually one-sided and associated with nausea or vomiting. Occasionally migraine sufferers develop a temporary partial paresis of the third nerve of the affected side instead of the usual scotoma. With repeated attacks the paresis may become more marked and in rare cases permanent (ophthalmoplegic migraine). Some observers believe that these cases are not genuine migraines but are symptomatic of organic intra-cranial trouble, e.g. aneurysm of the circle of Willis.

TREATMENT: This is within the province of the physician rather than the ophthalmologist, and the first essential step is to persuade the patient to reform his life and to avoid unnecessary tension and stress. Any refractive error should be corrected in order to relieve the patient of possible additional strain.

Colour-blindness:[1] True colour-blindness is always congenital and usually only partial. Complete colour-blindness, where all colours appear to be greys of a varying degree of brightness, is exceptionally rare, so much so that some authorities doubt its existence. In those few cases where it is said to occur it is associated with congenital nystagmus or other abnormalities. Partial colour-blindness, the condition with which the oculist is chiefly concerned, occurs in all degrees of severity. It is an inherited characteristic occurring most commonly in males. The commonest and most clinically important is red-green blindness, which is a serious defect in such occupations as aviation, navigation, railway employment, etc. Colour-blindness occurs in three forms:

PROTANOPES, where the red spectrum limit is shortened and reds appear less bright than normal. In these patients the red sensation is lacking.

---

[1] N.B. The student is at this stage advised to refresh his memory as to Young–Helmholtz's, Hering's and Hartridge's theories of colour vision. In past years lively discussions by supporters of these theories have taken place at meetings of various learned societies. These have always generated more heat than light! No one theory explains all the facts.

DEUTERANOPES, where there is a similar defect for green. These patients are green blind.

TRITANOPES, where the defects affect yellow-blue vision. These cases are, however, exceedingly rare.

It should be clearly understood that all cases of colour-blindness do not fall into these clear-cut divisions. There are many anomalous cases in all these groups where defects are not complete. Cases of acquired colour-blindness are always much vaguer. They occur in such pathological conditions as partial optic atrophy, choroidal disease, tobacco amblyopia, etc. The area of colour confusion is usually in the form of a scotoma, or of a constriction of the fields to reds or greens, as is typically seen in tobacco amblyopia.

DIAGNOSIS:

1. ISHIHARA'S TEST: Consists of coloured printed plates, some of which may be read only by the colour-blind and others which can only be read by normal individuals. It is a good test, simple, inexpensive and reliable, but is rather too exacting. These charts when not in use should always be kept in a case in the dark as they are liable to fade.
2. EDRIDGE GREEN'S LANTERN TEST: Consists of a lantern which shows differing colours in varying-sized apertures. The diagnosis is made by the correctness or otherwise of the patient's replies. A good lantern is a somewhat expensive instrument, but is essential for tests for the armed services since Ishihara's charts are too exacting and good recruits with trivial colour anomalies have been refused.
3. WOOL-MATCHING TEST: As its name implies, this test consists in giving the patient some wool skeins and asking him to pick out from a large assortment of skeins the colours that match. This test takes longer and is less reliable than the other two. It is seldom used now.

Night-blindness:

'Thrice as blind as any noon-tide owl.' TENNYSON, *Idylls of the King—The Holy Grail*

Various diseases cause this symptom, especially retinitis pigmentosa and xerosis. It may occur temporarily owing to vitamin A deficiency in patients who have undergone severe privations or who for other reasons are victims of malnutrition.

Occasional night-blindness may be due to retinal fatigue, e.g. after exposure to bright sunlight without protective glasses. This type is due to natural fatigue resulting in deficiency of visual purple. It must be remembered that vitamin A is essential for the formation of visual purple, hence its administration is the first essential in the treatment of this symptom. Occasional night-blindness is feigned by malingerers.

Word-blindness: A congenital condition, the patient being brought to the oculist because of inability to read—a fact which the parents usually attribute to defective eyesight. In spite of normal visual acuity, absence of ocular disease and refractive error, the child is quite unable to read the simplest words. In other respects he may be normal and even above average in intelligence, oral work and often arithmetic being very good. These cases are of psychological origin and punishment can bring nothing but harmful results. Much patience in teaching with individual attention is the only possible treatment.

Malingering:

'There's none so blind as they that won't see.' JONATHAN SWIFT, *Polite Conversations*, Dialogue 3

Blindness or diminished visual acuity is feigned in certain conditions such as when attempting to avoid military service or some other unpleasant duty; or when hoping to obtain a pension or compensation payment if the 'blindness' can be attributed to an injury. Rarely is bilateral blindness feigned, for it is easily detected by careful watching. One of the authors (C. M.-D.) had a case of this type under his observation in hospital. The patient was endeavouring to substantiate a claim for a war pension. When examined he professed to see hand movements only and on leaving the consulting room he carefully groped for the door. Later the same evening he was seen by the Ward Sister (whom he thought to be off duty) playing a very skilful game of darts with some fellow patients! If deliberate malingering is suspected it is often worth requesting one's secretary to follow the patient for a few minutes after he has left the consulting room. More than once a 'blind' patient has been seen to hail and stop a bus and to mount it without the least hesitation or difficulty. Feigned unilateral blindness is harder to detect, but one or more of the undermentioned tests will nearly always reveal it:

1. A prism is placed before the 'good' eye and the patient is told to look at a spotlight at 6 m. If he sees two lights, malingering is obvious.
2. A high convex lens is placed before the 'good' eye, thus completely fogging its vision. If the test type is read, vision must be present in the 'blind' eye.
3. The F R I E N D test is useful. In this test the letters forming the word FRIEND are printed alternately in red and green. Red glass is placed before the 'good' eye and the patient is asked what he sees. If the whole word is read out the eye is not blind, for when looking through a red glass the green letters are invisible.

Great care should be taken before malingering is diagnosed, for it is a very serious accusation to make and real malingerers are very few and far between. Far more common is the exaggeration (not always deliberate) of symptoms, which is often due to psychological causes combined with the fear that insufficient notice is being taken of what to the patient is a serious and often a vital matter. Due allowances for such cases should always be made and they should not be accused of malingering.

Hallucinations: Are of two types:
1. PHOTOPSIAE or FLASHES OF LIGHT: These may be due to pressure on the eyeball, contusion, or local ocular disease, e.g. chronic glaucoma, precursory symptoms before retinal detachment, etc. They are due to local stimulation of the retinal end-organs. The scintillating scotoma of migraine which has already been discussed is of cortical origin, probably due to temporary anaemia following arterial spasm.
2. INTEGRATED HALLUCINATIONS of a complicated nature occur in a variety of conditions: Delirium due to high temperatures, delirium tremens, morphinism, mental disease, arteriosclerosis and senility. These are usually due to cortical stimulation by toxins, emboli, etc.

DISTURBANCES OF VISUAL FIELDS (*Fig.* 2)[1]

Numerous diseases of the central nervous system cause field change of differing types, hence perimetry is of fundamental importance in diagnosis. These changes nearly always take the form of hemianopia, of which the following varieties occur:

Homonymous Hemianopia (*Fig.* 3): Occurs when either the right or the left half of the binocular field is lost, e.g. in right homonymous hemianopia the nasal half of the left field and the temporal half of the right field is missing. The visual result is as though there was a vertical curtain dividing the field, everything on the left of the cornea being clearly seen, but no object on the right of it is visible. Homonymous hemianopia is the commonest form of field loss and may be due to a lesion anywhere between the occipital lobe and the chiasma. Sometimes patients may be unaware of the lesion because the fixation point is often spared. In other cases the right field defect may cause great difficulty in reading, whereas a patient with left homonymous hemianopia is unable to see his fork when sitting at the dining-table.

Bitemporal Hemianopia (*Fig.* 4): The loss of the temporal field of each eye. The classic field found in pituitary disease. It is caused by

---

[1] In order to grasp the significance of the visual field changes which will now be discussed the student is advised at this stage to revise his knowledge of the undermentioned fundamental anatomical details: (1) The visual paths from the retina to the cortex; (2) The chiasmal region, including the relations of the chiasma, pituitary gland, internal carotid arteries, sphenoidal sinuses, etc.

pressure on the chiasma which destroys the fibres from the nasal half of each retina. Bitemporal hemianopia may also result from basal meningitis, syphilis, sphenoidal disease and traumatic involvement of the chiasma.

Binasal Hemianopia: The nasal half of each field is missing. A great rarity, so rare that many doubt whether it has ever occurred. Its presence

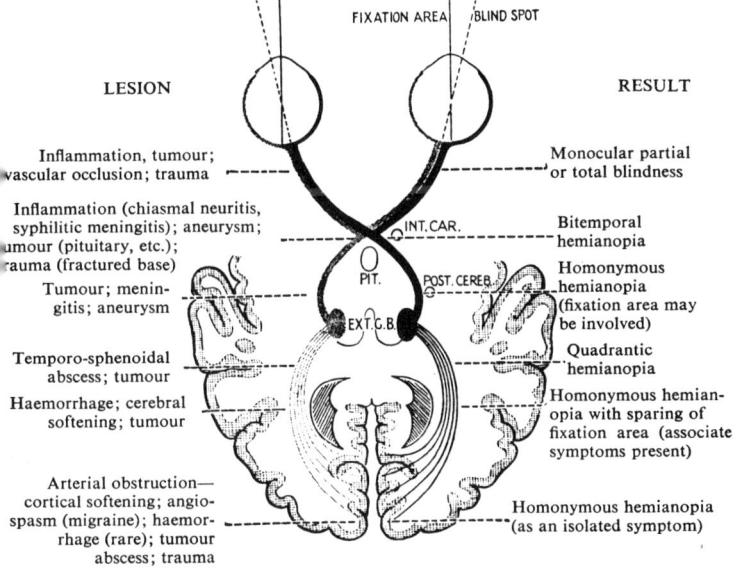

Fig. 2.—Course of visual fibres. On the left side are shown the common lesions in the various parts of the course of the fibres, on the right the results of the lesions. INT. CAR., Internal carotid artery; PIT., Pituitary body; POST. CEREB., Posterior cerebral artery; EXT. G. B., External geniculate bodies. (*Diagram constructed by Mr. A. McKie Reid.*)

must postulate two simultaneous lesions, one on each side of the chiasma. The only disease that could possibly fulfil these conditions would be atheroma of the two internal carotid arteries.

Altitudinal Hemianopia: Also very rare. In these cases the dividing line is horizontal. May be caused by pressure from a suprasellar tumour.

Quadrantic Hemianopia (*Fig.* 5): Rare. In this condition the corresponding quadrants of each field have been lost, e.g. the upper half of one

194 A SYNOPSIS OF OPHTHALMOLOGY

temporal and one nasal quadrant. May be due to lesions in the occipital cortex involving the calcarine fissure.

Other causes of field defects, e.g. glaucoma, pigmentary retinopathy, etc., will be found under their respective headings.

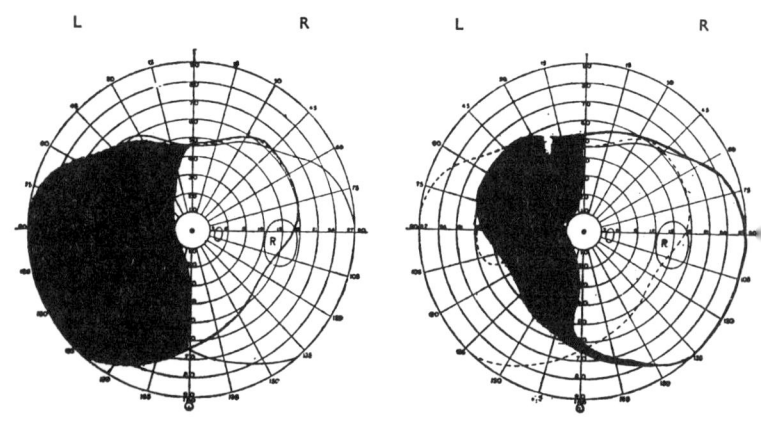

Fig. 3.—Left homonymous hemianopia. Tumour right parietal lobe; male, aged 50 years. Visual acuity: right and left eyes 6/6. Fixation area spared. Perimetry with white object 5 mm in diameter—daylight. (*Constructed by Mr. A. McKie Reid.*)

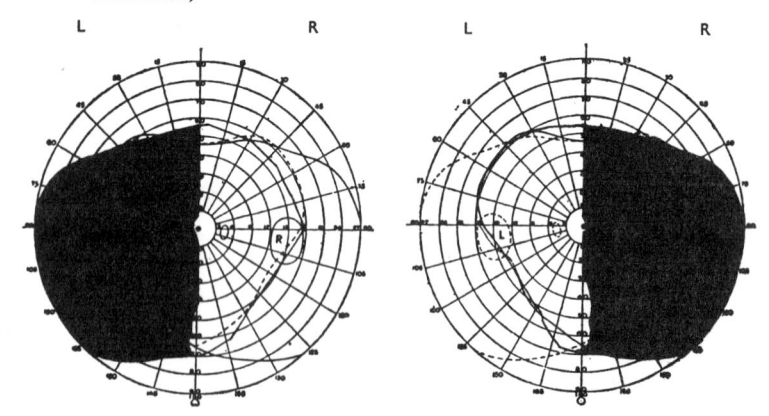

Fig. 4.—Bitemporal hemianopia. Pituitary tumour, six years' history. Visual acuity: right eye 6/9, left eye 6/24. Sparing of fixation area. Perimetry with 5-mm white object—daylight. (*Constructed by Mr. A. McKie Reid.*)

| L | R | L | R |

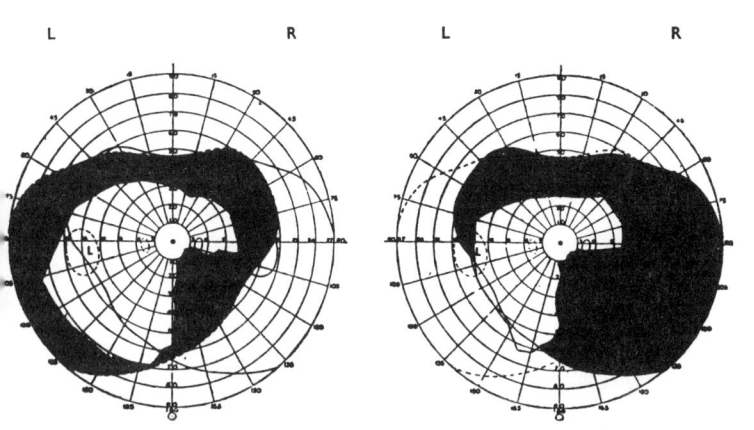

Fig. 5.—Quadrantic hemianopia. Subcortical haemorrhage left parietal lobe; male, aged 58 years. Accompanied by weakness of right arm and leg and blurring of speech. Visual acuity: right eye 6/12, left eye 6/9. Perimetry four months after onset with 2-mm white object—daylight. (*Constructed by Mr. A. McKie Reid.*)

Chapter XIX

OCULAR SIGNS OF GENERAL DISEASE

'A physician may be defined as: a medical man with diarrhoea of theory and constipation of action.' Source unknown

IT may be said without fear of contradiction that eye signs are so common in many general diseases that an ophthalmoscope has for years been an essential part of the armamentarium of every competent physician, and that no physical examination is really thorough or complete without an examination of the fundi. Reference has already been made under the appropriate headings to the eye signs found in such diseases as diabetes, nephritis, arteriosclerosis, etc. Apart from these it is in the field of diseases of the nervous system that ophthalmoscopic examination is so helpful. It will be apparent that lack of space prevents any description of the *general* signs and symptoms of the undermentioned diseases. These remarks deal solely with their *ocular* manifestations.

It must be understood that in some of the undermentioned diseases the ocular signs are complications and occasionally rare complications. Therefore, the ocular manifestations are occasionally absent altogether and seldom are more than one or two of the signs enumerated seen in any one case.

Acne Rosacea: Marked chronic conjunctivitis and keratitis frequently accompany this skin complaint.

Acrocephalosyndactyly: This is a congenital malformation with pointed skull and syndactyly. Ocular signs include exophthalmos, ophthalmoplegia and occasionally dislocated lenses.

Acromegaly: In this pituitary gland dysfunction, the most obvious sign is gigantism and a variety of eye signs can accompany it, including bitemporal hemianopia, squint, exophthalmos, papilloedema followed by optic atrophy. Occasionally the Foster Kennedy syndrome is seen (q.v.).

Albinism: This congenital complaint is obvious by the patient's almost white hair. The eye signs associated with it are photophobia, amblyopia, nystagmus, absence of pigment in iris and choroid and occasionally cataracts.

Amaurotic Familial Idiocy: *See* Tay–Sachs Disease (p. 213).

Anachrodactyly: This hereditary disease is manifested by long tapering fingers, 'double' joints and dolichocephaly. The eye signs can include buphthalmos, megalocornea, ptosis, unequal pupils, sometimes subluxation or coloboma of lens and coloboma of choroid.

Arterial Hypertension: *See* Arteriosclerotic Retinopathy (p. 77).

Autism: In this strange psychiatric disease of early childhood, some visual symptoms are often present. These include failure to comprehend simple pictures and a tendency to observe minor details without comprehending the scene as a whole. These children behave as though the peripheral fields were functioning but central vision lost, e.g. they tend to look sideways at objects and moving things attract attention while they fail to notice still objects. These symptoms may be present when there is no abnormality of refraction or fundus.

Banti's Disease (Splenic Anaemia): This disease sometimes shows gross congestion of retinal veins, with retinal haemorrhages and papilloedema.

Battered Baby Syndrome: Ocular damage in this syndrome is becoming increasingly common as indeed is the syndrome itself. It is difficult to diagnose as a really thorough ophthalmoscopic examination in any infant requires a general anaesthetic and a battered one is terrified at the slightest approach by anyone wearing a white coat and holding an instrument. In every suspected case two separate examinations are required:

1. A general external examination during which the surgeon should try to regain the baby's confidence in humanity by jangling a key-ring or showing a toy to interest the baby. While doing this he should note whether a squint is present, if ocular movements are normal, whether there is blood in the anterior chamber, the size, shape and reactions of the pupils.
2. After a mydriatic, an examination under anaesthetic should be made. The lens must be noted for possible subluxation, cataract, etc. The anterior chamber and vitreous must be looked at for haemorrhages and finally a careful search of the whole of the retina for haemorrhages, holes or detachments.

Any abnormality must be carefully noted and the prognosis should be guarded as haemorrhages at the time of trauma can lead on to retinal scarring or vitreous organization. It must also be remembered that intra-ocular haemorrhages can be associated with a subdural haematoma. If these unfortunate infants survive, many turn out to be mentally retarded, some have convulsions and others may be blind or partially sighted due to a developing optic atrophy which could not be diagnosed until a considerable lapse of time after the injury.

Blood Diseases: Retinal haemorrhages are seen in any form of blood disorder including pernicious anaemia, polycythaemia and in secondary anaemia from malignant disease. They are also common in the reticuloses such as leukaemia. In the purpuras and haemophilia, subconjunctival and orbital haemorrhages may be found in addition. Finally, it must be remembered that optic atrophy may be a late complication from prolonged and repeated haemorrhages from the uterus, bowel, etc.

Cerebral Abscess: Usually occurs in the temporal lobe as a complication of chronic middle-ear disease, but it may occur in any situation as a pyaemic infection from elsewhere, e.g. sinusitis, orbital cellulitis, etc. Forty per cent of cases show papilloedema, usually ipsilateral, associated with a partial third-nerve paralysis. When these signs are associated with a contralateral hemianopia, cerebral abscess is a likely diagnosis.

Cerebral Aneurysm: These occasionally cause papilloedema since they are space-taking intracranial lesions. Sometimes an aneurysm may burst when very acute cerebral symptoms occur: dizziness, headache, vomiting, followed by coma. Subarachnoid haemorrhage may occur also as the result of an aneurysm leaking into the subarachnoid space. This gives signs of acute meningeal irritation, subhyaloid retinal haemorrhages, vitreous haemorrhage and proptosis with varying ocular palsies. Blood is present in the cerebrospinal fluid. Cerebral aneurysm is rarely diagnosed by ocular signs before rupture, but if suspected they can frequently be demonstrated by angiograms (Mooney).

Cranial Arteritis: *See* Temporal Arteritis (p. 206).

Cytomegalic Inclusion Disease is a disease of infancy. It is a virus infection found in premature or underweight infants characterized by gastroenteritis, jaundice, splenic and hepatic enlargement, fever and anaemia, with a tendency to bleeding. Cerebral calcification is found on X-ray examination. Associated with these general signs are ocular manifestations which vary from membranous conjunctivitis with scleral ulceration to uveitis and acute choroiditis. Sometimes dacryocytitis is seen. Cytomegalic inclusions are found in the urine and in some severe cases in the intra-ocular fluid aspirated from the anterior chamber. Toxoplasmosis (which, it will be remembered, causes similar eye signs and cerebral calcification) is often associated with the virus that causes this disease. Diagnosis depends upon finding cells with inclusion bodies in the urine.

Diabetes: This causes a variety of eye signs. A frequent feature in diabetic eyes is the tendency to haemorrhages in different forms. This is especially noted during cataract or iridectomy operations. The following eye signs can be found:
1. Spontaneous hyphaema.
2. Rubeosis of iris (*see* p. 51).
3. Iritis.
4. Iridocyclitis.
5. Lenticular myopia.
6. Cataract.
7. Vitreous haemorrhages.

OCULAR SIGNS OF GENERAL DISEASE

8. Retinopathy, either of the exudative or haemorrhagic types. The latter often show micro-aneurysms.

Diphtheria can cause membranous conjunctivitis in the early stages of the disease, but it is sometimes forgotten that paralytic sequelae can also result: paralysis of accommodation and, more rarely, external rectus paralysis.

Encephalitis Lethargica: Diplopia or ptosis of sudden onset is one of the earliest symptoms of this disease. These ocular pareses are usually the only signs and their occurrence at the outset of a febrile illness should arouse the physician's suspicions.

Erysipelas of Face: This can cause abscess of lids, orbital cellulitis and by backward extension can lead to thrombosis of orbital veins and even of the cavernous sinus.

Erythema Multiforme Exudativum: An acute disease of the skin and mucous membranes with fever, arthritis, ulceration of the mouth, anus, etc. Occasionally there is a purulent conjunctivitis, keratitis leading to iridocyclitis. Sometimes vitreous abscess occurs.

Erythema Nodosum: This is characterized by dermatitis with general malaise and scattered tender red nodules. The eye signs include paresis of external muscles. Nodules can occur on the conjunctiva and sclera. Keratitis, iridocyclitis and possibly hypopyon occur.

Fabry's Disease: This is a sex-linked skin disease with tiny angiomata over the 'bathing trunks' area. It is often associated with nephritis or chronic vascular disease with fatal results in early adult life. The fundi show marked dilatation of vessels with aneurysms and the conjunctival vessels are also very dilated especially in the fornices.

Friedreich's Ataxia: This hereditary disease commences in early childhood and shows spinal sclerosis, ataxia, scoliosis and muscular paralysis. The eye signs found in this condition can include nystagmus, squint, ocular paresis usually of external rectus, and optic atrophy.

Glomerulonephritis: *See* Renal Retinopathy (p. 73).

Gonorrhoea: *See* Gonococcal Conjunctivitis (p. 10).

Gout: This is an inborn error of purine metabolism. The eye signs can include tophi in the lids, irritable conjunctivitis, episcleritis and scleritis.

Haemophilia and allied diseases. These are hereditary male diseases due to lack of coagulation factors in the blood. Exophthalmos due to orbital haemorrhages is sometimes seen as also are haemorrhages in the lids, conjunctivae, anterior chamber and retinae. Secondary optic atrophy due to pressure from orbital haematoma can occur.

Herpes Zoster: *See* Herpes Ophthalmicus (p. 37).

Hodgkin's Disease (Lymphadenoma): In this disease there is chronic progressive enlargement of lymphoid tissue with fever, anaemia, and wasting. Occasionally cystic orbital tumours are found causing exophthalmos. Iridocyclitis sometimes occurs.

Hyperadrenalism (Cushing's Syndrome): These patients are usually hypertensive, diabetic and suffering from osteoporosis. The eye signs are those of hypertensive retinopathy with papilloedema.

Hypertension: The ocular changes in this condition are described on p. 72. It is important to remember that it is often during a routine fundus examination that the presence of hypertension is first discovered.

Hyperthyroidism: In addition to the well-known medical textbook signs, i.e. Möbius, von Graefe, Stellwag and Dalrymple, this condition is complicated by chemosis, exophthalmic ophthalmoplegia and exposure keratitis.

Inborn Metabolic Errors produce eye signs as follows:

Alkaptonuria	Pigmentation of sclera and cornea
Amaurotic familial idiocy	Optic atrophy
Cystinosis	Crystals in cornea
Galactosaemia	Cataracts
Gargoylism	Corneal opacities
Myotica atrophica imperfecta	Cataracts
Osteogenesis imperfecta (or osteosclerosis)	Blue sclerotics

Intracranial Tumours: As in the case of abscesses, intracranial tumours give rise to eye signs as the result of pressure from their space-taking habits. The ocular signs are threefold: (1) Papilloedema; (2) Field changes; (3) Muscular paralyses. Since any part of the brain, pre-central, post-central, temporosphenoidal, subcortical, thalamic, cerebellar, pontine or ventricular regions, can be affected, it will be obvious that localization by eye signs alone is almost impossible. To make matters more confusing, by no means all cases of cerebral tumour develop these signs. Pontine lesions often occur without papilloedema and ocular paralyses are comparatively rare. Homonymous hemianopia when present is suggestive but by no means diagnostic of an occipital lobe lesion. The accurate localization of space-taking intracranial lesions is one of the many difficult and highly skilled tasks of the neurosurgeon.

Leprosy: The majority of lepers have one or more of the following eye complications: interstitial keratitis, nodules on eyelids, conjunctiva or sclera, iritis.

Leukaemia: Haemorrhages occur in the conjunctiva and vitreous. The retinae show gross venous congestion with scattered haemorrhages which have white centres. Subretinal haemorrhages sometimes occur, also exudates and papilloedema.

Lichen Planus: This is an inflammatory papular skin disease occurring in patches. Occasionally superficial punctate keratitis occurs and, more rarely, iridocyclitis and choroidoretinitis.

Lupus Erythematosus: Patients with this complaint usually have mild fever, leucopenia, enlargement of spleen, arthritis and nephritis in addition to skin eruptions. The condition can be complicated by iridocyclitis, retinal haemorrhages with exudates, perivasculitis, papilloedema and optic atrophy.

Malaria: Occasionally paralysis of any of the external ocular muscles occurs. Ptosis is not uncommon. Paralysis of accommodation, keratitis, iridocyclitis, retinal thrombosis and optic neuritis can also occur.

Measles: Mucopurulent conjunctivitis sometimes leading to corneal ulceration.

Meningitis: Apart from syphilitic basal meningitis, eye signs may occur in the following varieties:
   TUBERCULOUS MENINGITIS: Occasionally tubercles are visible in the choroid, but this is a late sign. Partial paralyses are common and conjugate deviation of the eyes may occur.
   CEREBROSPINAL MENINGITIS: One eye sign is said to be almost diagnostic of this disease—viz. widely opened eyes and infrequent blinking. If this is associated with papillitis, conjugate deviation of the eyes, a partial paralysis of the third or sixth nerves, together with symptoms of meningeal irritation, the diagnosis is certain.
   PURULENT MENINGITIS: May occur as a pyaemic manifestation. Its ocular signs are varying and unreliable except when the disease is complicated by abscess formation, etc.

Molluscum Contagiosum: This complaint is due to a virus of the poxvirus group. It shows scattered pedunculated nodules which can occur anywhere in the skin including the eyelids and even the cornea. It is spread by direct contact, towels, brushes, etc. Nodules should be incised, expressed and carbolized. Medication with sulphadiazine is said to help this condition.

Mongolism: These children usually have high refractive errors, epicanthus, nystagmus, iris hypoplasia, and sometimes endocrine punctate cataracts.

Multiple Sclerosis: Caused by demyelinating process affecting the medullary sheaths of the nerves while the axis cylinders escape. For this reason remissions are frequent and restoration of sight is possible. Nearly half the cases of multiple sclerosis have lesions in the visual paths. As has been mentioned, the typical sign in multiple sclerosis is retrobulbar neuritis, but higher lesions between the chiasma and the cortex may cause haemianopic changes. Recurrent attacks of retrobulbar neuritis are the rule, with a high degree of visual recovery when the attack has passed off. With each succeeding attack, however, the visual acuity is usually somewhat diminished. Permanent blindness is very rare, but partial optic atrophy is common. Ophthalmoscopic changes are usually absent unless the axis cylinders are attacked, when signs of optic atrophy may be present. Nystagmus is present in many cases and spinal myosis is occasionally seen. Transient ocular pareses occur if the lesions affect the nuclear region.

Mumps is a generalized virus infection; thus one would expect some structures in addition to the parotid glands to be involved. Almost every extra- and intra-ocular structure can be involved in exceptional cases. Occasionally the lacrimal glands are involved without necessarily the parotids. This causes considerable orbital pain and oedema with redness of the lids. Retrobulbar or optic neuritis is occasionally seen, but most cases improve spontaneously and normal vision is regained within 3 weeks. Transient pareses of the ocular muscles also occur. In rare cases, keratitis of very acute onset is seen. This is an early symptom accompanied by marked lacrimation and gross loss of vision. Fortunately, there is no corneal vascularization and the condition clears up in 2–3 weeks. Viral uveitis is occasionally seen.

Myasthenia Gravis: A disease of young people affecting various muscles and especially those concerned with swallowing, mastication and respiration. Great fatigue is present, but no muscular atrophy. One of the first signs is bilateral ptosis, slight in the mornings but increasing progressively as the day goes on and the patient becomes more tired. With this there is associated insufficiency of convergence due to weakness of the internal recti muscles, which causes difficulty in reading. The diagnosis of myasthenia gravis is clinched in a very simple manner: at a time when the ptosis is at its worst, 2 ml of neostigmine are injected intramuscularly. If myasthenia gravis is present a truly dramatic improvement in the ptosis (and incidentally in all the other affected muscles) occurs within a few minutes. A patient with almost complete bilateral ptosis is able to open the eyes with ease. The improvement is, of course, only temporary.

Myxoedema: The eyelids show marked oedema and alopecia. There is deficiency of tear secretion with a troublesome dry keratoconjunctivitis. Occasionally cataracts occur.

Nasal Sinusitis: By reason of its proximity to the nasal cavities the orbital tissues can become infected in nasal diseases and this infection can lead to orbital cellulitis, a condition which seldom, if ever, requires incision and exploration. It usually responds rapidly to antibiotic treatment. Proptosis without acute orbital infection is also frequently seen in chronic cases.

Neuromyelitis Optica or Devic's Disease: This disease causes bilateral optic neuritis with attacks of amaurosis. It is of sudden onset with pain on ocular movements. During the amaurotic stage, the pupils are dilated and non-reacting. Generally speaking, complete recovery can be expected.

Ophthalmoplegia: Although by no means necessarily due to syphilis, it will be convenient to discuss this important eye sign here. Ophthalmoplegia may be total or partial. In the former case, all the external and internal muscles are involved. Partial ophthalmoplegia is termed 'internal' or 'external' according to the situation of the paralysed muscles. The condition may be of sudden or gradual onset and may be unilateral or bilateral. Non-syphilitic cases may be due to a toxin or infection, e.g. lead, ptomaine, diphtheria, etc. Ophthalmoplegia can also occur in migraine (*see* p. 189). Exophthalmic ophthalmoplegia (q.v.) has already been described and is of a totally different pathology. Lastly, ophthalmoplegia can occur as a rare hereditary disease.

Paget's Disease: The characteristic changes are in the skull. A generalized arteriosclerosis is present which shows itself in the retinae. Angeoid streaks and central choroidal sclerosis are not uncommon. Occasionally brown-coloured opacities appear in the cornea. Exophthalmos and optic atrophy may be present.

Pemphigus: This skin complaint is characterized by bullae and itching spots which tend to become pigmented. Oedema of the lids frequently occurs, also xerosis of conjunctivae choroiditis.

Pertussis: Orbital and conjunctival haemorrhages can occur and in rare cases haemorrhages are seen in the anterior chamber, vitreous, or retina. Very occasionally ocular paresis occurs.

Pink Disease affects young children. It is characterized by peripheral vascular phenomena with erythema and polyneuritis. The eye signs include severe photophobia, excessive lacrimation and gross conjunctivitis.

Polyarteritis Nodosa: This widespread and severe disease can involve numerous tissues of the body. It is due to lesions in the smaller arteries. Hemianopia and ocular palsies can occur, also oedema of the lids and conjunctiva, choroiditis, iridocyclitis, haemorrhages into the anterior chamber vitreous. Embolism of the central artery sometimes complicates the picture, leading to optic atrophy.

Polycythaemia Rubra Vera: This disease shows gross increase in blood viscosity with enlargement of the spleen. Conjunctival chemosis with haemorrhages is often seen. Congested irides assume a dark red colour. There is gross retinal venous congestion with haemorrhages.

Purpura Haemorrhagica: Haemorrhages occur in the lids, conjunctiva, anterior chamber and retina.

Relapsing Fever: This is a spirochaetal infection which shows numerous eye signs including muscular paralysis, oedema of the lids, cellulitis of the orbit, exophthalmos, retinopathy, papilloedema and optic atrophy.

Rheumatic Fever: Eye signs are uncommon, but episcleritis and iridocyclitis have been observed.

Rheumatoid Arthritis: Eye symptoms are common in this condition. It is one of the recognized causes of chronic conjunctivitis. Choroiditis, iridocyclitis, hypopyon sometimes occur. Sjögren's syndrome (q.v.) is not infrequent.

Rubella: Ocular damage to the fetus includes abnormalities of the globe such as anophthalmos, microphthalmos, buphthalmos, etc. Corneal opacities sometimes result. Congenital cataracts are frequent; optic atrophy and occasionally glaucoma are seen.

Rubeola (Measles): Severe conjunctivitis with photophobia is common. Occasionally orbital cellulitis, corneal ulceration with perforation may occur. In the worst cases, panophthalmitis can occur.

Sarcoidosis (*see* p. 58).

Schilder's Disease: A demyelinating process occurring in infants which affects scattered areas throughout the brain, commencing in the occipital lobes. It causes blindness of cortical origin, but with normal fundi and reacting pupils. The disease leads to deafness, convulsions and imbecility, and is invariably fatal. The oculist should remember this possibility whenever confronted with a blind infant without ophthalmoscopic signs. Very late in the disease optic atrophy may set in if the demyelinating process has affected the axis cylinders.

Scleroderma: This is a chronic disease with atrophy of the skin and subcutaneous tissues and gross dermal thickening. These cases frequently show keratitis with ulceration, iridocyclitis and sometimes secondary cataract.

Subarachnoid Haemorrhage: This trouble, which seems to be increasing in recent years, shows a number of ocular signs including orbital pain, diplopia, ophthalmoplegia and ptosis. Preretinal or subhyaloid haemorrhages are seen, also vitreous haemorrhages and optic oedema.

Subdural Haematoma: The eye signs in this traumatic condition include homonymous hemianopia, unilateral facial palsy, ipsilateral mydriasis, retinal haemorrhages and papilloedema.

Syndactyly: This genetic skeletal disorder shows a number of congenital ophthalmic abnormalities, including aniridia and microphthalmos.

Syphilis: The disease *par excellence* for eye manifestations. Mention has already been made of keratitis, iritis and choroidoretinitis due to this disease, but there are three other eye signs that deserve special mention:

1. THE ARGYLL ROBERTSON PUPIL, which is diagnostic of cerebral syphilis, shows 'spinal myosis', unequal and irregular pupils, but no synechiae. The characteristic of the Argyll Robertson pupil is that it reacts normally to accommodation but not to light. This condition is usually bilateral.

    It must be carefully distinguished from *Adies's myotonic pupil*, the pathology of which is unknown but syphilis plays no part in it. In this condition the pupil fails to react to light and reacts so slowly to accommodation that it is often hard to observe. It occurs

OCULAR SIGNS OF GENERAL DISEASE 205

in healthy young people, is usually unilateral and is associated with diminished or absent tendon reflex. The myotonic pupil is usually larger than normal.

As a general medical examination invariably includes a careful examination of the pupils, the appended table gives details of abnormal pupillary reactions:

NAME	PUPILLARY ABNORMALITIES AND OTHER EYE SIGNS	PATHOLOGY OR OTHER CHARACTERISTICS
ADIES'S MYOTONIC PUPIL	May react to light. Very slight reaction to accommodation. Often unilateral	Absent or diminished tendon reflexes
ARGYLL ROBERTSON PUPIL	Unequal pupils. No reaction to light. Normal reaction to accommodation. Invariably bilateral	Absent knee-jerks and other signs of cerebral syphilis
HORNER'S SYNDROME	Unilateral myosis. Normal pupil reactions. Unilateral slight enophthalmos. Narrowing of palpebral fissure	Paralysis of cervical sympathetic
WERNICKE'S HEMIANOPIC PUPIL[1]	Unilateral brisk reaction when half of the retina is illuminated by a tiny spot of light from the slit-lamp. When the other half is illuminated, the reaction is feeble	Lesion of the optic tract

[1] N.B. Wernicke's sign is difficult to elicit and is not wholly reliable. It is, however, necessary to know it for examination purposes.

2. PRIMARY OPTIC ATROPHY: Very frequent in cerebral syphilis, and especially in tabes. It usually occurs in the fourth or fifth decade of life before ataxic symptoms supervene. The only symptom is the progressive failure of vision culminating in total blindness, which usually occurs within 3 or 4 years of the onset of symptoms. Primary optic atrophy is usually bilateral, but one eye is affected before its fellow. The signs are pallor of the optic disc and increasing peripheral constriction of the visual fields.

   PATHOLOGY: This disease starts as a peripheral degeneration in the bulbar end of the optic nerve, and it is on account of this that the peripheral field is lost before the central one, the reverse of what occurs in multiple sclerosis, etc. It is not possible to make any estimate of the patient's vision by the appearance of the discs.

3. OCULAR PARALYSIS: Varies from a paresis of one muscle to a total ophthalmoplegia and occurs in any form of cerebral syphilis.

The occurrence of a sudden ptosis or unexplained diplopia should always put the physician on his guard against syphilis. These pareses may or may not clear up on treatment. The prognosis is best when they occur early in the disease before ataxic symptoms are apparent.

Syringomyelia: A rare disease due to an irregular enlargement of the lumen of the spinal cord with consequent pressure symptoms. Since the cervical region is commonly affected, unequal dilatation of the pupils may be present owing to involvement of spinal dilator fibres. Nystagmus is present in this condition, occasionally ophthalmoplegia and optic atrophy. Sometimes Horner's syndrome is seen: small pupil, narrowing of the palpebral fissure and enophthalmos —the famous triad which he described as early as 1869.

Temporal Arteritis: Giant-cell arteritis is a chronic granulomatous inflammation which may affect any artery but is most commonly found in the carotid area and especially in its temporal branches. In classic cases there is pain and swelling over the thickened superficial temporal vessels which have become pulseless and occluded. The inflammatory process involves the ophthalmic, retinal and ciliary vessels, leading to sudden loss of vision. There are some cases when sudden loss of vision is the first symptom without central retinal arterial occlusion. Occasionally the presenting symptom is a sudden attack of transient diplopia. This with temporal pain in an elderly patient is very suggestive. The fundi may look normal except for slight swelling of the optic discs. In these cases occlusion has occurred farther back in the ophthalmic artery. In all cases there is marked increase in the sedimentation rate and a biopsy of the temporal artery will confirm the diagnosis. Large doses of steroid therapy are indicated over a prolonged time, in order to prevent involvement of the second eye. The actual cause of blindness in these cases is ischaemia of the optic nerve.

Tetanus: The eye signs include mydriasis, blepharospasm, paralysis of the accommodation and ophthalmoplegia.

Thromboangiitis Obliterans (Buerger's Disease): This disease gives rise to acute inflammation of the arteries and veins of the extremities often with superficial phlebitis. Associated with it may be vitreous haemorrhages, retinal vasculitis, retinopathy and thromboses.

Toxaemia of Pregnancy: *See* Hypertensive Retinopathy (p. 72).

Toxocara Infestation: Infestation by toxocara larvae is uncommon but leads to serious trouble. The patient is usually in the 4–6-year age group and the presenting symptoms may be either squint, a white pupil or defective vision. The trouble is uni-ocular and there is a history of close contact with puppies. The toxocara is a nematode parasite frequently found in dogs (and less often in cats) during their first 6 months of life. The signs and symptoms of infestation are fever, eosinophilia, lung infiltration, enlarged liver and encephalopathy. Eye involvement is late in the disease, long after the general symptoms have disappeared. The trouble is spread through ova excreted by the puppy and reaching the child's intestinal tract by contaminated fingers. In the gut the ova develop into larvae which never reach the adult worm stage but bore their way through the gut, entering a blood vessel and thus becoming scattered throughout the body, The eye is entered through the central retinal artery.

OCULAR LESIONS: The larvae may lodge in the retina or migrate through the retina to the ora and the anterior chamber causing any of the following lesions:

VITREOUS: An inflammatory retrolental membrane may be formed leading to chronic endophthalmitis.

ORA: Circumscribed lesions extend into the vitreous and the occurrence of hypopyon is not uncommon.

INTRARETINAL: White circumscribed granulomata occur usually at the posterior pole. Sometimes these granulomata extend into the surrounding retina.

PATHOLOGY: Greer found that these granulomata consisted of scar tissue with embedded larva and infiltration by eosinophils, lymphocytes, plasma and giant cells. The mass causes puckering of the adjacent retina which may protrude into the vitreous. It is firmly adherent to Bruch's membrane.

DIAGNOSIS: This is not easy. There is a superficial resemblance to Coats's disease and retinoblastoma. At present there is no easy or reliable immunological test. Research is being undertaken at the present time and future developments are probable.

Toxoplasmosis: This is an infection of the body by a protozoan parasite which enters and multiplies in any cell which possesses a nucleus. Multiplication continues until the cell is full of toxoplasms when it bursts, scattering new toxoplasms throughout adjacent tissues. In the less virulent forms, however, in spite of the cell bursting, a membrane forms around the toxoplasms which become encapsulated cysts. A toxoplasmic infection is difficult to detect, the most certain method being the inoculation of specimens of living tissue into mice. Apart from this, their demonstration is very uncertain, the method used being a complement-fixation and dye test. Toxoplasmosis is more widespread than was previously imagined and is found in numerous animals and birds in addition to human beings. The chief ophthalmic sign in every case is choroidoretinitis.

The mode of infestation is not certain. Greer considers that inhaling dust infected with dried excrement of cats, dogs, chickens, rabbits, cattle or pigs is one source. Also it can come through the alimentary canal by contaminated food, uncooked meat, etc. In 1972, workers in Seattle found that raw or undercooked meat was the chief source but there was a markedly higher incidence rate of the disease amongst those who kept cats, while keeping dogs did not show this high incidence rate. They therefore consider that contamination by cats' excreta to be a fairly common cause. Usually the infection is harmless and remains undetected. In congenital infection (the most important from the ophthalmic point of view) the mother becomes infected later on in pregnancy and, while most maternal lesions heal themselves, the infant is infected in utero.

SIGNS AND SYMPTOMS:
- CONGENITAL: In an infant born with active toxoplasmosis, jaundice and an enlarged liver and spleen are the most striking signs. Infection of the brain and eye is not likely to be noticed until later, when a characteristic triad appears—hydrocephalus, intracerebral calcification and choroidoretinitis.
- ACQUIRED TOXOPLASMOSIS: Enlargement of lymph glands with general malaise and loss of weight, very rarely encephalitis and myocarditis. Uveitis is not uncommon. Ophthalmologists in recent years believe that some unexplained cases of posterior uveitis may be due to acquired toxoplasmosis.
- EYE SIGNS: The clinical appearance does not help in the diagnosis during the acute stage of infection. When quiescent, rounded lesions of posterior uveitis are seen at the macula in the region of the disc. Sometimes they are more widely disseminated. In the adult, such lesions can be either a recurrence of a prenatal infection or may be the result of an acquired attack. The most frequent appearance is that of a punched-out hole near the macula resembling a coloboma. Diagnosis is difficult and must depend upon immunological tests.

TREATMENT: If toxoplasmosis is suspected, dye test titres should be carried out. Work done in the University of Ghent suggests that a course of pyrimethamine, sulphadiazine and penimepicycline is the most helpful line of treatment. This should be combined with systemic steroid therapy.

Tuberculosis: The following ophthalmic conditions are believed by some ophthalmologists to be either manifestations of tuberculosis or the allergic reactions in the eye to tuberculosis foci elsewhere in the body:
1. Sclerosing keratitis (*see* p. 94).
2. Uveoparotid fever (*see* p. 58).
3. Miliary choroidal tuberculosis.
4. Polypoid conjunctival granules (*see* p. 21).
5. Phlyctenular conjunctivitis (*see* p. 12).
6. Anterior uveitis.
7. Choroiditis.
8. Sarcoidosis (*see* p. 58).

It must be admitted that the evidence of tubercular origin of several of the above is very slender.

Tuberous Sclerosis (*see* p. 83).

Tularaemia: This is a bacterial infection with the *Pasteurella tularensis*. The eye signs include orbital cellulitis, oculoglandular conjunctivitis, keratitis with ulceration and iridocyclitis.

Typhoid: Numerous eye signs are visible in this condition. Various muscular palsies, paralysis of accommodation, orbital haemorrhage, oedema of the lids, proptosis, corneal ulceration, iridocyclitis, hypopyon, retinal haemorrhages, thrombosis and embolism, and panophthalmitis.

Typhus: Although very rare in Great Britain this disease can be complicated by corneal ulcers, iritis and optic neuritis.

Ulcerative Colitis: Occasionally oedema of the lids, episcleritis and iritis are seen.

Weil's Disease: This is a spirochaetal infection which occasionally produces ocular palsies and ptosis, jaundice of the sclerotics, keratitis, iridocyclitis with secondary cataract, vitreous opacities, retinal haemorrhages and retinopathy.

For the student who is working for his Higher Ophthalmic Diploma it will not be out of place to include an alphabetical list of syndromes together with their pathology, ocular and other associated signs (*see* pp. 210–214).

ALPHABETICAL LIST OF OCULAR SYNDROMES

SYNDROME OR DISEASE	PATHOLOGY	OCULAR SIGNS	GENERAL SIGNS
Albers-Schönberg's disease (osteopetrosis)	Hereditary. Increased calcium deposits in bones	Narrowing of optic foramen causing optic atrophy	Heavy brittle bones
Alport's syndrome	Hereditary. Progressive nephropathy with proteinuria and haematuria	Cataracts; posterior lenticonus	Deafness
Batten-Mayou disease	Degeneration of rod and cone layer starting in childhood	Macular stippling; optic atrophy	Mental deficiency, starting about 6 years of age Degenerative changes in cerebrum, cerebellum, etc.
Behçet's syndrome	Unknown	Iritis with hypopyon	Ulceration of mucous membranes
Bell's palsy	Paralysis of 7th nerve	Epiphora; inability to close lids; exposure keratitis	Nil
Bourneville's disease	Multiple cystic tumours	Retinal tumours (see PHAKOMATOSES, p. 82)	Multiple tumours (see PHAKOMATOSES, p. 82)
Cogan's syndrome	Uncertain	Non-specific interstitial keratitis (sometimes uveitis)	Cochleovestibular symptoms, increased sedimentation rate and leucocytosis
Crouzon's disease (dysostosis craniofacialis)	Congenital	Divergent squint; exophthalmos; optic atrophy	Gross facial deformity; sunken upper jaw, etc.
Duane's syndrome	Unknown	Deficiency of abduction; retraction of globe on adduction	Nil
Ehlers-Danlos syndrome	Mesodermal maldevelopment	Keratochromia, dislocated lens and angeoid streaks	Hyperelasticity of skin; hyperlaxity of joints. Tendency to haematomata

ALPHABETICAL LIST OF OCULAR SYNDROMES—continued

SYNDROME OR DISEASE	PATHOLOGY	OCULAR SIGNS	GENERAL SIGNS
Fanconi's syndrome	Dysfunction of cystine metabolism	Photophobia; cystine crystals in cornea, conjunctiva and iris	Rickety dwarfism; thirst and polyuria
Gaucher's disease	Unknown	Pigmented pingeculae	Hepatic and splenic enlargement
Greig's disease (hypertelorism)	Congenital	Divergent squint; wide pupillary distance	Retroussé nose; deformity of frontal and maxillary bones; sometimes syndactyly and undescended testes
Harada's syndrome (see p. 58)	Unknown	Alopecia of lids; iridocyclitis; retinal oedema; sometimes detachment	Alopecia; skin eruptions; deafness; lymphocytosis
Heerfordt's disease	Uncertain, possibly tuberculous	Uveitis	Bilateral parotitis; paralysis of 7th nerve; pyrexia
von Hippel's syndrome	Multiple angiomatosis	Retinal angiomatosis (p. 82)	(See PHAKOMATOSES, p. 82)
Horner's syndrome	Paralysis of cervical sympathetic	Unilateral enophthalmos; myosis; narrowing of palpebral fissure	Nil
Hurler's disease (gargoylism)	Familial dysostosis with lipoid metabolic dysfunction	Infiltration of cornea with metabolic dysfunction	Dwarfism; coarse hair; large head; lipoid deposits in viscera
Laurence–Moon–Biedl's syndrome	Hypopituitarism	Pigmentary retinal degeneration	Polydactyly; mental and gonadal retardation; obesity
Leber's disease (hereditary optic atrophy)	Familial	Retrobulbar neuritis, leading to optic atrophy	Nil
Little's disease	Subdural haemorrhage due to difficult labour	Convergent squint	Spastic paralysis

ALPHABETICAL LIST OF OCULAR SYNDROMES—continued

SYNDROME OR DISEASE	PATHOLOGY	OCULAR SIGNS	GENERAL SIGNS
Lowe's syndrome	Hereditary metabolic error	Buphthalmos; nystagmus; corneal dystrophy; iris atrophy; cataracts, occasionally congenital glaucoma	Mental retardation; hypotonia; proteinuria; acidosis
Marfan's syndrome	Familial mesodermal dysfunction	Subluxation of lens	Arachnodactyly; sometimes widespread mesodermal defects in long skeletal bones, etc.
Marie–Strümpell's disease	Unknown	Iridocyclitis	Ankylosing spondylitis
Mikulicz's syndrome	Uncertain; has been attributed to leukaemia, tuberculosis, syphilis	Chronic bilateral enlargement of lacrimal glands	Bilateral enlargement of salivary glands
Morgnio's disease	Unknown	Sometimes optic atrophy	Osseous dystrophy of the whole of the skeleton except head and face
Niemann–Pick's disease	Widespread lipoid changes	Retinal degeneration; optic atrophy; yellow disc	Lipoid degeneration of liver, spleen, etc.
Parker's disease	Unknown	Uveitis	Alopecia vitiligo; poliosis; deafness
von Recklinghausen's disease	Multiple neurofibromatosis	(See PHAKOMATOSES, p. 82)	(See PHAKOMATOSES, p. 82)
Reiter's syndrome	Unknown; *not* gonococcal	Purulent conjunctivitis	Urethritis; multiple arthritis
Rieger's syndrome	Developmental abnormality	Iris hypoplasia; chamber angle abnormalities; glaucoma	Oligodontia; deformities of fingers and toes
Riley–Day syndrome	Neuro-ectodermal maldevelopment	Conjunctival alacrima; neuroparalytic keratitis	Autonomic dysfunction; retarded development; respiratory infection and excessive sweating

OCULAR SIGNS OF GENERAL DISEASE

ALPHABETICAL LIST OF OCULAR SYNDROMES—continued

SYNDROME OR DISEASE	PATHOLOGY	OCULAR SIGNS	GENERAL SIGNS
Romberg's syndrome	Mesodermal maldevelopment	Fifth nerve neuralgia; neuroparalytic keratitis; epiphora; ocular palsies; Horner's syndrome and heterochromia	Hemifacial atrophy
Schilder's disease	Demyelinating degeneration	Blindness with normal fundus; optic atrophy occurs late	Vomiting; convulsions; apathy; paralysis; deafness
Schüller–Christian syndrome (xanthomatosis)	Familial lipoid dysfunction, causing areas of rarefaction in bones	Proptosis due to lipoid deposits	Lipoid deposits in bones and viscera; diabetes insipidus; hypopituitarism
Sjögren's disease	Secretory dysfunction of lacrimal and other glands	Diminished lacrimal secretion; dryness of conjunctiva	Arthritis; dysphagia; huskiness of voice; achlorhydria
Stargardt's disease	Hereditary	Macular degeneration	Sometimes idiocy, paralyses, etc.
Stevens–Johnson's syndrome	Unknown; probably virus	Membranous conjunctivitis forming symblepharon; sometimes iritis	Acute respiratory catarrh; stomatitis; erythema multiforme; balanitis
Still's disease	Infantile rheumatoid arthritis	Keratitis with band opacity; iridocyclitis; secondary cataract	Fusiform joint swelling; enlarged lymph glands and liver
Sturge–Weber syndrome	Congenital (phakomatous) calcification of orbital and cerebral vessels; one side only involved	Glaucoma; buphthalmos (See PHAKOMATOSES, p. 82)	Naevus flammaeus one side of face; hemiplegia; convulsions (See PHAKOMATOSES, p. 82)
Tay-Sachs disease (amaurotic family idiocy)	Degeneration of ganglion cells	Retinal degeneration; optic atrophy	Idiocy in infants, usually Jewish

ALPHABETICAL LIST OF OCULAR SYNDROMES—*continued*

SYNDROME OR DISEASE	PATHOLOGY	OCULAR SIGNS	GENERAL SIGNS
van den Hoeve's syndrome	Unknown	Blue sclerotics	Fragilitas ossium; otosclerosis
Vogt–Koyanagi's syndrome	(*See* PARKER'S DISEASE, *above*)		
Waadenburg's syndrome	Hereditary ectodermal maldevelopment	Anomalies of the internal angle of eyelids and base of nose; punctum displacement; heterochromia	Deafness, white forelock
Werner's syndrome	Hereditofamilial disorder, commencing at adolescence	Cataracts and bullous keratopathy	Progeria loss and greying of hair; atophic dermatoses; ulceration of legs
Wilson's disease	Hepatolenticular degeneration	Kaiser-Fleischer's ring in cornea; 'sunflower' cataracts	Tremors; rigidity; hepatic enlargement
Wolfram–Tyrer's syndrome	Uncertain	Congenital optic atrophy; defective eye movements	Juvenile diabetes; ataxia; defective intelligence

Chapter XX

OCULAR SIDE-EFFECTS OF SYSTEMIC MEDICATION

Toxic effects in the eyes are occasionally observed resulting from: (1) Side-effects of systemic medication; (2) Following local treatment. These results can occur almost immediately or after an appreciable lapse of time as the result of a build-up of the drugs.

It must be stressed that ocular side-effects are comparatively rare and are usually due either to individual idiosyncrasy or to taking excessive quantities of the particular drug over a long period of time. The following effects have been observed:

Acetazolamide (Diamox): In susceptible patients, this drug has caused transient myopia and occasionally oedema of the retina.

Anthelmintics, such as Santonin and Felix Mas, can cause xanthopsia, toxic amblyopia and optic atrophy.

Antibiotic Therapy: Streptomycin and chloramphenicol have been known to lead to optic neuritis with gross impairment of vision.

Antihypertensive Drugs: Some of these, especially methonium compounds, have caused permanent blindness due to retinal ischaemia following the sudden lowering of blood pressure. In less serious cases cyclopeglia occurs. Adrenergic drugs (e.g. Bretylium tosylate) can produce diplopia, ptosis, transient myopia and rarely occlusion of central retinal artery.

Anti-Parkinsonian Drugs not infrequently produce dilatation of the pupil, paralysis of accommodation resulting in blurred vision, and occasionally closed angle glaucoma. This applies to the drug L-dopa. It is a wise precaution to prescribe pilocarpine drops while patients are undergoing treatment.

Antirheumatic Drugs: Phenylbutazone and indomethazine can cause retinal haemorrhages or toxic amblyopia.

Antispasmodic Drugs: Anticholinergic drugs such as atropine used in a number of tablets and mixtures for diarrhoea can cause mydriasis, difficulty with reading and even closed angle glaucoma.

Antithyroid Drugs, e.g. radioactive iodine, have been known to cause severe exophthalmos, ophthalmoplegia, visual hallucinations and toxic amblyopia.

Atropine is a very common cause of intense local irritation and the same is true though less frequently of other alkaloids such as eserine and pilocarpine. In these cases when it is essential to continue with local treatment the eyelids and surrounding areas should be covered with petroleum jelly before applying the drops.

216 A SYNOPSIS OF OPHTHALMOLOGY

Cardiovascular Drugs have caused a variety of ocular side-effects. Overdosage with digitalis has resulted in haloes and subjective visual sensations. Quinidine has caused loss of vision in very rare cases of idiosyncrasy. Hydrodiuril has been known to cause oedema of the retina. Apresoline causes ciliary spasm.

Central Nervous System Depressants such as barbiturates, phenothiazine, tranquillizers, etc. can lead to blurred vision and diplopia. These symptoms clear up promptly on the withdrawal.

Chlorpromazine can cause anterior capsular cataract, dilatation of the retinal vessels, pink optic discs, oculogyric crises and pigment deposits in the cornea, sclera and skin of lids.

Corticosteroids when used systemically over a long period have produced posterior subcapsular cataracts. It has long been known that prolonged high doses of corticosteroids, e.g. in rheumatoid arthritis, cause lens opacities and eventual cataract formation. If this does occur there is no reason why the cataract should not be extracted.

Glaucoma can be caused by local use of steroid drops. Their topical use in cases of open angle glaucoma, or even when there is a strong family history of glaucoma, is liable to cause a considerable rise of tension.

Ethyl and Methyl Alcohol: Chronic addiction especially when associated with heavy smoking can lead to amblyopia which is sometimes irreversible unless the patient is strong willed enough to abstain from both drugs. The reversal process is accelerated by generous intake of vitamin B complex. In neglected cases, optic atrophy supervenes.

Ganglion-blocking Agents, such as stramonium derivatives, hexamethonium, etc. can cause optic neuritis.

Heavy Metal Therapy: Arsenic is seldom used in these days of antibiotics and chemotherapy, but it has caused optic atrophy in former days when used in the treatment of syphilis. Local treatment with gold, silver, copper and mercury can cause metallic deposits in the conjunctiva and cornea, e.g. argyrosis (q.v.). Thallium and lead have caused optic neuropathy.

Hormone Therapy:
1. ACTH and steroids can cause subcapsular cataracts, glaucoma, and papilloedema.
2. Female sex hormones. Some ocular complications have been reported after oral contraceptives including perivasculitis and central artery occlusion. Hemianopia and other scotomata have occurred. It cannot at this stage be proved that all such cases are the direct result of the drugs.

Iodides cause amblyopia, keratitis and occasional iridocyclitis and hypopyon. Cases of retinopathy or pigmentary retinal degeneration have been reported following their prolonged use.

Isoniazid when administered through the spinal route has caused optic atrophy. Pyridoxine should be administered at the same time to counteract this possibility.

Oxygen Therapy in premature infants has frequently caused retrolental fibroplasia (q.v.).

Parasympathomimetic Drugs can cause considerable conjunctival irritation which responds well to local steroid therapy.

Penicillin: This used to give marked local reaction when used as drops or ointment. It is seldom seen now as tetracycline, streptomycin or neomycin is used instead.

Phenothiazine can cause oculogyric crises as well as diplopia. Some drugs in this group have produced irreversible pigmentary changes in the retina with blurred vision and night blindness. Barsa and Saunders have found that when this drug has been taken over a prolonged period of time, lenticular and even corneal opacities have resulted. It must therefore be used with caution and periodic eye examinations are necessary.

Practolol (or 'Eraldin'): sometimes causes progressive dryness of the eyes leading to filamentary or punctate keratitis which may result in impairment of vision. Tarsal involvement can cause scarring, symblepharon or entropion.

Quinine Derivatives as used in protozoan infection have been responsible for gross narrowing of the visual fields and blindness following optic atrophy. Quinacrine, chloroquine and amodioquin can produce central scotoma, corneal oedema, retinal degeneration, as well as optic atrophy. Plaquenil as used in the long-term treatment of rheumatoid arthritis and lupus erythematosus has caused transient corneal oedema, occasionally paralysis on accommodation, retinal changes including pigmentary degeneration and optic atrophy. If the retinal changes are detected early they are reversible on withdrawal of the drug, therefore all patients on this treatment should have 3-monthly ophthalmic examinations, including visual fields.

Salicylates have been known to cause retinal haemorrhages.

Sulphonamide Therapy: In rare cases this has produced severe conjunctivo-corneal signs, similar to those of the Stevens–Johnson syndrome (q.v.). This has led to corneal opacification and blindness. Very occasionally retinal oedema and haemorrhages or toxic amblyopia are seen.

Sympathomimetic Drugs such as adrenaline, ephedrine, amphetamine, etc. result in dilatation of the pupil which in turn can cause angle blockage glaucoma.

Travel Sickness Drugs may contain hyoscine or antihistamines. Their effects can be similar to those described under antispasmodics.

Finally, in any puzzling or unexplained eye condition the ophthalmologist should make careful inquiries as to whether the patient is having any systemic treatment.

Chapter XXI

CONTACT LENSES

'He clapped the glass to his sightless eye.' SIR H. NEWBOLT, *Admirals All*

THE first time in history that a patient was fitted with a contact lens was in 1887 when Dr. Saemisch fitted a blown glass lens to a patient who had already lost one eye and whose remaining one was endangered through exposure since the upper lid was destroyed. This was a complete success and saved the eye, the patient dying some 20 years later. Ever since that date isolated ophthalmologists and optical firms have been experimenting with contact lenses and more particularly have attempted grinding optical lenses on to a contact glass with a view to correcting refractive errors as well as affording protection. For years all these efforts met with only partial success. Tribute must be paid to the Carl Zeiss Co., of Jena, for persistent efforts over many years, but the name that will come down to posterity for having first efficiently treated numerous eye diseases with the contact lens is that of Dr. Josef Dallos, of Budapest and later of London. Dallos, after years of patient research and experiment, achieved the honour of having made these lenses a sound practical possibility.

The contact lens is so called because it is in contact with the eye in just the same way as a denture is in contact with the mouth. There are two types of contact lenses:

1. **Corneoscleral Lenses,** which, as their name implies, are in contact with both the corneal and scleral surfaces of the eye. The corneal part is intended to provide an optical correction to abolish corneal irregularities or to protect the underlying cornea according to the nature of the case. The scleral part is concerned solely with the fitting of the lens and the maintenance of its position on the eye.
2. **Microcorneal Lenses** are much smaller, being literally the size of the patient's cornea and having no scleral flange. The circumference of these lenses coincides with that of the patient's cornea.

The majority of surgeons now favour the microcorneal lenses except for those patients where it is necessary to cover the cornea completely to protect it. It is probably too early to form a final judgement, but some ideas as to the advantages and otherwise of both types can be gained from the table blow.

The latest technical advance in contact lenses is their manufacture in soft pliable material. These are known as hydrophylic or 'soft' lenses. They are more comfortable to wear and they adapt themselves to the shape of the cornea. They have disadvantages as they are more difficult for the optician to 'work' and as they are soft and assume the shape of the eye they do not abolish corneal astigmatism as hard lenses do. They are therefore contraindicated when any marked degree of astigmatism is present. At present most surgeons prefer to order hard lenses but it is probable that there may be a change of opinion after further trial and research.

	CORNEOSCLERAL LENSES	MICROCORNEAL LENSES
ADVANTAGES	1. Cannot fall out 2. Easy to handle by poor-sighted patients 3. More comfortable to wear initially	1. Smaller and less bulky 2. Less interference with circulation through aqueous veins 3. More comfortable for prolonged wear
DISADVANTAGES	1. Bulky when in situ 2. Cause pressure on aqueous veins and can cause rise of tension in narrow angle cases 3. Less comfortable for prolonged wear	1. Fall out easily 2. Initially more irritable to wear 3. More liable to cause limbal ulceration

When a hard contact lens is worn, the tiny space of 0·1 mm between the cornea and the lens is filled with normal saline, thus abolishing all corneal astigmatism (of greatest benefit in cases of conical cornea), and filling in corneal facets or irregularly reflecting surfaces due to nebulae, etc. It is hardly necessary to point out what a boon this type of lens can be when in addition to the above advantages a spherical lens can be incorporated, providing the patient with the necessary optical correction.

Indications for Contact Lenses:
1. FOR OCCUPATIONAL USE where conventional glasses cannot be worn, e.g. theatrical, ballet professions, etc.
2. FOR PROTECTION OF THE CORNEA in various diseases of the eye, e.g. entropion with trichiasis, lagophthalmos, neuroparalytic keratitis, etc.
3. CONICAL CORNEA: In these cases an otherwise uncorrectable astigmatism is abolished.
4. CORNEAL NEBULAE, FACETS, ETC. FROM ANY CAUSE: Probably the best indication is mustard-gas keratitis.
5. CERTAIN REFRACTIVE ERRORS: More especially:
    HIGH MYOPIA, where it is impossible to get the posterior surface of the correcting lens close enough to the cornea to give good vision.

SEVERE ASTIGMATISM where conventional lenses fail to give satisfactory visual acuity.

ANISOMETROPIA: In selected cases binocular vision can be obtained by means of a contact lens.

UNILATERAL APHAKIA in young persons. Binocular vision can be restored in these cases.

In addition to these indications there is scope for contact lenses in the diagnosis and treatment of certain eye diseases such as:

6. PREVENTION OF SYMBLEPHARON following burns, injuries, etc.
7. FOR THE PROTECTION OF THE EYE during X-ray treatment, the shell in these cases being covered on the outside with lead.
8. FOR LOCALIZATION of intra-ocular foreign bodies.

Advantages of Contact Lenses:
1. In selected cases a contact lens may bring the visual acuity to 6/12 or even better where ordinary spectacles are a comparative failure, giving a visual acuity of 6/60 or less. This is especially true in cases of conical corneae and old keratitis, and it is always worth considering in any case of irregular corneal astigmatism.
2. In unilateral aphakia a contact lens reduces the disparity in size of the retinal images and thus makes binocular vision possible. This is of real advantage in some cases, most especially in traumatic aphakia in young persons.

Disadvantages of Contact Lenses:
1. These lenses are very expensive, and they entail several visits before an adequate fit can be obtained.
2. Some patients are intolerant, and even when the finished article is a perfect fit they may not be able to wear them for more than an hour or two a day without discomfort: 4 or 5 hours of daily wear would be a fair average; 6–8 hours is good, but quite a number of patients can wear them for the entire day. Microcorneal lenses are better tolerated than corneoscleral ones.

In conclusion, it must be emphasized that contact lens work is a very skilled and specialized craft. To be a success the lens must be made for the patient with painstaking thoroughness which demands not merely collaboration between the ophthalmic surgeon and the technician, both of whom must have experience of the work, but it also demands a cooperative patient who is prepared to 'go through with it' even though many sessions for fitting may be necessary. Given these factors, the case will have a very fair chance of success.

Chapter XXII

THE EYES IN MALNUTRITION

Nutritional Retinopathy in Prisoners of War: While it has been a recognized fact for many years that vitamin deficiencies can cause corneal manifestations, it was not until the Second World War that it dawned upon ophthalmologists that these deficiencies could have such far-reaching and permanent effects as severe amblyopia or even optic atrophy. In developed countries such cases were rarely seen, but they were common enough amongst prisoners of war in the Far East who endured great privations and were fed on a diet without any regard to vitamin content or calorie value and who in many cases were treated with great barbarity and compelled to do forced labour from dawn to dusk. Most of these patients were fed on boiled carbohydrates, usually a poor quality polished rice, supplemented by mixed vegetable soup. The meat ration if given at all was very small, and seldom was it possible to get such things as eggs, fresh fruit, etc. It will, therefore, be realized that such a diet lacked adequate quantities of vitamins A, B and C.

Harold Ridley examined about 500 of these cases and he found that the commonest ocular symptom in these patients was partial visual failure, usually bilateral and of sudden onset. Their visual acuity varied from 1/60 to 6/9 with correction, and gross central scotomata were often present. Many of these patients showed symptoms of pellagra, beri-beri, etc. and quite a number of amblyopic patients became nerve-deaf. The pupils in the more severe cases were dilated, but no abnormalities were found in the fundi except in severe or long-standing cases where a pathological temporal pallor of the disc was noted. Optic neuritis was never found and the retinal vessels were normal in all cases. No cases showed xerosis or Bitot's spots, but over 90 per cent of them had a fine limbal capillary plexus with superficial opacities, and many of the limbal capillaries showed great variation in size, some with aneurysmal dilatations. Stannus considers these cases of amblyopia to be due to a deficiency of vitamin B_2, but the fact remains that all these patients were deprived of proteins and fats as well as vitamins, and thus it is not improbable that general malnutrition rather than a deficiency in one particular vitamin may have been responsible. The site of the lesions is still unknown. Nutritional retrobulbar retinopathy is only too common in the mid-twentieth century in underdeveloped and underfed countries.

TREATMENT: Full normal diet with all possible supplementary vitamins, including thiamine, riboflavin, ascorbic and nicotinic acids, with aneurin and halibut-liver oil.

PROGNOSIS: Uncertain. Some degree of visual improvement may occur, but by no means always. After two years on a normal diet any defect in visual acuity must be considered permanent.

Vitamin A Deficiency: Deficiency of this vitamin gives rise to three cardinal signs and symptoms: (1) xerophthalmia, (2) keratomalacia and (3) defective dark adaptation.

1. XEROPHTHALMIA: A dry lustreless condition of a conjunctiva. White triangular patches (Bitot's spots) are found on the outer and inner sides of the corneae. Night blindness is usually present and epidermoid changes occur in the epithelium, causing inability to secrete mucus and consequent dryness. It should be remembered that xerosis can result from local ocular disease, trachoma, burns, exposure, etc. as well as from vitamin A deficiency. Xerophthalmia is still a major cause of blindness in young persons in Asia, Africa and Latin America.

2. KERATOMALACIA: This is a corneal disease occurring nearly always in young children who are wasted, rickety and apathetic. The condition is bilateral. It commences with a dryness and lack of corneal lustre, frequently associated with night-blindness and followed by infiltration and eventually even necrosis. The cornea is insensitive and no gross inflammatory changes are present.

3. DEFECTIVE DARK ADAPTATION: The student is reminded here that vitamin A is an essential factor in the formation of visual purple, a photosensitive pigment present in the rods of the retina. Any gross deficiency of this vitamin is bound to have an adverse effect on night vision, for which this purple pigment is essential.

TREATMENT: All the above cases call for a diet rich in milk, cod- or halibut-liver oil, butter, etc. In dry corneal conditions, hyaluronidase (Benger) 10 units per ml used as eye drops may give prompt relief.

Vitamin B Deficiency: This is a very complex vitamin of which there are at least twelve known factors, and others previously unknown are in the habit of springing up almost overnight. The most important factors from the oculist's point of view are B_1 and B_2, aneurin and riboflavin respectively. An arbitrary division of the signs and symptoms due to lack of these two factors is impossible, for a patient is scarcely ever deprived of one without the other. In addition to the amblyopia and other symptoms discussed in the beginning of this chapter, it is known that riboflavin deficiency leads to a sodden conjunctival epithelium with irritable burning eyes and photophobia.

Eventually a circumcorneal vascularization of a characteristic type occurs. The vascularization is always bilateral and involves the entire circumference of both corneae. Slit-lamp examination shows that from the apices of the normal vascular loops fine vessels run towards the cornea, each in turn anastomosing with its neighbour and forming further apical loops, thus causing a slow but progressive subepithelial vascularization of the cornea. To clinch the diagnosis is the response to riboflavin treatment: this is striking and often dramatic. Daily administration of 10 mg of riboflavin causes a complete recovery in 3–4 weeks. Stern considers that ariboflavinosis *always* causes this vascularity of the cornea if it has been present long enough to cause a low concentration of riboflavin in the blood. He further considers that any vascularization of the above type is pathognomic of ariboflavinosis.

Vitamin C Deficiency: No dramatic eye signs follow vitamin C deficiency comparable with those that have been described as being due to other vitamin deficiency, but it must be remembered that normally the cornea, the intra-ocular fluid, and lens of the human eye all have a high ascorbic acid content and the theory has been advanced that since none of these tissues can get oxygen direct from the blood, vitamin C plays some role in their respiration. In support of this theory is the fact that the lens, which normally contains much ascorbic acid, shows a diminishing concentration in old age and a complete absence if cataract supervenes. Since it is known that an opaque lens is one that has been deprived of oxygen, it is reasonable to assume that ascorbic acid is concerned with its respiration, but the exact part it plays has yet to be discovered. Consideration of these facts, and bearing in mind that corneal ulceration is of frequent occurrence in scurvy, makes it safe to draw this conclusion: an adequate concentration of ascorbic acid is essential for the maintenance of the health of the eye and especially of those parts which are dependent upon an auto-oxidation system for their nourishment.

VITAMIN C TREATMENT: Many authorities have stressed the therapeutic value of ascorbic acid, either intravenously or orally as an adjunct to antibiotic treatment in a number of pathological conditions such as severe inflammatory conditions of the cornea and hypopyon ulcer. Observers claim that this treatment is beneficial even in those cases where there is no demonstrable deficiency in the blood ascorbic acid content. Unfortunately, there is no evidence whatever to suggest that ascorbic acid treatment has any effect in the prevention or cure of cataract.

Vitamin K Deficiency: Although it is by no means true that cases of unexplained retinal or vitreous haemorrhages are necessarily due to hypoprothrombinaemia, vitamin K is well worth a trial in their treatment. Hypoprothrombinaemia is sometimes the result of drugs such as sulphonamides, salicylates, quinine, dicoumarol, etc. If ever an intra-ocular haemorrhage occurs in any patient who has been having such treatment, vitamin K therapy in large doses is definitely indicated.

Chapter XXIII

OPHTHALMIC OPERATIONS

'Honour hath no skill in surgery, then?' W. SHAKESPEARE, *King Henry IV*, Part 1

IN a synopsis which aims at giving a bird's-eye view of the whole of ophthalmology in one volume, lack of space naturally precludes a description of the various ophthalmic operations. Details of operative technique have therefore been omitted and emphasis has been put on the principles underlying and the indications for the various operative procedures in common use. These are set out in alphabetical order, and, in addition to this list, the reader is reminded that the indications for several operations have been discussed, in passing, under the various diseases they were designed to alleviate.

Cataract Extraction: The first recorded cataract extraction was done by Daviel, a Frenchman, at a date uncertain but well over 200 years ago. It was done through a section through the lower half of the cornea. Samuel Sharp of London first performed extraction operation with a knife by puncture and counter puncture as is done today. The operation may be performed in two ways:

1. INTRACAPSULAR, whereby the cataract is removed complete in its capsule. With modern anaesthesia and suturing techniques the operation is best performed under general anaesthesia, or failing this, a neuroleptalgesic technique.

    The classic approach is by Graefe section but even in the hands of an accomplished operator perfect control of the section is not possible, especially in very soft eyes and shallow anterior chambers. A better method is to effect the section by a razor-blade fragment knife after reflecting a limbal-based conjunctival flap (the occasional operator is advised to use the keratome and scissors approach). The advantage of this method is its precise placement and that the incision can be stepped and sutures pre- or post-placed according to the surgeon's wishes. Peripheral iridectomy is performed, and the lens removed with a cryo-probe. Zonulysin may be used prior to extraction in the younger patients. A slow delivery of the lens enables some moulding to take place in the wound and therefore the section can be smaller than the usual 180°. Adherent hyalocapsular ligament can also be stripped off with a cellulose sponge swab. The wound is then closed with sufficient 10/0 Perlon sutures to render the whole watertight, and the anterior chamber is reformed with Ringer's solution or normal saline.

INDICATIONS:
- *a.* Immature cataracts.
- *b.* Hypermature cataracts.
- *c.* Some cases of dislocated lens.

ADVANTAGES OVER THE EXTRACAPSULAR OPERATION:
- *a.* Better cosmetic result.
- *b.* No capsule to require needling.
- *c.* Less postoperative inflammatory reaction.

2. EXTRACAPSULAR, i.e. when the lens is removed but the capsule is left behind.

INDICATIONS:
- *a.* Complicated cataracts.
- *b.* Brown cataracts.
- *c.* In conjunction with some intra-ocular implants.
- *d.* Mature cataracts and the occasional operator.

The majority are performed as 'failed' intracapsular extractions. The extracapsular method is essentially the same except that the capsule of the lens is incised, the nucleus removed with extracapsular forceps (or expressed) and cortical matter washed out.

Cataract Extractions with Intra-ocular Implants: These are occasionally indicated in unilateral aphakia and are of two different types:

1. ACRYLIC LENS: In 1951, in a paper at the Oxford Ophthalmic Congress, Mr. Harold Ridley described what was then a revolutionary treatment for uni-ocular cataract. In order to overcome the anisometropia following unilateral cataract extraction, Mr. Ridley inserted in the place of the extracted lens a Perspex lens of the same size and refractive index as the human lens. His technique was to perform an extracapsular operation and to place the implant behind the iris resting on the posterior capsule. These lenses promised much but, unfortunately, an undue proportion of them seem to cause marked inflammatory reactions and postoperative iritis. In a number of cases they have had to be removed within a few days of the operation. Another drawback in some of these cases is the difficulty in performing a needling operation if this proves necessary. The Ridley implant cannot, of course, be used in intracapsular cases as they rely upon the posterior lens capable for the support. Also a number of much later complications have been reported including secondary glaucoma and keratopathies which have occurred as late as four years after operation.

2. ANTERIOR CHAMBER IMPLANT: In view of the inflammatory reactions following the Ridley lens, Barraquer, Strampelli and their co-workers in 1954 tried an anterior chamber implant placed in front of the iris and behind the cornea. More recently Mr. Choyce at Southend General Hospital has improved upon these

techniques. This type of implant can be inserted at a later date after the cataract has been removed and the eye has settled down. An additional advantage of the Choyce implant is that it can be inserted after intracapsular operations. In a series of 100 of these operations, Mr. Choyce reports 10 per cent of disappointments, the majority being due to iritis, secondary glaucoma or corneal endothelial changes. Binocular vision was restored in 75 per cent of his cases.

3. IRIS CLIP IMPLANTS: These fix on anterior surfaces of the iris like a collar stud. The lenticule is held in place by the iris sphincter, which takes on a square shape but additional security can be attained by a Perlon suture anchoring wire loop to iris. Rupture of the hyaloid face is the commonest operative hazard but is usually plugged by the in situ implant and the small amount remaining in the anterior chamber can be mopped away with a cellulose sponge before re-forming the anterior chamber. At the moment these forms of lenticular implant have largely supplanted the anterior variety but who knows what man's ingenuity and the future will provide?

4. PHACO-EMULSIFICATION: Kelman (*Trans. ophthal. Soc. U.K.*, 1970, **90**, 13) has described a technique for the removal of cataracts which may well be the method of choice in the future. The technique demands only a small limbal incision followed by a cystitome incision of the capsule, the emulsifier consisting of a hollow titanium needle surrounded by a concentric plastic tube. The needle vibrates at high frequency producing local emulsification of the cataract, whilst the concentric tubes maintain a computer-controlled aspiration–suction action on the anterior chamber contents. All types of cataracts except hypermature and brown cataracts have been successfully removed with encouraging results to date. Convalescence is short and complication-free. Its disadvantages are its high cost and expensive maintenance.

Conjunctivo-dacryocystostomy (Stallard's Operation): Involves the stitching of the lacrimal sac into the conjunctiva near the inner canthus.

INDICATIONS: Absence or destruction of the lower punctum or canaliculus.

Corneal Transplantation (Keratoplasty): The removal of a small disc of a clear cornea from a donor eye and its implanting into a window of similar size removed from the recipient's opaque cornea. The trephined disc varies in size from 4 mm to 8 mm but occasionally larger grafts are used. The graft may be of partial thickness (lamellar) or full thickness (penetrating). Most surgeons use a circular trephine but square or rectangular grafts can be obtained with a twin-bladed knife. It is important that the graft be cleanly cut to avoid damage to the endothelium. The graft is positioned with deeply placed,

10/0 Perlon sutures in either an interrupted or a continuous pattern. The anterior chamber is re-formed with normal saline.

INDICATIONS: It is a very useful operation for blindness due to opaque corneae when there is reason to believe that the rest of the eye is healthy; or, of course, it is equally satisfactory for a unilateral opaque cornea when the remaining eye is blind for any reason. It is of value in perforating (or impending perforation) ulcers of the cornea. In skilled hands this operation has been markedly successful, but unfortunately in a number of cases the implanted graft becomes opaque in the process of time, thus causing the patient heartbreaking disappointment.

Corneal Prosthesis: In some cases the damage to the cornea is so extensive that corneal grafting is doomed to failure. In an endeavour to give these unfortunate patients some useful sight, several surgeons have designed intracameral acrylic implants to act as an artificial cornea. The prosthesis consists of an acrylic cylinder retained in position by an intralamellar flange and an anterior 'button' projecting externally.

Curette Evacuation: Is undertaken for the purpose of washing out soft lens matter from the anterior chamber. It is most commonly performed on young adults for traumatic cataract or after needling for other forms of cataract. This operation was first performed by von Graefe in 1867. In 1967 Rice described an operation for dealing with congenital or traumatic cataracts in patients under 30 years of age. Under microscopic control, a capsulotomy is performed with a Barkan's goniotomy knife. A blunted No. 17 needle, mounted on a 2-ml syringe, is passed along the knife tract and into the capsular opening. Lens matter is alternately aspirated and irrigated with Ringer's solution until all lens matter is removed. Its great advantage lies in that it is a single operation and avoids the damaging postoperative inflammation of repeated needlings. It is likely that the incidence of detachment will be markedly reduced.

Cyclodialysis: Aims at effecting a communication between the anterior chamber and the suprachoroidal lymph space.

INDICATIONS:

1. Chronic glaucoma with limited rise of tension.
2. Buphthalmos.
3. Secondary glaucoma.
4. Glaucoma following cataract extraction.

Dacryocystectomy: The excision of the lacrimal sac. Its only indication is in chronic and recurrent dacryocystitis. It has one rather marked disadvantage—there is certain to be some resulting epiphora, since there is no means of communication between the conjunctival sac and the nose. The tears, however, after operation are not infected and the discharge from the eye is always 'clean' water and not 'dirty'

OPHTHALMIC OPERATIONS

water. This operation has now been discarded by most surgeons in favour of dacryocystorhinostomy.

Dacryocystorhinostomy: Aims at making a passage to drain the tears into the nose by means of a manufactured canal through the lacrimal bone and the nasal mucosa.

INDICATION: Occlusion of the nasolacrimal duct which cannot be overcome by probing.

It has the great advantage that in successful cases there is no resulting epiphora and a good drainage is established between the conjunctiva and the nose. It must be frankly admitted that there are still a number of failures but the results of this operation seem to improve year by year.

Detachment Operations: *See* p. 89 for description of diathermy, scleral resections and vitreous implant operations.

Discission (or Needling): Is indicated:
1. In young persons under the age of 30 as an operation for congenital or lamellar cataract.
2. At any age when necessary to make an opening in the capsule which may persist after a cataract operation.

This operation is sometimes known as 'capsulotomy'.

Enucleation: The removal of the globe from the orbit.

INDICATIONS:
1. In cases of malignant intra-ocular tumours.
2. For chronic painful blind eyes, e.g. absolute glaucoma, etc.
3. To prevent the onset of sympathetic ophthalmia, q.v.
4. Severe trauma.

A refinement of this operation is the insertion of an implant. This prosthesis is sutured to the four recti muscles after the globe is removed, thus enabling the artificial eye to move more or less normally.

Evisceration: The curetting of the contents of the globe, leaving its scleral coat intact.

INDICATIONS:
1. Panophthalmitis.
2. For the removal of a badly injured, perforated and collapsed eye.

Exenteration of Orbit: Reserved for malignant neoplasms with extra-ocular extension. It involves the removal of the entire orbital contents, including the lids and the lining periosteum, the cavity being lined with skin usually obtained from a pedicle graft.

Glaucoma Operations:
1. BUPHTHALMOS: The operation of choice is *goniotomy*. The operating miscroscope, Worst's gonioprism and Barkan's knife are used. About one-quarter of the filtration angle is stripped of mesodermal tissue at a single operation. If the corneal diameter exceeds 14 mm, the canal of Schlemm is likely to be absent or

atrophic and an alternative procedure is indicated. Postoperative control is likely if tearing and photophobia is absent.
2. NARROW ANGLE GLAUCOMA: Here the operation of choice is peripheral iridectomy if the angle shows less than 80 per cent peripheral anterior synechiae. The other eye also requires prophylactic iridectomy, and both operations can be performed at one sitting. Sector iridectomy is sometimes indicated in cases which fail to respond to intensive miotics, and an angle closure demands a filtering operation.
3. WIDE ANGLE GLAUCOMA: There is a monumental amount of literature devoted to the operative control of this disease—in itself a monument to the surgeon's failure to understand or control the condition.
   a. IRIDENCLEISIS: A wick of iris is incarcerated in an anterior sclerectomy incision, allowing aqueous to drain subconjunctivally and thus relieve excess pressure. The methods of Lagrange and Stallard are commonly employed.
   b. SCHEIE'S OPERATION: 'A Preziosi operation on a broad front'. Today this is the most popular operation performed for glaucoma, in that it is quick, simple and effective in about 75 per cent of cases. A limbal-based conjunctival flap is made, Tenon's membrane stripped back and an *ab externa* anterior sclerectomy is carried down to the deeper scleral layers. Cautery is now applied to the posterior lip of the wound, causing it to retract. The sclerectomy is now completed, peripheral iridectomy performed and the conjunctival flap sutured.
   c. TRABECULAR SURGERY: It is probable that the basic lesion in wide angle glaucoma lies in resistance to outflow in the trabecular network. Taking this hypothesis, several surgeons have directed their attention recently to techniques designed at overcoming this defect at source rather than by-passing it with filtering operations. Of these procedures, that of Cairns promises to be the most successful and is briefly described below.
      Trabeculectomy: Under microscopic control, a half-thickness, 5-mm square, scleral trapdoor is fashioned extending from the limbus posteriorly. A paracentesis needle enters the anterior chamber, lowering the intra-ocular pressure and filling Schlemm's canal with blood for ease of identification. Next a 4×1-mm trapdoor incision is performed extending from the scleral spur to Schwalbe's line. The flap is reflected posteriorly and excised, thus removing a 4-mm strip of trabecular meshwork and adjacent Schlemm's canal. The wound is closed in layers. To date, the operation is complication-free and successful in about 70 per cent of cases, but a number turn themselves into filtering operations.

d. MISCELLANEOUS:
   Cyclodialysis: Useful in aphakia and can be repeated.
   Cyclo-diathermy (*Cryotherapy*): The last resort in cases such as thrombotic glaucoma, but the operation of choice in Negroes.
   Iridotomy: Puncture of the iris for the relief of iris bombé causing secondary glaucoma.

Inferior Oblique Myomectomy: Is undertaken on the contralateral muscle for the relief of ocular torticollis. Exposure of the muscle can be made by one of two routes: (1) through the skin of the lower lid; (2) transconjunctivally (Chevasse's operation) with the lower lid everted.

Iridectomy: The first iridectomy operation by pulling out part of the iris and snipping it off with scissors was performed by Beer in 1798. This is done for the following reasons:
   1. As a preliminary to various intra-ocular procedures.
   2. For the relief of acute narrow angle glaucoma.
   3. For the removal of a prolapsed iris.
   4. For the removal of an iris tumour.
   5. For optical purposes, e.g. in cases of central corneal opacity with a clear periphery.

Lacrimal Prosthesis Operation: Mr. L. H. G. Moore of Dudley has described (personal communication) a very simple quick and satisfactory operation for cases of lacrimal obstruction. It consists of inserting a plastic prosthesis between the nasolacrimal duct and the sac. Mr. Moore considers it ideal in mucocele cases but contraindicated where there is heavy and repeated infection. One of the authors (C. M.-D.) has watched Mr. Moore perform these operations and he is impressed with the technique and simplicity of the procedure. There is no doubt, however, that a successful dacryocysto-rhinostomy operation gives better results. Mr. Moore himself agrees with this. In cases in which the sac and canaliculi are destroyed, conjunctivo-rhinostomy can be performed incorporating a plastic tube (Lester Jones) sutured to the conjunctiva.

Muscle Transplant (Sixth Nerve Palsy): The usual method of dealing with this problem is by a recession and resection with transplantation of slips of muscle from superior and inferior recti, preferably before secondary overactions occur. Recently we have undertaken a similar approach, but the transplantation consists of the whole superior rectus only. The results are, we feel, better and, surprisingly, there is no impairment of elevation.

Partial Cyclectomy: Pioneered by Stallard, this operation was devised for malignant melanoma of the iris spreading into the angle and ciliary body. A limbal incision some 10 mm long is carried backwards and radially to effect a posteriorly hinged scleral trapdoor approach. The extent of the lesion is circumscribed with diathermy, the anterior portion of the neoplasm is drawn out of the limbal incision and excised much as a sector iridectomy whose pillars extend posteriorly as far back as the limits of the neoplasm. The end-result is a sector iridectomy, partial cyclectomy and excision of a portion of pars plana. In spite of its extensive nature and 'eyeball to eyeball' confrontation with the vitreous body, the operation is surprisingly easy and complication-free generally. More recently this approach has been successfully employed in small choroidal malignant melanomata.

Resection and Recession: The first operation for squint was undertaken by Dieffenbach in 1839. It consisted of free tenotomy of the internal rectus and it certainly was successful inasmuch as it turned a convergent squint into a divergent one! The idea spread with such rapidity that in 1840 one surgeon alone at the Royal Westminster Eye Hospital did 356 operations in less than seven months. This operation has been replaced by resection and recession.

RESECTION is the operation usually performed on the antagonistic muscle to the one recessed. It consists in the removal of a portion of the muscle tendon for the purpose of shortening it. This operation is sometimes called 'advancement' because part of the muscle tendon near its insertion is removed and the remainder of the muscle is advanced and sutured to its normal insertion.

RECESSION of an extra-ocular muscle is frequently performed for the relief of squint. It involves the removal of a tendon from its insertion and stitching it to the sclera at a desired position posterior to its normal insertion. It has the effect of lengthening the muscle.

INDICATIONS FOR RECESSION AND RESECTION OPERATIONS: These are chiefly employed for squints of an angle of 20° or more. In an internal squint the external rectus is resected and the internal recessed. The reverse is true in cases of divergent squint. The amount of resection and recession necessary to cure a squint of any given angle may be seen from the table.

ANGLE OF SQUINT	RESECTION (mm)	RECESSION (mm)
10	7	0
15	7	2
20	7	3
25	8	3
30	9	4
35	10	4
40	10	5
45	12	5

For squints of less than 15° operation on one muscle only (i.e. either recession or resection) will usually suffice. All six muscles can be tackled in this way, but due to its relative avascularity the superior oblique is better 'tucked'.

'A' and 'V' phenomena can also be dealt with by 'slant' recessions and resections but often have to be followed by further surgery on the obliques.

Scleral Resection: (*See* p. 90.)

Tattooing of Cornea: Is performed for cosmetic purposes when a disfiguring leucoma is present. Two per cent platinum chloride is the pigment usually used, followed by hydrazine hydrate. A small circular area is tattooed to resemble a pupil. A contact lens with a black pupillary area is probably a better proposition.

Vitreal Surgery: (*See* p. 91.)

The authors are only too conscious of the inadequacy of this chapter. It would have been comparatively easy to have written a whole volume in the Synopsis series on ophthalmic operations, but such details are far beyond the scope of this book. It is for this reason that no mention is made of the less common operations or of those for which the indications are obvious, such as plastic surgery of the lids, operations for epicanthus, ptosis, ectropion, entropion, division of synechiae, occlusio pupillae, implantation of radon seeds, removal of non-magnetic foreign bodies, exploration of the orbit, etc.

Chapter XXIV

SYMPATHETIC OPHTHALMIA

THIS is a rare but very severe form of iridocyclitis which affects a previously sound eye as the direct result of a penetrating injury to the other one. The injured eye is called the 'exciting' eye and the uninjured one the 'sympathizing' eye.

Aetiology: The one *sine qua non* in the diagnosis of sympathetic ophthalmia is a perforating injury to one eye. This perforation may be accidental or it may follow a surgical incision, e.g. cataract extraction. Very rarely indeed a sarcoma of the choroid acts as an exciting eye to produce sympathetic ophthalmia in the other, but such an occurrence is not likely to be seen more than once in a lifetime. Wounds resulting in a retained foreign body or a protrusion of uveal tissue are the most likely to develop sympathetic ophthalmia and those involving the ciliary body are the most dangerous of all, particularly if they occur in childhood. Frank suppuration (including perforating ulcers) in an eye renders the occurrence of sympathetic ophthalmia unlikely. The lapse of time gives no immunity from this disease, for it may occur at any time from 3 weeks to 40 years after the injury.

Signs and Symptoms:

THE EXCITING EYE, instead of settling down normally, after 10–14 days the injured eye shows much irritation with lacrimation, photophobia and ciliary flush. A chronic iridocyclitis with KP eventually develops. In sympathetic ophthalmia of very late onset the exciting eye may be blind and even shrunken, but some signs of irritation and ciliary flush are usually seen.

THE SYMPATHIZING EYE develops a diastic iridocyclitis that cannot be clinically differentiated from any other attack of iridocyclitis. The first symptom is that of irritability and lacrimation, and the first discoverable sign is 'aqueous flare' visible with the slit lamp and caused by the presence of cells and excess proteins in the anterior chamber. Shortly after this sign ciliary flush follows and later KP and all the other dire results of plastic iridocyclitis. The disease runs a subacute course lasting from 6 to 24 months.

Pathology: The histological characteristic of sympathetic ophthalmia is the gross lymphocytic infiltration of the entire uveal tract with giant-cell formation. This infiltration is so great that the choroidal thickening is visible macroscopically. The retina usually remains unaffected and fibrinous exudates and polymorphonuclear leucocytes are conspicuous by their absence, thus distinguishing this condition

histologically from a septic endophthalmitis. The following theories have been advanced to explain its occurrence:
1. An infection from one eye to the other via the chiasma. This theory will not hold water because such an infection would appear as a neuroretinitis, whereas the optic disc and retina remain healthy although an intense uveitis occurs.
2. A virus infection via the bloodstream. This is a possibility that has been neither proved nor disproved.
3. An allergic reaction to uveal pigment which became dislodged at the time of the original injury. Sorsby (*Modern Ophthalmology*) accepts this view and gives convincing reasons for it.
4. A tuberculous manifestation, a view held by some Continental ophthalmologists. This theory is based upon the occurrence of giant-cell systems in both diseases, but it breaks down at one point: caseation never occurs in sympathetic disease no matter how long it has lasted.

The modern view represents a combination of the allergic and infective theories. It is believed that a saprophytic organism or virus (not a pathogenic one, because suppurating eyes scarcely ever cause sympathetic trouble) from the conjunctival sac enters the eye at the original injury and invades the bloodstream. At the same time some uveal pigment is dislodged, which acts as an antigen and produces a state of hypersensitivity in the uveal tract of the uninjured eye, hence the organism innocuous to other tissues lodges in the sensitized eye and produces sympathetic ophthalmia.

All these views are theories only. In spite of all efforts to discover the cause, the problem is still unsolved.

For another condition showing remarkable similarities to sympathetic ophthalmia *see* Vogt–Koyanagi–Harada's syndrome, p. 58.

Treatment:
1. PROPHYLACTIC TREATMENT: Most important of all. If the injured eye is excised within 14 days of the injury sympathetic ophthalmia will not occur. None the less, this fact should not lead oculists to excise every injured eye, like fools who often rush in where angels fear to tread. The following are positive indications for the removal of an injured eye:
    a. An eye that is so badly damaged that there is no chance of it ever becoming useful as an organ of vision.
    b. Any injured eye that shows no sign of settling down after 14 days and especially if KP appear or the iris assumes a greenish hue.

    Apart from these absolute indications for early excision, a particularly careful watch should be kept upon the following types of case:

i. Children are particularly liable and their treatment is a great responsibility. It is always wise whenever possible to get a colleague's opinion in cases of doubt.
ii. When the iris, ciliary body or lens capsule is caught up in the wound. Every effort should be made to free these structures, since no eye can be considered as safe while any such entanglement exists.
iii. As has been mentioned, the ciliary body is the 'danger area', and any wound exposing this structure must be regarded with grave suspicion.

Corticosteroid therapy has so altered the prognosis in what used to be the most dreaded of all eye diseases that some delay in the removal of a potentially exciting eye is not merely justifiable, but is often indicated. In all doubtful cases, however, the opinion of a colleague should be sought to share the onus of responsibility.

2. TREATMENT OF ESTABLISHED SYMPATHETIC IRIDOCYCLITIS: This presents many problems, too.
    a. If the case is seen early and the exciting eye has no useful vision, this eye should be excised forthwith. Early excision of an exciting eye is always beneficial to the sympathizing one, but late excision is useless.
    b. If the exciting eye has some useful vision and the inflammation in the sympathizing one is severe, expectant treatment is indicated since the visual end-result may well be better in the exciting eye than in the sympathizing one.
    c. If sympathetic ophthalmia is well established, no good whatever will result from removing the exciting eye.
    d. Apart from the above considerations the treatment of sympathetic disease is the same as that of any other form of iridocyclitis, but corticosteroid therapy is more effective in this than in any other form of eye inflammation. Intensive and energetic therapy is therefore called for by injection, by mouth, locally to the eye in ointment form and by subconjunctival injection. Treatment must be continued until well after all signs of ocular inflammation have ceased.

Prognosis: Modern steroid therapy has completely altered what used to be the exceptionally grave prognosis of this disease. In all cases where treatment is started really early the outlook is now good. If treatment is delayed until the disease is well established the prognosis is much less favourable.

Chapter XXV

CHEMOTHERAPY AND ANTIBIOTICS IN EYE DISEASES

'What drugs, what charms, what conjuration and what mighty magic.'
W. SHAKESPEARE, *Othello*

It would be difficult to exaggerate the advances in treatment made in the past quarter century by the discovery of chemotherapeutic and antibiotic treatment. These advances have revolutionized treatment in many branches of medicine and surgery and not the least in ophthalmology. Before their discovery, surgeons depended upon antiseptics to kill bacteria. This they were able to do, but unfortunately an antiseptic strong enough to kill bacteria was also strong enough to kill the tissues invaded by them. Chemotherapy and antibiotic drugs on the other hand inhibit bacteria and prevent them from multiplying but do not kill either the bacteria or the tissues. This bacteriostatic action is the greatest possible help, for it enables the phagocytes, the scavengers of the bloodstream, to cope with invading organisms which they would be unable to do if the organisms spread and multiplied unhindered. The use of these drugs, therefore, gives the natural defences of the body the chance to cope with the situation. It follows that, if the drug is withdrawn too soon, the remaining bacteria will start to multiply again and the infection will recur. This premature withdrawal of antibiotics is a common mistake.

In considering the use of the various antibiotic drugs in eye diseases it is important to stress the difference between ocular *infections* and *inflammations*. The vast majority of the former respond to chemotherapy, whereas the latter prove resistant and disappointing. Take ophthalmia neonatorum as an instance of an infection: This responds to almost any form of chemotherapy or antibiotic treatment either local or general, and the condition vanishes under treatment like snow in May, but in an inflammation, e.g. iritis, iridocyclitis, etc., there may be no response whatever and the disease may run the same course whether antibiotics are used or not.

When confronted by any eye lesion that might require chemotherapy, the oculist should ask himself two questions: (1) Is this case a genuine infection or an inflammation? (2) If the former, is the organism causing it one that is likely to respond to chemotherapy or antibiotics?

Unless the surgeon has gone into these two points the use of such treatment is more likely to be an abuse of it, but unfortunately for the public this abuse is rarely attended by harmful results.

In making a decision as to the respective merits of chemotherapeutic and antibiotic drugs the following facts must be considered: (1) When given systemically antibiotics are usually less toxic than drugs of the sulpha group; (2) The presence of pus makes sulpha drugs ineffective; (3) General chemotherapy is indicated in severe infections when a quick and high intra-ocular concentration is desired. It should be given in conjunction with local antibiotics; (4) The choice of any particular antibiotic drug is made more difficult by the fact that many firms produce identical preparations (often a combination of antibiotics) under many different proprietary names and at varying prices. In our present state of knowledge and with new preparations being marketed almost every day, it would be invidious to comment on any particular make and if this were attempted this chapter would probably become out of date before leaving the printer's hands.

Finally, it must be borne in mind that neither chemotherapeutic nor antibiotic drugs are anything more than bacteriostatic agents. They are not in themselves curative and, therefore, they do not replace any other general or local treatment that may be indicated.

Chemotherapeutic Drugs:

1. SULPHONAMIDES: This group of drugs was originally discovered and marketed under the name of Prontosil, but this particular drug was rather toxic in its effect. The same applies to sulphapyridine (M and B 693). Since then, numerous drugs of the sulpha group have been marketed. In ophthalmology those most favoured at the present time are:

    Sulphamerazine
    Sulphadimidine
    Sulphadiazine

    Also some drugs that have a more prolonged action such as sulphamethoxypyridazine and sulphaphenazole.

    These are favoured because (1) they are less toxic than other drugs, (2) they readily penetrate the blood/aqueous barrier and produce a rapid blood concentration when given in adequate doses and (3) they are excreted slowly, hence, once an adequate blood concentration is reached, a comparatively infrequent maintenance dose is sufficient. Drugs in this group have a wide spectrum range. They are effective against:

    Coliform bacilli
    Diplobacilli
    Gonococci
    Influenza bacillus
    Meningococci
    Pneumonococci
    Staph. aureus
    Streptococci

CHEMOTHERAPY AND ANTIBIOTICS IN EYE DISEASES

The effectiveness is greatest against haemolytic streptococci and is least against *Staph. aureus*.

Sulpha drugs are ineffective against brucellosis, leprosy, syphilis, tuberculosis, tularaemia and virus infections.

There are, however, three common viruses of ophthalmic interest that are exceptions to this rule. Trachoma, inclusion blennorrhoea and lymphogranuloma venereum. All these are sensitive to sulpha drugs.

Drugs in the sulphonamide group are suitable for general or local use. Systemic administration is very effective in acute ocular diseases since it produces a high concentration in the intra-ocular fluid. (This is not the case with systemic penicillin treatment.) It is essential to give an adequate initial dose to produce a high blood concentration if it is to be effective in the intra-ocular fluid. In conjunctival and corneal infections, the best *local* sulpha preparation is sodium sulphacetamide 10–30 per cent drops, or 2–6 per cent ointment, but it must be remembered that local broad-spectrum antibiotic treatment is more effective. Thus local chemotherapy has been largely replaced by local broad-spectrum antibiotics: chloramphenicol, tetracycline, etc.

2. PAS (Para-amino-salicylic acid) or ISONIAZID (Isonicotine acid hydrazide): This is used in conjunction with streptomycin exclusively for tuberculous infections, whether intra- or extra-ocular.

Antibiotic Drugs: These date from the discovery of penicillin by Fleming in 1929. In recent years so many antibiotics have been marketed that it is difficult to keep pace with them, and new preparations seem to spring up overnight. These different preparations are of value according to their range of antibacterial action ('spectrum'). The most important, up to date, are shown in the appended table (p. 241).

1. PENICILLIN is still a very useful antibiotic in ophthalmology owing to its availability and cheapness. There are, however, a relatively large number of people who are hypersensitive to it. Its spectrum range includes most Gram-positive organisms and Gram-negative bacilli. It has, however (unlike sulphonamides), difficulty in penetrating the blood/aqueous barrier, thus sulpha drugs are indicated in intra-ocular infections and penicillin for those that are extra-ocular. In cases of deep-seated infections of the lids and orbit, it should be given parenterally, but in superficial infections it is best given as drops or ointment. To maintain an adequate blood concentration, a dose of 500 000 units is recommended daily, unless one of the long-acting varieties is used. Some or these long-acting penicillins retain their effectiveness for several days. Penicillin is also available in the form of capsules, tablets or syrup for children. But penicillin by mouth is less effective. The chief indications for general penicillin are such conditions as

orbital cellulitis, acute dacryocystitis and panophthalmitis, etc. Local penicillin can be administered in the following ways:

   a. DROPS OR OINTMENT: This is effective in Gram-positive infections but most surgeons now prefer chloramphenicol on account of its broader spectrum in the Gram-negative range.
   b. SUBCONJUNCTIVAL INJECTION: This is a useful method of treatment for anterior segment infections. It produces an immediate and high concentration in the anterior chamber and its action is prolonged. Penicillin thus used must be freshly prepared from the pure (white) penicillin crystals. The yellow amorphous variety is impure and irritating. This treatment was very popular but in the past decade it is less commonly employed.
   c. PURE PENICILLIN CRYSTALS: These may be placed on a corneal ulcer after cocainizing. This is an excellent and safe method of treatment for hypopyon ulcers. It rapidly produces a high penicillin concentration in the anterior chamber. Only the pure crystals may be used in this way.
   d. INJECTION INTO THE ANTERIOR CHAMBER: In very serious infections of the anterior segment, a few minims of intra-ocular fluid can be withdrawn with a needle and syringe and penicillin 10 000 u/ml can be substituted. This method should be reserved for serious cases where subconjunctival injection has been tried and failed. This treatment is seldom undertaken now.
   e. INTRA-VITREOUS INJECTIONS: These have been attempted in serious cases of panophthalmitis, but the reports are very discouraging. It is a heroic measure not to be recommended, and only to be attempted when there is no hope of vision remaining in the affected eye. The eye is a 'write-off' so far as vision is concerned so the patient would be cosmetically better off if it was removed and a good artificial one fitted.
2. STREPTOMYCIN: This has a fair spectrum, especially against tuberculous and some Gram-negative infections. Its most important action is, of course, against the tubercle bacillus. It has the disadvantages of being toxic and necessitating a prolonged course. It is most effective when given in conjunction with PAS.
3. BROAD-SPECTRUM DRUGS: These are effective against a wide variety of bacteria and against some of the larger viruses. In ophthalmology they are unable to produce an adequate concentration in the intra-ocular fluid except when administered locally in ointment form. The broad-spectrum drugs in frequent use are:
   a. CHLORAMPHENICOL is widely used for local application in ophthalmology. It is very effective and its spectrum is more comprehensive than that of penicillin. In fact as far as local treatment is concerned, chloramphenicol could justifiably say to penicillin

in the words of a popular song, 'Anything you can do, I can do better!'

b. TETRACYCLINE: This is a valuable antibiotic and is used under various names, such as achromycin, aureomycin, neomycin, and tetramycin, etc. It is one of the most effective so far as spectrum is concerned. A large number of Gram-positive and Gram-negative organisms respond to it. It is also effective against the virus of trachoma, inclusion blennorrhoea and lymphogranuloma. It has, however, much difficulty in penetrating the blood/aqueous barrier or even entering the anterior chamber through the conjunctival sac. Its use is therefore limited to superficial ocular and lid infections.

c. THE POLYMYXINS: These are chiefly effective against Gram-negative infections. It is, however, one of the few antibiotics which include *Ps. pyocyanea* in its spectrum range. In these infections it is best used in the form of drops or conjunctival injection.

d. SOFRAMYCIN is a comparatively recent antibiotic which includes most Gram-positive cocci and Gram-negative bacilli in its

PROPRIETARY NAME	MAKER	THERAPEUTIC INGREDIENT(S)
Achromycin	Lederle	Tetracycline
Albucid	British Schering	Sulphacetamide
Aureomycin	Lederle	Chlortetracycline
Benadryl	Parke Davis & Co.	Diphenhydramine
Brolene	May & Baker	Dibromopropamidine
Chloromycetin	Parke Davis & Co.	Chloramphenicol
Cortucid	British Schering	Sulphacetamide. Hydrocortisone
Dendrid	Alcon	Idoxuridine (IDU)
Framygen	Fison	Framycetin sulphate
Gantrisin	Roche	Sulphafurazole
Genticin	British Schering	Gentamicin sulphate
Isoptocetamide	Alcon	Sulphacetamide
Kerecid	Smith, Kline & French	Idoxuridine (IDU)
Myciguent	Upjohn	Neomycin
Neosporin	Burroughs Wellcome & Co.	Neomycin and Polymyxin B. Gramicidin
Nivemycin	Boots	Neomycin
Ocusol	Boots	Sulphacetamide and zinc
Otrivine-Antistin	Ciba	Xylometazoline hydrochloride. Antazoline sulphate
Polyfax	Burroughs Wellcome & Co.	Polymyxin B. Bacitracin
Soframycin	Roussel	Framycetin
Sulfomyl	Bayer	*p*-Sulphonamide benzylene
Terramycin	Pfizer	Oxytetracycline
Terramycin Polymixin B	Pfizer	Oxytetracycline. Polymyxin B
Vasocon-A	Smith, Miller & Patch	Chloramphenicol. Polymyxin B
Vasosulf	Smith, Miller & Patch	Sulphacetamide

spectrum. It is particularly effective against *Ps. pyocyanea* and, being non-irritating, it is an excellent drug for subconjunctival injections, as well as for use in the form of ointment.

4. ANTIVIRAL DRUGS: So far, those put on the market have not stood the test of prolonged clinical trial. Indeed, many have proved most disappointing. Experimental work is still going on and it is possible that there may be a dramatic breakthrough in the near future in this exciting new field of therapeutics.

To sum up: chemotherapy and antibiotics in ophthalmology are most effective in eye infections caused by one or more of the organisms mentioned in the list below. It is also of value in the hands of an expert in serious deep-seated infections, especially those of a fulminating type.

SPECTRUM TABLE OF ANTIBIOTICS

	PENICILLIN	STREPTOMYCIN	TETRACYCLINE	CHLORAMPHENICOL	ERYTHROMYCIN	POLYMYXIN	BACITRACIN	SULPHACETAMIDE	NEOMYCIN
Staph. aureus	A	A	A	A	A	X	A	X	A
Dip. pneumoniae	A	A	A	A	A	X	A	X	X
Strep. pyogenes	A	A	A	X	A	X	A	X	X
Cl. welchii	A	X	A	X	A	X	A	—	X
Cl. tetani	A	X	A	X	A	X	A	—	X
Kl. pneumoniae	X	A	A	A	X	X	X	A	A
Esch. coli	X	A	A	A	X	X	X	A	A
H. influenzae	X	X	A	A	X	X	X	A	X
Ps. pyocyanea	X	X	X	X	X	A	X	X	A
Morax lacutanus	X	A	A	—	—	—	—	—	—
Proteus vulgaris	X	A	X	X	X	X	X	X	A
N. gonorrhoeoe	A	A	A	A	A	A	A	A	X
Tr. pallida	A	X	A	A	—	X	A	X	—
M. tuberculosis	X	A	X	X	X	X	—	X	X

A denotes *in vivo* activity.

X denotes no *in vivo* activity.

— denotes no reliable information available.

In connection with the above it should be noted that this table should be taken only as a guide to clinical usage. The activity of various antibiotics in clinical usage is variable according to the site of the infection, the change in the sensitivity of the infecting organism and the presence of other antibiotics. It should not be inferred that *in vivo* activity necessarily means that these antibiotics will be active when instilled into the conjunctival sac, for this route of administration is affected by many factors. (The authors acknowledge indebtedness to the Professional Services Department of Messrs. Smith, Miller & Patch for help in preparing this table.)

CHEMOTHERAPY AND ANTIBIOTICS IN EYE DISEASES 243

The 'in-between' cases, which are more of the nature of an inflammation than an infection and prove the greatest problem to the oculist, are not influenced by this modern treatment. Local therapy is also of undoubted value in preoperative cases where operation has had to be postponed owing to the presence of pyogenic organisms in the conjunctival sac. Likewise, it is used by many surgeons postoperatively as a prophylactic measure against infection.

In the list on page 241 the authors have tried to include most of the proprietary antibiotics and chemotherapeutic agents used in ophthalmology, together with the name of the maker and the therapeutic ingredients.

Chapter XXVI

CORTICOSTEROIDS IN OPHTHALMOLOGY

'Be not the first by whom the new are tried,
Nor yet the last to cast the old aside.' ALEXANDER POPE, *An Essay on Criticism*

IN 1949 Hench and other workers from the Mayo Clinic reported that two hormones, one from the cortical portion of the suprarenal gland, and the other from the pituitary gland, had had remarkable success in the treatment of rheumatoid arthritis. These compounds are dehydrocorticosterone and the adrenocorticotrophic hormone, and are known as cortisone and ACTH respectively. Later, experiments were made in the treatment of numerous other diseases and they were found to be outstandingly successful, particularly in allergic conditions. These discoveries led other workers to experiment in the sphere of ophthalmic therapeutics with very considerable success. Indeed it would be true to say that corticosteroid therapy has been the greatest single contribution to ophthalmology in recent years. Such widely differing diseases as sympathetic ophthalmia, iritis, tuberculous uveitis, interstitial keratitis, atropine irritation, spring catarrh, etc., have shown an improvement which can only be described as dramatic.

Mode of Action: The actual method whereby these hormones produce their therapeutic results is still unknown, but the *modus operandi* is as follows:

ACTH: Amongst other hormones the pituitary secretes the adrenocorticotrophic hormones. It has been shown that when ACTH is injected intramuscularly the suprarenal cortex gives a prompt response by increasing its normal hormone secretion. The use of ACTH, a powerful suprarenal stimulant, presupposes the presence of a normally functioning suprarenal gland, and its prolonged use would, at any rate in theory, run the risk of causing Cushing's syndrome (muscular weakness, hirsutism, hypertension and amenorrhoea).

CORTISONE, on the other hand, acts directly as other hormones do when injected (e.g. pituitrin), but its continued use is liable to cause suprarenal cortical atrophy. It can, however, be used in cases of suprarenal dysfunction (e.g. Addison's disease), where there would be no response to ACTH.

Method of Administration: ACTH cannot, of course, be used locally. It is given by injection only. Cortisone may be used either locally or generally.

Since Hench's original work, considerable advances have been made in this form of hormone therapy, largely due to the discovery of the following:

HYDROCORTISONE, which has proved to be more effective and powerful than cortisone when used locally.

PREDNISONE AND PREDNISOLONE: These preparations are preferable to ACTH for systemic use as they are less toxic and less liable to side-effects than ACTH. They can be used for any ophthalmic condition for which ACTH was indicated.

Contra-indications:
 1. Gross hypertension.
 2. Chronic nephritis.
 3. Unstabilized diabetes.
 4. Dendritic ulcer.
 5. Peptic ulcer.

General Remarks on Treatment: The immediate effect of steroid treatment is to reduce the exudative and inflammatory processes and to inhibit fibroblast formation and tissue repair. It decreases capillary permeability and reduces vascularization and fibrosis. All these effects, though highly desirable and helpful, are not in themselves curative, therefore steroid therapy should be regarded as an adjunct to whatever antibiotic or treatment may be required.

It is of greatest value in acute cases, and the more anterior the inflammation the more effective. Probably its greatest value lies in the fact that, unlike antibiotic drugs, it is effective in *inflammation* where no *infection* is present. Hence, it is of great value in ocular allergic conditions and in such inflammations as iritis, etc. In short, the function of steroid therapy in eye diseases is to help in checking acute inflammatory and exudative processes until such time as other factors (the natural defences of the body, antibiotics, etc.) overcome the cause of the trouble. This is a valuable contribution indeed when it is borne in mind how rapidly untreated exudative conditions can cause blindness.

Method of Treatment: Generally speaking, local treatment is the method of choice for anterior segment infections, and general treatment for infections of the posterior segments.
 1. LOCAL TREATMENT: Corticosteroids can be given as drops or ointment, or can be injected subconjunctivally if more prolonged action is required. It must, however, be remembered that prolonged local therapy is not without its dangers as it can produce a marked rise in tension, especially in patients with open angle glaucoma and even in those with a strong familial history of glaucoma. Therefore, patients on prolonged local treatment should have their tensions checked every 2 or 3 weeks.

2. GENERAL TREATMENT: Dosage of corticosteroids must be individually assessed for each patient, the golden rule being the smallest possible dose over the shortest possible period of time. In acute cases large doses should be given for the first 2 or 3 days only and this should be followed by a much reduced maintenance dose just sufficient to keep the inflammation under control.

All treatment, both local and general, should be stopped as soon as possible.

CORTICOSTEROIDS USED IN OPHTHALMOLOGY

PROPRIETARY NAME	MAKER	THERAPEUTIC INGREDIENT(S)
Betnesol	Glaxo	Betamethasone
Betnesol-N	Glaxo	Betamethasone. Neomycin
Chloromycetin hydrocortisone	Parke Davis	Chloramphenicol. Hydrocortisone
Codelsol	Merck, Sharp & Dohme	Prednisolone. Neomycin
Cortistab	Boots	Cortisone
Cortisyl	Roussel	Cortisone
Cortocaps	Boots	Hydrocortisone. Neomycin
Ef-Cortelan	Glaxo	Hydrocortisone. Neomycin
Ef-Cortelan-N	Glaxo	Hydrocortisone. Neomycin
Framycort	Ophthalmic Fison	Framycetin. Hydrocortisone
Hydrocortistab	Boots	Hydrocortisone
Hydrocortisyl	Roussel	Hydrocortisone
Hydrocortone	Merck, Sharp & Dohme	Hydrocortisone
Hydromycin-D	Boots	Prednisolone. Neomycin
Ledercort with Neomycin	Lederle	Triamcinolone. Neomycin
Maxidex	Alcon	Dexamethasone. Phenylephrine
Maxitrol	Alcon	Dexamethasone. Neomycin. Polymyxin B
Neo-Cortet	Upjohn	Neomycin. Hydrocortisone
Predsol	Glaxo	Prednisolone
Predsol-N	Glaxo	Prednisolone. Neomycin
Sofradex	Roussel	Dexamethasone. Framycetin. Gramicidin

In the list shown above the authors have tried to include most of the proprietary corticosteroid preparations more commonly used in ophthalmology, together with the name of the maker and the therapeutic ingredients.

Indications:
1. LOCAL TREATMENT: The following diseases normally respond to local corticosteroid treatment:
    Blepharoconjunctivitis
    Chemical burns of cornea and conjunctiva
    Dermatitis of lids
    Episcleritis

Iridocyclitis[1]
Iritis[1]
Keratitis in most forms
Phlyctenular conjunctivitis
Scleritis

2. GENERAL STEROID THERAPY is essential and invaluable in the following conditions:

    Posterior uveitis
    Sympathetic ophthalmia
    Temporal arteritis

    It is contraindicated in dendritic ulcers. Patients with non-granulomatous iritis and sarcoid uveitis may require oral steroids in addition.

3. GENERAL TREATMENT: This is of greatest value in sympathetic ophthalmia and should also be given in posterior uveitis and temporal arteritis.

In any chronic infection steroid therapy is unlikely to be of benefit, and in degenerative cases it is completely useless.

---

[1] These conditions may require oral treatment in addition.

Chapter XXVII

ALLERGY IN OPHTHALMOLOGY

ALL allergic manifestations are caused by a hypersensitivity to a specific antigen and the actual attack is precipitated by the contact of this antigen with the hypersensitive cells. While much of allergy is a tangled skein which requires the combined efforts of physician, pathologist, biochemist and ophthalmologist to unravel, a few threads have emerged which, if followed, may lead to some partial disentanglement. It is now known that this hypersensitivity is of three distinct clinical varieties: (1) Anaphylactic; (2) Pollen sensitivity; (3) Bacterial sensitivity.

The first two varieties of hypersensitivity are due to proteins and the reaction is prompt and characterized by urticaria, an increased capillary permeability, and contraction of smooth muscle. These phenomena are probably due to the liberation of histamine. Bacterial hypersensitivity is caused by contact of the tissues with living or dead bacteria or viruses. In this type the onset is not so sudden and it may take 24–48 hours to develop. The following allergic manifestations are seen in ophthalmology:

Lids: Probably the commonest form is seen in atropine or boracic irritation, but the subcutaneous oedema caused by exposure to primulas, *Rhus toxicodendron* and other plant pollens is well known.

Conjunctiva: Acute conjunctivitis is frequently associated with hay fever. Oedema, lacrimation and gross congestion with complete absence of mucopurulent discharge is characteristic of allergic conjunctivitis. Spring catarrh is almost certainly an allergic complaint.

Cornea: The modern tendency is to regard more and more corneal diseases as of allergic origin. Phlyctenular disease, recurrent marginal ulcers, superficial punctate keratitis and acne rosacea keratitis may be directly or indirectly due to hypersensitivity to viruses. The same may well be true of some of the deeper forms of keratitis which are associated with uveitis, e.g. tuberculous keratitis, insterstitial keratitis, etc.

Uveal Tract: The role played by uveal pigment acting as an antigen in sympathetic ophthalmia has already been discussed. Few observers noting the severe reaction seen in certain cases of iridocyclitis after tuberculin injections can account for them on anything other than an allergic basis. It is highly probable that chronic uveitis due to focal sepsis is an instance of bacterial allergy, and it may well be that the uncommon syndrome known as Behçet's syndrome may be a manifestation of ocular sensitivity to bacterial antigens found in the buccal ulcers with which it is associated.

Enough has been written to show that the diagnosis of ocular allergy is a complicated matter and when the vast gap in our knowledge has been bridged, as bridged it undoubtedly will be by careful observation and competent research, new fields will be opened up for treatment. Until that day the oculist should bear in mind that an allergic condition is an ever-present possibility and he should be prepared to cooperate with the physician and pathologist in an endeavour to make his contribution towards this end.

Treatment of Ocular Allergy:
1. ISOLATION: Most important of all is isolation from the allergen responsible for the condition. This involves an accurate diagnosis, and except in the more obvious conditions it is far from easy, and if the allergen is an unusual one it will tax the ingenuity of Sherlock Holmes and the patience of Job.
2. DESENSITIZATION: This presupposes that a specific antigen has been discovered. It is a long and wearisome process and is in the province of the allergist and beyond the scope of the practising ophthalmologist. It should be noted that the tuberculin treatment of iridocyclitis and phlyctenular disease almost amounts to a desensitization.
3. LOCAL TREATMENT: Local steroid therapy often gives prompt relief. It is best used in ointment or drop form.
4. ANTIHISTAMINE TREATMENT: This is very effective, particularly if the ocular condition is associated with urticaria or other skin eruption. This should be given in severe cases in addition to local steroids. Evidence at the moment points to the efficacy of these drugs in the pollen and anaphylactic varieties, but there is nothing to suggest that they influence allergy of bacterial origin.

Chapter XXVIII

SLIT-LAMP MICROSCOPY

During the 1914–18 War, when nearly all the nations of Europe were intent on destroying each other, the Swiss were fortunate in being able to concentrate on more peaceful things, and when the other nations emerged from the welter of bloodshed, they were confronted by an instrument that was destined to revolutionize the diagnosis of eye diseases more than any other discovery since that of the ophthalmoscope. Professor Vogt, of Zürich, had perfected the slit-lamp that was invented by Gullstrand in 1911.

The principle of the slit-lamp is simple. All are familiar with the appearance of a streak of bright light entering a darkened room such as sunlight through an open letter-box, and in his childhood days the reader must have been struck by the way this illumination shows up floating particles of dust, etc. This actual principle is utilized in slit-lamp examination, with one important addition: objects within the rays of the beam are examined under magnification. In perfecting the slit-lamp Vogt produced an instrument that could accurately focus a slit of light of variable thickness. With this, he combined a binocular microscope that could give stereoscopic vision together with a magnification from 9 to 103 diameters, and which was capable of being focused upon the slit of light. A head-rest to fix the patient's head completed his very ingenious instrument.

Technique of Slit-lamp Examination:
1. DIFFUSE ILLUMINATION: With the beam out of focus the entire cornea can be seen in bright illumination under magnification and stereoscopically.
2. DIRECT FOCAL ILLUMINATION: This consists in getting the image of the slit sharply focused on the object being examined. Direct focal illumination can be employed in two ways:
    a. WITH THE BROAD BEAM: This is an excellent method for examining gross lesions under bright illumination, e.g. corneal nebulae, iris nodules, etc.
    b. WITH THE NARROW BEAM (OPTICAL SECTION): This entails exact focusing of the slit image and it gives less illumination, but it is an excellent method of estimating the depth of a corneal lesion.
3. RETRO-ILLUMINATION: In this method the object is examined by light reflected backwards from structures posterior to it. It thus appears as a direct silhouette against a light background. This technique is very useful for examining the iris for atrophy of its pigment layer.

4. SPECULAR REFLECTION: In this examination, the microscope is directed along the path of the reflected light. It requires some practice to master this technique but once this is accomplished it is possible to examine the cellular details of the reflecting surface.
5. SCLEROTIC SCATTER: In this method the beam is focused obliquely on the corneoscleral junction. This produces a halo of light around the entire cornea and furthermore the light passes through the cornea by internal reflection. Any lesion affecting the corneal transparency is immediately obvious. Another advantage of this method of examination is that much less light enters the patient's eye, hence causing the minimum of discomfort.

With the above methods, it is possible to examine the eye as far back as the anterior portion of the vitreous, but the farther back the slit is directed, the more light is 'used up' and the less satisfactory is the result. There is one other important point to remember in slit-lamp examination: the question of magnification. It is obvious that the higher the magnification the more are the slightest ocular movements magnified. For this reason a really high magnification is impossible in the living eye. Those generally employed are $\times 9$, $\times 23$ and $\times 35$, and of these the $\times 23$ is the best for general use.

Examination of the Conjunctiva: Slit-lamp examination is of value in revealing aneurysmal dilatations of vessels, such as 'blood lakes' in old mustard-gas lesions.

Examination of Cornea: The limbal region should be examined in cases of suspected vitamin B_2 deficiency where vessels grow straight out from the limbal arches all around the cornea of each eye. Corneal corpuscles can be seen and wandering cells that have entered in response to inflammation. The corneal nerves are visible dividing dichotomously, and blood vessels otherwise invisible can be seen by retro-illumination in cases of interstitial keratitis. The exact depth of foreign bodies, corneal opacities, etc., can be ascertained by optical section. In addition to this, in suitable cases the following phenomena can be observed:

HASSEL–HENLE BODIES, which are proliferations of normal endothelium occasionally seen in elderly patients.

HUDSON–STAHLI LINE at the level of the closure of the lids. This is due to some form of chronic irritation.

DYSTROPHIES of various types where the whole of the substantia propria is altered, or in other forms where the endothelial or epithelial layers alone are affected.

KAYSER–FLEISCHER'S RING can be seen in hepatolenticular degeneration. It consists of a brown ring in the region of the arcus senilis and is diagnostic of Wilson's disease.

KERATIC PRECIPITATES can be studied as to shape, distribution, etc.

OEDEMA ('bedewing') is well seen by retro-illumination.

Examination of the Anterior Chamber: The normal anterior chamber cannot be examined because it is optically empty. Descemet's membrane should first be located and examined, because any abnormality in the anterior chamber (keratitis punctata, etc.) will manifest itself there. Its depth can easily be ascertained by optical section, and indeed slit-lamp examination is often useful in deciding whether an anterior chamber is present or not. Retro-illumination should always be used, for this reveals keratitis punctata at a glance; and if any doubt as to whether objects seen are keratitis punctata or corneal opacities, examination should be made with the optical section, which will reveal their exact situation at once. The pinhole instead of the slit beam is best used when looking for aqueous 'flare' which is due to proteins in the intra-ocular fluid and is a valuable and early sign of aqueous inflammation. If actual cells are present in large numbers, some of these may be seen also. Owing to heat convection the aqueous rises up by the iris and down by the cornea, hence cells which get caught in this thermal current are seen in a vertical line known as Turk's line. The slit-lamp is valuable in the early diagnosis of sympathetic ophthalmia. It shows in an injured eye whether suspected keratitis punctata are really keratitis punctata or aggregations of lens matter, and if the sympathizing eye shows aqueous flare or cells, it is high time to remove the exciting one.

Examination of the Iris: This is the easiest structure to examine. Diffuse and retro-illumination should both be employed. If an Argyll Robertson pupil is suspected, the slit-lamp will decide a problem which is often difficult and sometimes impossible to decide by any other method. This also applies to Wernicke's hemianopic pupil (*see* p. 205). Persistent pupillary membrane can be seen and synechiae may be visible which cannot be seen in any other way. Stereoscopic magnification of an iris nodule may reveal blood vessels, etc., and give the impression of solidity which will enable the diagnosis of a new growth to be made quite easily. In cases of traumatic mydriasis, a tear in the sphincter muscle can sometimes be seen. New vessels in some cases of iritis are only visible by the slit-lamp.

Examination of the Lens: Owing to the depth of the lens it is not easy to get the microscope and the light focused together, and it is best to commence with the broad beam and to locate the Y sutures. Next, the optical section should be used to reveal the zones of discontinuity. The light should be directed as nearly through the centre of the lens as possible, therefore the angle between the light and the

CLASSIFICATION OF LENS OPACITIES BY SLIT-LAMP

Types of Congenital Cataract	*Types of Acquired Cataract*
Punctate opacities (blue or white)	Endocrine (subcapsular) cataract
Crystalline opacities (endocrine type)	Dermatogenous cataract
Clefts	Heat ray cataract
Flat opacities	Diabetic cataract
Vacuoles	Senile cataract
Corkscrew opacities	Traumatic (stellate) cataract
Spiral opacities	Complicated cataract
Nummular cataract	
Lamellar cataract	
Suture cataract	
Axial cataract	
Equatorial cataract	
Reduplicated cataract	

microscope should be a narrow one. In the zone of specular reflection with the broad beam the coarsely granular appearance (shagreen) of the anterior surface and the finer posterior surface can be seen. Retro-illumination will reveal any opacity. Embryonic remains (stellar dust) can be seen on the anterior capsule, but for hyaloid remains a search should be made posterior and to the nasal side of the posterior Y suture. In traumatic cases Vossius ring may be visible. Lens opacities, congenital or otherwise, can be studied with a wealth of detail and can be classified with a greater degree of accuracy than is possible with any other form of clinical examination. The table above will give an idea of the varieties of classifications possible with the aid of the slit-lamp.

While under normal conditions slit-lamp examination is only used as far back as the anterior vitreous, there is a method whereby the posterior vitreous and even the central part of the fundus can be examined. If a contact lens with a flat anterior surface is placed on the patient's eye, the beam from the slit-lamp will reach the retina, and the central portion, including the disc and macula, can be seen binocularly and under high magnification. This is very useful in the diagnosis of unusual retinal cysts, holes, tumours, etc. Full dilatation is essential for this examination.

Gonioscopy: A further valuable function of the slit-lamp is the examination of the angle of the anterior chamber which is invisible by any other form of clinical examination. It is, of course, of paramount importance in the diagnosis of glaucoma. In order to see the angle, the patient must wear a Goldmann contact lens which contains a mirror set at an angle to deflect the slit-lamp beam on to the angle of the anterior chamber. By this means the whole of this most important region is brought into view and can be studied binocularly and under high magnification.

Enough has been written to show that a slit-lamp is as necessary a part of the modern oculist's equipment as his ophthalmoscope. Every student should take whatever opportunities present themselves for becoming familiar with the technique of this examination, for it is only by repeated use that its value becomes obvious and the interpretation of findings becomes accurate and helpful.

Chapter XXIX

RECENT ADVANCES IN OPHTHALMIC PRACTICE

DURING the past decade there have been a number of important advances in the diagnosis and treatment of some eye diseases. It will be appreciated that these are not yet available to many of the smaller hospitals and that much work has yet to be done in assessing their value and interpreting their results. A brief description of these trends is appended to enable the student to be aware of the general principles involved in ultrasound, fluorescein angiography and lasers.

ULTRASOUND IN OPHTHALMOLOGY
'The sound must seem an echo to the sense.' ALEXANDER POPE, *An Essay on Criticism*

Ultrasound examination is one of the more recent trends in ophthalmology. Although it is in a comparatively early stage it is possible to record the strength of echoes obtained from normal and pathological tissues in the eye. The strength of the echoes helps in differential diagnosis, giving some indication as to the density of the ocular tissues examined. Visual diagnosis, when possible, is much to be preferred but where this is not possible ultrasound is a useful accessory rather comparable with transillumination.

A metal object causes a much higher echo than blood or tumour tissue. On this principle differentiation can be made between various normal and pathological tissues which may be present.

As an aid to diagnosis this is helpful in cases of opaque media, subretinal lesions, foreign bodies invisible to X-rays, retrobulbar tumours, vitreous haemorrhages, etc. Diagnostic units are now available in portable form with rechargeable batteries. Sound probing is done through the globe or in the orbit behind the globe. It must be remembered that ultrasonic waves are liable to reflection, refraction and absorption, just as light waves are. Any changes in acoustic densities are recorded on an echograph and in cases of solid tumours, like carcinomata, the echoes differ from those given by fluid cysts, etc. At present the greatest practical use of ultrasound is in the location and removal of non-magnetic foreign bodies.

LASERS IN OPHTHALMOLOGY
Hazards from Exposure to Laser Beams:
'He saw; but blasted with excess of light,
  Closed his eyes in endless night' [Milton]. THOMAS GRAY, *The Progress of Poesy*

The word 'laser' is made up from the first letter of each principal word of the following sentence: Light Amplified by Stimulated

256 A SYNOPSIS OF OPHTHALMOLOGY

Emission of Radiation. The first laser was used in 1960 with a ruby crystal and since that date incredible progress has been made in its development and intensity. Lasers are now in daily use in many industries and laboratories. During the next few years they will no doubt become of greater importance and more widespread in use, thus adding another hazard to the human eye, but to offset this the ophthalmic surgeon has found in them another valuable therapeutic weapon. Some lasers can give an immensely powerful beam so dangerous that unless rigid precautions are observed the risk to sight and health can be very great indeed. It has been calculated that the intensity of a low-power laser beam on the retina is vastly greater than the intensity of the sun's image. The effect therefore of a high-power beam would be catastrophic. All establishments where such lasers are in use have every possible built-in safety device. For instance, nobody must enter the laboratory when the beam is on and opening the door of such a laboratory automatically switches off the beam. At the other end of the scale, a weak laser device is built into an ophthalmoscope handle which is comparatively harmless to anything other than the delicate ocular tissues. Experimental work chiefly in America has shown that exposure to lasers can produce a large number of pathological changes in various animals. Changes in the blood, brain, nervous system, skin, bone, teeth, cornea, iris, lens and retina can be produced. Therefore such a potent device demands the most wholesome respect as an infinitesimally short direct exposure could result in instant and irreparable damage to the macula similar to that seen in an eclipse burn. On the other hand, with reasonable precautions there seems so far to be no long-term bad results amongst those who work with lasers. One of the authors (C. M.-D.) has examined approximately 70 experimental officers working on lasers every year for more than 10 years and no untoward findings were recorded except in one patient who decided to look at a laser beam through a spectroscope! This of course was the height of folly and is not a normal risk.

Lasers in Ophthalmic Surgery: A description of lasers is highly technical and beyond the scope of this work. Suffice it to say that most lasers have a ruby beam. It has been found, however, that the argon beam has advantages in ocular surgery. In an editorial article in the *American Medical Association Journal* dated 18 November, 1968, there is a heading 'A Bright New Light Glows in Eye Surgery'. In this the claim is made that the intense blue-green light of an argon laser is readily absorbed by vascular tissues and haemoglobin. The red beam of the ruby laser is not absorbed so well and in patients treated for diabetic retinopathy the damage was less with the argon instrument. Argon radiation requires one-fifth of the energy of xenon and one-eleventh of the energy of the ruby laser. This involves less damage to the surrounding areas. A laser ophthalmoscope has been devised in which accidental damage to tissues being treated is largely eliminated. It consists of an optical system designed to illuminate the target with a beam of light. The system includes a reflector and light-transmitting region which can remove part of the beam to produce a dark aiming spot within the illuminated area. A laser beam can then be focused in the light-transmitting area and is directed to follow the same path as the illuminated beam so that the laser beam and the aiming spot are brought into a common focus. Unfortunately the cost of these laser ophthalmoscopes is very high indeed, hence they are not normally available to small clinics or hospitals. The indications for laser surgery are detailed under the various diseases to which such treatment may be helpful; these include detached retinae, melanomata, angiomatosis, Eales's disease, retinitis proliferans and most especially diabetic retinopathy.

The Dangers of Photocoagulation by Lasers are:
1. Field loss in treated areas.
2. Large arcuate scotomata in lesions treated near disc.
3. Macular damage by an accidental direct hit.
4. Haemorrhage from large vessels (e.g. angiomatosis retinae, etc.).

Fluorescein Angiography of the fundus is of increasing value in diagnosis and in assessing the results of treatment. Five ml of a 10 per cent solution are injected intravenously and the fundus examined and photographed at frequent intervals. Fluorescence of the choroid is seen very soon and later the arterioles and veins fluoresce. In normal retinae this disappears within half an hour. An undue amount of fluorescence is due to new vessel formation, increased permeability of capillaries and atrophy of the pigment epithelium. In diabetic retinopathy scattered fluorescent dots are present and large haemorrhages are seen as dark areas in a fluorescent background. Malignant choroidal melanomata fluoresce as also do some metastatic tumours. In cases of papilloedema the vascular nerve head shows well. Japanese ophthalmologists have been amongst the leaders in this field of research, doubtless aided by their technological skill in making fundus cameras. Professors Shikano and Shimizo of Tokyo have produced an *Atlas of Fluorescence Fundus Photography* illustrating the advantages of this new diagnostic method. In retinal fluoroscopy a really first-class fundus camera is a *sine qua non*. The difficulty in fluorographs is in the interpretation of results when pathological conditions are present but as an adjunct to the ophthalmoscope and the retinal camera it is helpful in the diagnoses of macular disorders, central retinopathy, fundus tumours and oedema of the optic nerve head.

HELPING THE BLIND TO SEE

'Bring forth the people who are blind, yet have eyes.' ISAIAH 43: 8 (RSV)

Blind people, especially those who were born blind or who became blind in childhood, have an almost uncanny ability to get about aided by echoes from tapping with a stick. When sight is lost, other senses become extra acute, especially the senses of hearing and touch. In past years one of the authors (C. M.-D.) used to take out boys from the Worcester College for the Blind to spend an afternoon and evening in his home. One boy (who had only visited the author's home twice previously) remarked: 'You live in the third road on the left past the Eye Hospital; don't you?' When asked how he knew this he explained that he 'heard' the breaks in the houses in built-up areas where sideroads joined the main one. What he 'heard' was the different echo as the car passed the sideroads. On another occasion the author was taking a car load of these boys back to the college late in the evening in a thick fog and at a very slow pace. On reaching a bifurcation of the road the author took the wrong turn when one of the boys remarked: 'Doctor, I believe you have taken the wrong turn.' The blind boy discovered this before the driver!

Technology is now taking a hand in aiding these remarkable innate gifts and in creating an awareness of obstacles in the path of blind people. Research has been going on in Nottingham since 1967 by Dr. Armstrong into electronic helps and this has been described in *Pulse*, 4 September, 1973, p. 13. These consist of a torch-shaped transmitter and receiver which sends out sonic waves that hit objects and bounce back. The rebound waves are transmitted to the ears and give the patient an impression of something ahead. The difficulty of course lay in the interpretation of the signals. The next move was to mount the aid by a strap to the forehead thus leaving the patient with two free hands and providing a steadier base for the aid. This was used with a longer and lighter cane than usual. Research is now being directed to producing a sonic beam that becomes louder as it nears the obstruction.

More recently, Kay of Canterbury University, Christchurch, N.Z., has designed a similar sonic aid that gives the blind non-visual perception by means of meaningful audible sound. This aid is mounted on a spectacle frame and sounds are conducted through earphones on the arms of the spectacle. These earphones do not block out natural sounds. Kay reports that after training patients have an enhanced environmental sense and greater confidence in getting about. It does not help in open spaces but is very useful in built-up areas where pedestrians abound and where traffic noises mask other auditory helps.

Unfortunately older people who become blind never develop this extra hearing sense and it is seldom possible to teach blind patients Braille if they are over 60 years of age. They could never cope with the new electronic aids. The 'talking book' and of course the radio are the only technological help for them.

AUTOMATIC SELF-OPERATED RECORDING PERIMETER

This instrument, known as the *Ocutron*, is very scarce at the time of writing and no detailed description or assessment of results is yet available. It is a hemispherical bowl with perforations through which lights are shown singly. The patient presses a button when the light is visible and the position is automatically recorded. The patient is supposed to be able to record his own fields but it would seem to the authors that accurate results would vary directly with the intelligence of the patient!

THE OPERATING MICROSCOPE

For many years aural surgeons have been using this valuable aid to surgery but their ophthalmic colleagues have been slow off the mark in adapting themselves to this new technique with the result that it has only been in fairly general use in recent years. Previously, eye surgeons have contented themselves with binocular loupes or prismatic spectacles which gave a magnification of not more than $\times 2$ to $\times 2.5$. They were hesitant to use a greater magnification owing to the resulting reduction in depth and width of the operating field. Another cause for this hesitation is the well-known fact that the greater the magnification the more the patient's movements are magnified. This fact is well known to anyone who has looked through a $\times 20$ pair of binoculars instead of the usual $\times 8$. It is difficult to hold them still enough to get a proper view. In these days anaesthetic techniques have advanced so rapidly that it is possible to ensure a good quiet general anaesthesia with the patients absolutely still.

Ophthalmic microscopes can be obtained with a zoom type of lens that can be altered at will from $\times 4$ to $\times 25$ magnification or for those who prefer a fixed magnification at $\times 10$ is usual. The operating distance averages 300 mm and the objectives vary from 125 mm to 200 mm, the latter being the more popular. Foot controls for focusing and magnification are essential as they leave the hands free for operating. Double microscopes are available for use by an assistant or for teaching.

Operating under magnification offers considerable advantages:
1. It makes it possible to use extremely fine suture material.
2. It gives a much better defined and more accurate view of pathological or damaged tissues hence making it easier to differentiate these tissues from the normal.
3. It gives an adequate view of structures previously considered too minute to deal with surgically.

Going from the general to the particular advantages, it greatly assists in the suturing of delicate structures such as corneal grafts, cataract sections, etc. It makes possible the removal of deep-seated corneal scars, lamellar grafts with much less risk of perforation than would formally have been the case. It greatly facilitates the removal of foreign bodies from the anterior chamber and any operative procedure in the anterior third of the eye. Filtration operations for glaucoma are better controlled since the canal of Schlemm and the trabeculae are much more clearly seen. Operations involving the lacrimal passages and canaliculi carry a greater prospect of success and a lessened likelihood of surgical damage.

All these advantages, however, demand new techniques from the surgeon. An operating microscope is rigid and immobile compared with the loupe and the surgeon's head movements are restricted, demanding more use of wrists and forearms in order to manipulate his instruments. This is helped by the built-in arm rests usually provided. Handling instruments in a smaller and magnified field is strange and awkward at first but these initial difficulties are soon overcome with practice. Vision outside the operating field presents problems to the presbyobic surgeon when he wants to select instruments from the table but this can be overcome with a special pair of half-glasses fitted well down the nose so as not to interfere with his use of the microscope. Finally, immobilization of the patient's head by appropriate head rests is essential whether the patient is under general or local anaesthesia.

Chapter XXX

THE SOCIAL ASPECTS OF BLINDNESS AND PARTIAL SIGHT

'The eye is the lamp of the body . . . if your eye is not sound, your whole body will be in darkness.' ST. MATTHEW 6: 23, 24 (RSV)

IN Great Britain the official definition of a blind person is 'a person so blind as to be unable to perform any work for which eyesight is essential'. This covers a wide range of visual disability from total and complete blindness to severe and deteriorating partial sight. Most ophthalmologists consider that a vision of 3/60 or less in the better eye should be reckoned as blind. Also blindness is assumed to exist even if the visual acuity is fair but the patient has, in addition, 'tunnel vision', i.e. the fields consisting only of a tiny area around the fixation point. Such blindness has to be officially certified by an ophthalmic surgeon on the form BD 8 and when this form is sent in the local authorities take every possible step to help the patient. A specially trained welfare officer is sent to the patient's home to make inquiries and assess the requirements of each individual patient. This officer makes recommendations as to special needs, requirements and training.

Blind people can be classified into one of the following groups each of which vary greatly in their personal social and other problems:

GROUP 1: Those who have been born blind or whose blindness occurs in early infancy.

GROUP 2: Those who have become blind in early childhood or during their school days.

GROUP 3: Those who have become blind during their active and working years.

GROUP 4: Those who become blind late in life.

There are, of course, physical, psychological and social aspects of every blind person and these vary greatly according to the age group at which they become blind.

Groups 1 and 2 find it comparatively easy to come to terms with their disability. Most have only dim memories (if any) of sighted life and they are easy to train for a large variety of useful jobs that enable them to make a valuable contribution to society in all sorts of vocations. There are residential nursery schools for those under 5 years and other residential schools for the 5–16 age group. For those with academic ability there is the College for the Blind at Worcester for boys and the Chorley

Wood College for girls. When they reach adult life, guide dogs are invaluable for those in these two groups.

Group 3 presents the greatest difficulties of all. Their first reaction is unbelief: 'It cannot possibly happen to me', etc. This is followed by a period of depression when much help and encouragement are required if the patient is to avoid the worst of all reactions—self-pity. Later follows a determination to adapt to their handicap. It is particularly important for this age group to learn braille, touch typing and some handicraft in order to keep an interest in life and if possible to get a new job. The greatest fear in this group is that of poverty. This can be dispelled at once for social security, etc., makes sure that such a person can look forward to a future of reasonable comfort even though the patient is unable to learn a new trade. Residential training and guide dogs greatly help this group especially if blindness occurs before middle life.

Patients in group 4 after some initial depression usually learn to come to terms with their trouble and to accept it. Talking books and, of course, the radio give much pleasure to these older people. Their greatest need of all is for people to visit them for a chat and to read the paper to them.

Local authorities through their welfare officers do everything possible to provide help in mitigating the effects of blindness and by helping in rehabilitation, teaching means of communication (braille, etc.) and handicrafts in their own homes, if necessary, but nothing quite takes the place of residential courses if this can be arranged. The Department of Employment and the Royal National Institute for the Blind assist in finding suitable employment in industry, where possible.

In all age groups—children, adult life and old age—every blind patient should be encouraged to be as active and independent as possible. Relatives and friends must remember that the one thing the average blind patient dislikes more than anything else is being fussed over. In infancy and childhood it is all too easy for mother love to develop into 'smother' love with undue protection and a tendency to restrict movements unnecessarily. Too much waiting on a blind patient is not helpful and the worst thing of all is to try to lead them about. It is far better to walk by the patient's side giving a verbal warning of steps ahead and saying how many. The arm should only be taken for the actual negotiation of the steps, pedestrian crossings, etc. These remarks apply equally to adult blind as well as children. They all like to be treated as far as possible as normal people with the minimum of proffered help and no fussing, and never any show of pity. Their attitude can be summarized by a remark made recently to one of the authors (C. M.-D.) by a young blind teacher of English at a girls' public school who was talking about the way some strangers treat her: 'I may be blind but I can cope with that but the one thing I cannot stand is being treated as though I am daft.' *Verbum sapientis satis est.*

SOCIAL ASPECTS OF BLINDNESS AND PARTIAL SIGHT

PARTIAL SIGHT

'I see men as trees walking.' ST. MARK 8: 24 (RSV)

Partial sight also presents problems both of a personal and social nature. These problems largely depend upon the following considerations:

1. The age at which partial sight commences; and
2. Whether the condition is stationary or progressive.

Of these two considerations that of age of incidence is the most important. From the point of view of patients' particular needs and problems, they can be classified into three groups:

GROUP 1: Those who become partially sighted during childhood or school life.

GROUP 2: Those affected in active working life.

GROUP 3: Those affected during retirement or old age.

The difficulties of each of these age groups vary so much that each will be considered separately:

Group 1: Those in this group find the least difficulty in adjusting their lives to the disability but their education depends very largely upon whether the condition is progressive. If it is, eventual blindness must be anticipated and their education arranged accordingly, e.g. no sighted reading must be allowed and braille should be taught at the earliest possible stage. In these cases education at a special school is required. If, however, the condition is not likely to worsen (e.g. congenital nystagmus) normal reading with low visual acuity aids, if necessary, should be encouraged and the child can be educated at a normal school.

Group 2: The problems here arise chiefly from the nature of their occupation and from the prognosis regarding the sight that remains.

OCCUPATION: Those most affected are: (1) Those whose work involves concentrated near vision, e.g. compositors, draughtsmen, engineers using micrometers, etc., and (2) Those requiring perfect distance vision, e.g. railwaymen, drivers, etc.

On the other hand, there are vast numbers of occupations where good near or distance vision is not involved, e.g. agriculture, horticulture, watchmen, storekeepers, shop assistants, some factory work, etc. Many partially sighted patients who have to give up their normal work can find useful employment in some such work where good sight is not essential. It must also be remembered that employers are required by law to employ 3 per cent of disabled persons and they are glad to offer work to the partially sighted or blind if they are otherwise fit and suitable. There is therefore great scope for the partially sighted to find new employment and the welfare officers gladly liaise with others to find suitable re-employment.

It is surprising, however, how a determined and active person can go through life with few but his own family knowing of the disability. One of the authors (C. M.-D.) had a patient who was a master at a grammar school who worked until retiring age although he was unable to see to read anything from the age of 45. His wife used to read his pupils' homework out to him and he assessed the marks. Few of the staff or pupils suspected this, they merely thought he was 'a bit short-sighted'! Another patient was the manager of a large branch of an insurance company. He succeeded in reaching retiring age although he was unable to read any but the largest print for years. None of his staff suspected this possibly because much of his time was spent interviewing clients.

Of course, every partially sighted person must be clearly told that driving a car is out of the question. Many refuse to accept this at first saying that they can see perfectly well enough.

PROGNOSIS: If the patient's condition is likely to lead to actual blindness the patients should be told so that he can be taught braille (if he is not too old) and otherwise come to terms with his trouble. None the less he must be encouraged to remain in his present job for as long as possible. Again the welfare officers are most helpful in sorting out any individual problems and in helping patients to adjust themselves to their new circumstances.

Group 3: Partial sight in old age is usually due to macular changes, cataract or glaucoma. Many such patients progress to blindness eventually but in many cases the progress is so slow that their remaining vision enables them to carry on reasonably well for the remainder of their allotted span of life. Such old folk find it a great comfort if their oculist can truthfully assure them that they are unlikely to become blind enough to be dependent upon other people and that they can still expect to do housework and to go out of doors. These assurances can be quite true even if they require to be certified as blind eventually. Inability to read is the greatest hardship and for such the 'talking book' is invaluable. It must also be remembered that most public libraries have a section containing books with very large print which can be read by all but the severely partially sighted.

INDEX

Ablepharon, 150
Accommodation, physiology of, 167–8
Acetazolamide, ocular side-effects, 215
Acne rosacea, 32
— — ocular signs of, 196
Acrocephalosyndactyly, ocular signs, 196
Acromegaly, ocular signs, 196
Acrylic lens, 226
— — complications with, 226
ACTH administration, 244
— mode of action, 244
Adies's myotonic pupil, 204–5
Adrenergic drugs, ocular side-effects, 215
'After' cataract, 119
Albers-Schönberg disease, 210
Albinism, nystagmus in, 187
— ocular signs, 196
— partial and total, 61
Alcohol amblyopia, 85
— ocular side-effects, 216
Alkaptonuria, ocular signs, 200
Allergy(ies), cellulitis of eyelids due to, 144
— conjunctivitis due to, 12, 18
— episcleritis due to, 93–4
— non-granulomatous uveitis due to, 57
— ocular, treatment, 249
— in ophthalmology, 248–9
— steroid therapy in, 244, 245
Alport's syndrome, 210
Amaurosis, anaemic, 71–2
— in Devic's disease, 202
— fugax, 188
— uraemic, 74
Amaurotic family idiocy, 81–2, 213
— — — ocular signs, 196
Amblyopia in anisometropia, 172
— hysterical, 188
— in malnutrition, 221, 222
— strabismus, 178–9
— toxic, 84–5, 188, 216
— treatment, 181, 182, 183
Amblyopic eye, 98
Ammonia burns of conjunctiva, 24
Amsler's charts, 65
Anachrodactyly, ocular signs, 196
Anaemia, papilloedema due to, 99
— splenic, ocular signs, 197
— vitreous haemorrhage due to, 105
Anaphylactic allergy, 248
Angeoid streaks, retinal, 81
— — — in Paget's disease, 203

Angiograms in cerebral aneurysm, 198
Angiography, fluorescein, 257
Angioma, orbital, 138
Angiomatosis retinae, 78, 82–3
— — laser surgery for, 257
Angular conjunctivitis, 14
Aniridia, 54, 204
Anisometropia, 172–3
— contact lens for, 220
Ankyloblepharon, treatment, 152
Ankylosing spondylitis, acute iritis with, 49, 51
'Annular' scleritis, 94
Anterior capsular cataract, acquired, 30, 114
— — — congenital, 112
Anterior chamber, depth of, 6
— — examination of, 6
— — — by slit-lamp, 252
— — foreign body in, 107
— — implant, 226–7
Anthelmintics, ocular side-effects, 215
Antibiotic drugs, broad-spectrum, 240
— — comparison with chemotherapeutic drugs, 238, 242–3
— — proprietary list, 241
— — spectrum table, 242
— — suitable in ophthalmology, 239–43
— therapy in blepharitis, 142
— — conjunctivitis, 9–10, 11
— — eye diseases, 237–43
— — — infections, 237
— — ocular side-effects, 215
— — in uveitis, 48
Anticholinesterase, 43
Antihistamine treatment of ocular allergy, 249
Antihypertensive drugs, ocular side-effects, 215
Anti-Parkinsonian drugs, ocular side-effects, 215
Antirheumatic drugs, ocular side-effects, 215
Antispasmodic drugs, ocular side-effects, 215
Antithyroid drugs, ocular side-effects, 215
Antiviral drugs in eye diseases, 242
Aphakia, 113, 172
— contact lens for, 220
Aqueous 'flare', 252
Arachnodactyly, megalocornea with, 40

INDEX

Arachnoid sheath, 96
Arcus juvenilis, 38
— senilis, 38
Argyll Robertson pupil, 204–5, 252
'Arrowhead' rents of retina, 88
Arterial embolism, 203
— hypertension, ocular signs, 196
— obstruction of retina, 69
— spasm of retina, 69
Arteriosclerosis, amaurosis in, 188
— retinal arterial obstruction in, 69, 72
— — venous thrombosis in, 71
— vitreous haemorrhage in, 105
Arteritis, giant-cell, 206
— temporal, ocular signs, 206
— — steroid therapy in, 247
Ascorbic acid deficiency, ocular signs, 223
Astigmatism, 171–2
— contact lens for, 219, 220
Astrocytoma, 162
Atopic cataract, 114
Atropine, 43
— contra-indication, 71
— occlusion for squint, 181
— ocular side-effects, 71, 215
— in secondary glaucoma, 54
Autism, ocular signs, 197
Automatic self-operated recording perimeter, 259
Avitaminosis, 221
— optic atrophy due to, 102
— papilloedema due to, 99

Bacterial sensitivity, 248
Bacteriostasis, 237, 238
Band opacity of cornea, 38
Banti's disease, ocular signs, 197
Batten–Mayou's disease, ocular signs, 82, 210
Battered baby syndrome, ocular signs, 197
'Bedewing', 252
Behçet's syndrome, 210
— — acute iritis in, 49, 53
— — allergy in, 248
Bell's palsy, 210
Biber opacities, 40
Bifocal lenses, 169
Binocular vision and diplopia, 175–6
Bishop Harman loupe, 66
Bitot's spots, 222
'Black eye', 151
Blaskowicz's operation for ectropion, 146
— — ptosis, 147
Blepharitis, 4, 142–3
— chronic, causes, 142
Blind people, classification of, 261
— — helping, 262
— — — them to see, 258–9

Blind people, training for employment, 261–2
Blindness due to anaemic amaurosis, 71
— — arterial obstruction, 69
— — drugs, 215
— — malignant myopia, 165
— — optic atrophy, 101–2, 205
— — primary glaucoma, 122, 123
— — scleromalacia perforans, 95
— — toxic amblyopias, 84–5, 217
— — xerophthalmia, 222
— in Batten–Mayou's disease, 82
— corneal graft for, 228
— in hereditary choroideremia, 61
— infantile, 204
— in renal retinopathy, 74
— social aspects of, 261–2
— sudden complete, 69, 99
— in Tay–Sach's disease, 81
— transitory, 188
Blinking, infrequent in cerebrospinal meningitis, 201
Blood diseases, ocular signs, 197–8
— lakes, conjunctival, 251
'Blow-out', orbital, 139, 140
'Blue dot' cataract, 114, 115
— sclerotics, 95, 200
Bony orbital tumours, 138
Books, large print, 264
— talking, 259, 262, 264
'Bookworms', 167
Bourneville's disease, 83, 210
Bowman's membrane, 25
— — destruction in pannus degenerativus, 38
— — in trachoma, 16
Braille, 258, 263, 264
Broad-spectrum antibiotics, 240–2
— — list of, 241
Bruch's membrane, angeoid streaks in, 81
— — in melanoma of choroid, 160
— — Tay's choroiditis, 65
Buerger's disease, ocular signs, 206
Buphthalmos, 129, 130, 131
— haemangioma in, 148
— operations for, 228, 229–30
— in Sturge–Weber disease, 83
Burns, chemical, steroid therapy in, 246
— conjunctival, 24, 246
— contact lens following, 220
— of eyelids, 151
— retina, 78

Canaliculus, 154
— blockage of, 157
Canalization of nasolacrimal duct, delayed 157–8
Capsulotomy, 229

INDEX 267

Carcinoma of choroid, 159
— eyelid, 149
— lacrimal gland, 153
— orbit, 138
Cardiovascular drugs, ocular side-effects, 216
Carotid insufficiency, retinal embolus in, 69
Cataract, acquired, 112, 114–19, 253
— 'after', 119
— after angiomatosis, 82
— — choroiditis, 63
— — retinitis, 78, 81
— anterior capsular, 30, 112, 114
— atopic, 114
— axial, 253
— 'blue dot', 114
— chain-maker's, 115–16
— clefts, 253
— complicated, 253
— congenital, 112–14, 187, 204, 253
— coronary, 112–13
— dermatogenous, 253
— diabetic, 198, 253
— endocrine, 253
— equatorial, 253
— extraction, 225–7, 228
— — extracapsular, 226
— — intracapsular, 225
— — — indications, 226
— — by phaco-emulsification, 227
— — with intra-ocular implants, 226–7
— fusiform, 113
— 'heat-ray', 115–16, 253
— lamellar, 113, 253
— metabolic, 114–15, 200
— mongolian, 115
— myotonic, 115
— 'needling' for, 229
— nuclear, 113
— nummular, 253
— parathyroid, 115
— pathogenesis of, 111–12, 116
— polar, 107
— posterior capsular, 114, 216
— punctate, 114, 201, 253
— radiation, 115–16
— reduplicated, 253
— rubella, 114
— secondary, 116, 204, 209
— senile, 116–18, 253
— — operation for, 117–18
— signs and symptoms, 111
— stages of, 111
— stellate, 253
— suture, 114, 253
— tetany, 115
— toxic, 118

Cataract, traumatic, 118–19, 120, 253
— — foreign body, 108
— types of, 112
— varieties, 112
— visual acuity in, 111, 113
Caterpillar hairs, ophthalmia nodosum due to, 19
Caustic burns, 24
Cautery for dendritic ulcer, 36
— ectropion, 146
— entropion, 145
Cavernous sinus thrombosis, 134
— lymphangioma, 138
Cellulitis, causes and treatment, 133–4
— of eyelids, 144
— orbital, 199, 204, 209
Central areolar atrophy, 65
— nervous system depressants, ocular side-effects, 216
Cerebral abscess, ocular signs, 198
— aneurysm, ocular signs, 198
Cerebromacular degeneration, 82
Chain-makers' cataract, 115–16
Chalazion, 143
Chemotherapeutic drugs, comparison with antibiotics, 238–43
— — list of, 238–9
Chemotherapy in eye diseases, 237–43
'Cherry red' spot, 69, 82
Chevasse's operation, 231
Chicken-pox contacts of herpes ophthalmicus, 37
China foreign body, 108
Chlamydia, trachoma due to, 16
Chloramphenicol, 240–1, 242
Chloroma, orbital, 138
Chlorpromazine, ocular side-effects, 216
'Choked disc' in papilloedema, 99
Cholesterol crystals in vitreous, 104
Cholinergic drugs, 43
Chondroma, orbital, 138
Choriocapillaris absent in retinitis pigmentosa, 80, 81
Choroid, anatomy of, 46
— bone formation in, 56
— carcinoma of, 159
— coloboma of, 60–1
— congenital abnormalities of, 60–2
— degenerations of, 64–6
— — due to iridocyclitis, 56
— detachment of, 66
— diseases of, 60–6
— inflammations of, 62–4
— melanoma of, 160–2
— — metastasis in, 161
— rupture of, 86
— sarcoma of, retinal detachment in, 87
— tuberculosis of, 163

268 INDEX

Choroid tumours, 66 (*see also* Intraocular neoplasms)
Choroidal sclerosis, 66, 81, 203
— veins, 48
Choroideremia, 61–2
Choroiditis, 45, 203
— acute suppurative, 62
— chronic non-suppurative, 62
— clinical varieties of, 63–4, 65
— metastatic, 64
— tuberculous, 208
Choroidoretinitis, 200
— cataract in, 116
— causing optic atrophy, 100
— due to toxoplasmosis, 79, 207
Choyce implant, 226–7
Cilia, 141
— adherent in blepharitis, 142
— — trichiasis, 145
Ciliary abnormality, 150
— arteries, 46
— body, anatomy, 45–6
— — diseases of, 56–60, 63
— — exposure of, causing sympathetic ophthalmia, 236
— — melanoma of, 162
— flush, 5, 49, 59
— muscle, 46
— region, examination of, 5–6
'Circinate degeneration of the retina', 77 81
Coats's disease, 78, 163
Cogan's syndrome, 210
Cole–Marshall charts, 89
Coloboma, 187
— of choroid, 60–1
— disc, 102–3
— eyelid, 150
— iris, 61
— lens, 119
Colour-blindness, 189–90
— in Leber's disease, 98
Commotio retinae, 85–6
Concomitant divergent squint, 183–4
— — — consecutive, 185
— strabismus, 178–86
Conjunctiva, anatomy and physiology of, 8
— bacteriology of, 8
— burns, 24
— — steroid therapy in, 246
— cysts of, 22
— degenerative changes of, 21–2
— diseases of, 8–24, 93
— essential shrinkage of, 20
— examination of, 4–5
— — slit-lamp, 251
— sarcoid of, 21
— spring catarrh, 17–18, 248

Conjunctiva, syphilis of, 21
— tuberculosis of, 20–1, 208
— tularaemia of, 21
— tumours of, 22–3
— wounds of, 23–4
Conjunctival sac, bacteriology of, 8
Conjunctivitis, acute, 9
— — differential diagnosis, 59
— allergic, 248
— angular, 14
— chronic, 13–14, 203
— due to ectropion, 146
— — irritants, 18–19
— eczematous, 12
— follicular, 15
— gouty, 199
— membranous, 11–12
— mucopurulent, 9–10, 201
— oculoglandular, 209
— phlyctenular, 12–13
— purulent, 10, 199
— syndrome, 19–20
Conjunctivo-dacryocystostomy, 227
Contact lens(es), 218–20
— — advantages and disadvantages, 219, 220
— — in albinism, 61
— — for anisometropia, 173
— — in aphakia, 172, 220
— — cicatricial entropion, 146, 219
— — for corneal abnormalities, 40
— — corneoscleral, 218
— — hydrophylic, soft, 218–19
— — indications for, 219–20
— — for leucoma, cosmetic, 233
— — microcorneal, 218
— — in pemphigus, 20
— — senile cataract, 117
— — Sjögren's syndrome, 20
— — in slit-lamp examination of vitreous, 253
— — — gonioscopy, 253
— — in trichiasis, 145, 219
Convergence, 174, 175
— insufficiency, 186
Copper foreign body, 108
Cornea, anaesthetic in herpes ophthalmicus, 37
— anatomy and physiology of, 25
— conical, 5, 40, 219
— diseases of, 25–42
— examination of, 5
— — slit-lamp, 251–2
— ground-glass, 59, 122, 123
— pathology of, 25
— respiratory mechanism of, 25
— steamy, 59, 122, 123
— in trachoma, 16

INDEX 269

Cornea, wounds of, 41–2
— — complications, 41
Corneal burns, 42
— — chemical, steroid therapy for, 246
— congenital abnormalities, 40
— — — contact lens for, 40
— crystals, 200
— degeneration, 38–9
— dystrophies, 39–40
— fistula, 29, 30
— infiltrations, 32–5
— inflammations, 27
— oedema, 27
— opacities, 26, 27, 187
— perforation, 29–30
— — complications of, 30, 128
— prosthesis, 228
— scarring in herpes ophthalmicus, 37
— tattooing, 233
— transplantation, 227–8
— trauma, 27
— ulcers, 5, 24, 27–32, 204
— — complications of, 28–30
— — in scurvy, 223
— vascularization, 26–7
— virus diseases, 25–8
Corneoscleral junction, wounds involving, 41–2
Coronary cataract, 112–13
Corticosteroids (*see also under* Steroid)
— contra-indications, 245
— indications, 246–7
— method of administration, 244–5
— — treatment, 245–6
— ocular side-effects, 216
— in ophthalmology, 244–7
— — list of, 246
— in sympathetic ophthalmia, 236
Cortisone administration, 244
— mode of action, 244
'Cotton-wool' patches, 73, 74
Cover test for heterophoria, 185
— — squint, 178
Cranial arteritis, 198, 206
Crookes lenses, 170–1
Crouzon's disease, 210
Cryosurgery for detachments, 90
— glaucoma, 231
Cryotherapy, 83
Cryptophthalmia, 150
Cupping in glaucoma, 123, 126, 130
Curette evacuation for cataract, 228
Cushing's syndrome, ocular signs, 200
Cyclitis, 45, 49
— cataract in, 116
Cyclodialysis in glaucoma, 228, 231
Cyclo-diathermy, 231
Cycloplegics, 43

Cyst(s), conjunctival, 22
— of iris, implantation, 55
— — retinal epithelial, 55
— — serous, 55
— meibomian, 4, 143
— orbital, 137–8, 199
— — parasitic, 138
— in phakomatoses, 82–3
— retention, of lacrimal gland, 154
— of retina, detachment in, 87
— tarsal, 143
— toxoplasms, 207
— with microphthalmos, 137–8
Cystic hygroma, 138
Cystine disease, 39
Cystinosis, ocular signs, 200
'Cytoid bodies', 74
Cytomegalic inclusion disease, ocular signs, 198

Dacryo-adenitis, 153
Dacryocystectomy, 228–9
Dacryocystitis, 155–6
Dacryocystorhinostomy, 156, 158, 229
Dacryops, 154
Dalrymple's sign, 136, 200
Dark adaptation, defective in vitamin A deficiency, 222
Dark-room test for glaucoma, 123
Dazzling in cataract, 111
Deafness in quinine amblyopia, 85
— Vogt–Koyanagi–Harada syndrome, 58
Degenerations of choroid, 56, 64–6
— conjunctiva, 21–2
— cornea, 38–9
— iris, 55–6
— myopic, 66
— of retina, 79–82, 86, 166
— Saltzmann's nodular, 39
— senile macular, 65
— steroid therapy useless in, 247
Dendritic ulcer, corneal, 35–6
Dermatosis, cataract due to, 114
Dermoids of conjunctiva, 22–3
— eyelids, 148
— orbit, 138
Descemet's membrane, 25, 252
— — rupture of, in marginal atrophy, 38
— — split in buphthalmos, 129
Descemetocele, 29
Desensitization in allergic conditions, 249
Detachment of choroid, 66
— operations, 88–91, 256–7
— of retina (*see under* Retina)
Deuteranope(s), 190
Deviation, conjugate in tuberculous meningitis, 201
— in paralytic strabismus, 176

270 INDEX

Devic's disease causing retrobulbar neuritis, 97–8
— — ocular signs, 202
Diabetes, acute iritis in, 49, 51
— ocular signs, 198
— retrobulbar neuritis in, 97
— rubeosis, 51
— vitreous haemorrhage in, 105
Diabetic cataract, 114–15
— retinopathy, 74–6
— — fluorescein angiography in, 257
— — laser surgery in, 257
— — lipaemia in, 75
— — malignant, 74–5
Diamox, ocular side-effects, 215
Diathermy for detachment surgery, 89–90
Diphtheria, ocular signs, 199
Diplopia, binocular vision and, 175–6
— in encephalitis lethargica, 199
— strabismus, 176
— subarachnoid haemorrhage, 204
— syphilis, 206
— temporal arteritis, 206
— uniocular, in cataract, 111
Discission (needling), 229
'Disc, choked', in papilloedema, 99
— coloboma of, 102–3
— congenital holes in, 103
— cupping of, 101, 123, 126, 130
— lesions of, 101, 108
Disciform keratitis, 33, 36
Dis-insertions, retinal, 88
Dislocation of lens, 120
Distichiasis, 150
Drainage of intra-ocular fluid, 121
— tears, obstruction of, 155
Driving car, 264
Drowsiness in papilloedema, 99
Drugs affecting intra-ocular muscles, 43–4, 46
— indicated by wearing dark glasses, 171
— ocular side-effects in medication, 215–17
Duane's syndrome, 210
Dura mater, 96
Dysostosis craniofacialis, 210
Dystrophy, corneal, 5, 251
— pigmentary retinal, 79, 81

Eales's disease, 68–9, 78
— — laser surgery for, 257
— — vitreous haemorrhage in, 105
Eccentric fixation, 179, 182, 183
Echo location, 258
Ectasia of sclera, 94, 95
Ectopia pupillae, 55
Ectropion, 4, 146
— uveae, 49, 56
Eczematous conjunctivitis, 12

Edridge Green's lantern test for colour blindness, 190
Education of the blind, 261–2
— partially sighted, 263
Ehlers–Danlos syndrome, 210
Electronic aids, 258–9
Emmetropia, 168
— squint in, 180
Encephalitis lethargica, ocular signs, 199
— paralytic strabismus in, 177
Encephalocele, orbital, 138
Endophthalmitis, 62, 207
— due to lens wound, 119
— subacute, causing pseudoglioma, 106
Endothelial dystrophy of cornea, 39–40
Endothelioma, 139
Enophthalmos, causes, 133
Entropion, 4, 145–6
— cautery for, 145
— cicatricial, 146
Enucleation of eyeball, 229
— — dangers of, 48
— — and implant insertion, 229
— — in tuberculous choroiditis, 64
Epicanthus of eyelid, 150
— in mongolism, 201
Epiphora, 6, 154–5
— in ectropion, 146
— infantile, 157–8
Episcleritis, 5, 93–4, 203, 209
— steroid therapy in, 246
Epithelial dystrophy of cornea, 39–40
Epithelioma of conjunctiva, 23
Erysipelas of face, ocular signs, 199
Erythema multiforme, ocular signs, 199
— nodosum, ocular signs, 199
Erythromycin, 242
Eserine, 43, 124
— ocular side-effects, 18, 215
Esophoria, 184
Ethmoiditis, 135
Evisceration of eyeball, 48, 106
— — indications, 229
Examination, general, 7
— ocular, of battered baby, 197
— — external, 4
— — routine, order of, 1–7
— — for squint, 180
Excision of eye in absolute glaucoma, 125
— — foreign body present, 109
— — in melanoma, 161
— — to prevent sympathetic ophthalmia, 235–6
— — in retinoblastoma, 163
Exciting eye in sympathetic ophthalmia, 234–6
Exenteration of orbit, 229
— — in melanoma, 161, 163

INDEX 271

Exenteration of orbit in retinoblastoma, 163
Exophoria, 184
Exophthalmic goitre, 136
— ophthalmoplegia, 136-7
Exophthalmos, bilateral and unilateral, causes, 133, 199, 203
— due to orbital haematoma, 139
— pulsating, 136
— in tumours of optic nerve, 139
Exposure keratitis, 32, 146
Exudative retinitis, 78
Eye drops, use of, 26, 128
— enucleation of, 48, 64, 224
— excision of, 109, 125, 161, 163, 235-6
— foreign body in, 107-9, 140, 220, 255
— inflammations, differential diagnosis, 59
— strain, 184
Eyelids, anatomy, 141
— cellulitis of, 144
— congenital abnormalities of, 150
— dermatitis, steroid therapy in, 246
— dermoid cysts of, 148
— diseases of, 141-52
— — inflammatory, 142-5
— examination of, 4
— glands of, 141
— gross deformities due to trachoma, 17
— injuries of, 150-2
— malposition of, disorders due to, 145-7
— margins, 141
— muscles, 141
— nodules on, 200
— oedema of, 11, 202, 203, 209
— — allergic, 248
— syphilis of, 144-5
— tumours of, 148-9

Fabry's disease, ocular signs, 199
Facial palsy, 204
Familial dystrophy of cornea, 40
Fanconi's syndrome, 39, 211
Fascicular ulcer, 31
Fibroma, orbital, 138
Filamentary keratitis, 35
Fixation, eccentric, 179, 182, 183
Flashes of light in choroiditis, 62
— — hallucinations, 192
— — retinal detachment, 87
Fleischer's ring, 40
Flint foreign body, 108
Floating specks, 104, 165
'Fluid' vitreous, 105, 166
Fluorescein angiography, 161, 257
Focus, errors of, 164-73
Follicular conjunctivitis, 15
Foramen, anterior and posterior scleral, 93
Foreign body(ies), intra-ocular, 107-9

Foreign body(ies), intra-ocular, localization, contact lens for, 220
— — location and removal by ultrasound, 255
— — orbital, 140
— — tracks of, in cornea, 5, 107
— — types of, 108
Forster's areolar choroiditis, 63
Foster Kennedy syndrome, 99, 196
Fovea centralis, 67
— — red spot at, 69, 82
Fractures of bony orbit, 139
Fragilitas ossium, blue sclerotics in, 95
Friedreich's ataxia, ocular signs, 199
'Friend' test for malingering, 191
Fuchs corneal dystrophy, 39-40
Fundus, examination of, 7
— — in cataract, 112
— photography, 7, 257
— 'striped', in retinitis pigmentosa, 80
— tumours of, diagnosis by fluorographs, 257
Fungal infections, 8, 157
Fusiform cataract, 113

Galactosaemia, ocular signs, 200
Ganglion-blocking agents, ocular side-effects, 216
Ganglion-cell toxins, 84-5
— — causing optic atrophy, 100
Gargoylism, ocular signs, 200, 211
Gaucher's disease, 211
Giant cells in sympathetic ophthalmia, 235
Glass foreign body, 108
Glasses (lenses), in anisometropia, 184
— bifocal, 169, 181
— correcting, 168-9
— multifocal, 169-70
— occupational, 169
— for phorias, 185-6
— squint, 180
— tinted, 170
Glaucoma, absolute, 123, 125
— acute narrow angle, 122
— — — — differential diagnosis, 59, 123, 130
— capsulare, 129
— cataract in, 116
— chronic, 125-8
— corticosteroid treatment, dangers of, 245
— 'haloes' in, 122, 123, 130
— infantile, 129, 131
— in melanoma of ciliary body, 162
— narrow angle, 121-5
— — — acute, 122
— — — — congestive, 124-5
— — — — chronic, 123

272 INDEX

Glaucoma, narrow angle, treatment, 124–5, 230
— open angle, 125, 130
— operations for, 228, 229–31
— optic atrophy due to, 101
— pain in, 122–3
— primary, 121–8
— proprietary drops used for, 128
— secondary, 128–31
— — to angiomatosis, 82
— — atrophy of iris, 56
— — causes, 128–9, 166, 204, 216
— — to foreign body in eye, 108
— — iritis, 49, 54
— — retinitis, 78
— — scleritis, 94
— — traumatic cataract, 119
— simplex, 125–30
— — treatment, 127, 230
— tension, intra-ocular in, 122–3, 126, 130
— thrombotic, 70
— tonometry in, 123–4
— visual fields in, 130
Glial tissue in retinitis pigmentosa, 80
Glioma, 138–9
— diagnosis from retinoblastoma, 139
— — — tuberculous choroiditis, 64
— endophytum, 163
— exophytum, 163
— of retina (*see* Retinoblastoma)
— in Sturge–Weber disease, 83
Globe encirclement, 90
— lesions causing optic atrophy, 101
Glomerulonephritis, ocular signs, 199
Goitre, exophthalmic, 136
Goldmann contact lens in gonioscopy, 253
Gonioscopy, 7, 253
— for glaucoma, 123, 253
Goniotomy for buphthalmos, 130, 131, 229–30
Gonococcal conjunctivitis, 10, 11
— iritis, 49, 50, 53
Gout, ocular signs, 199
Graefe section (cataract extraction), 225
von Graefe's sign, 136, 200
Graft for ankyloblepharon and symblepharon, 151–2
Granuloma(ta) of conjunctiva, 23
Greeves's operation, 147
Greig's disease, 211
'Grey line', 141
Groenouw opacities of cornea, 40
'Ground glass' cornea, 59
Guide dogs, 262
Gumma(ta) of eyelids, 144
Gummatous nodules, differential diagnosis, 50

Haemangioma, cavernous, 148
— of eyelids, 148
Haematoma of eyelids, 151
— orbital, causing exophthalmos, 139
— subdural, ocular signs, 204
Haemophilia, ocular signs, 197, 199
Haemorrhage, intra-ocular, due to perforated ulcer, 30
— — glaucoma due to, 128
— — ocular, in battered baby, 197
— — blood diseases, 197–8, 200, 203
— — diabetes, 198
— — pertussis, 203
— — subarachnoid haemorrhage, 204
— — vitamin K treatment for, 223–4
— optic atrophy due to, 102
— — nerve sheath, into, 103
— orbital, 209
— in papilloedema, 99
— pulsating exophthalmos, 136
— retinal, 68, 77, 209
— — in arteriosclerosis, 73
— — diabetes, 75, 115
— — renal cases, 73
— vitreous in diabetes, 115
— — syphilis, 77
Haidinger's brushes, 182
Hallucinations, causes, 192
'Haloes' in glaucoma, 122, 123, 130
Harada's syndrome, 58, 211
Hassel–Henle bodies, 251
Hay fever, 248
Head tilt in strabismus, 176
Headaches in heterophoria, 184
— hypermetropia, 164
— papilloedema, 99
— severe in migraine, 189
— — retinopathy, 73
'Heat-ray' cataract, 115–16
Heavy metal therapy, ocular side-effects, 216
Heerfordt's disease, 58, 211
— — enlargement of lacrimal gland in, 153
Hemianopia, 203, 205
— altitudinal, 193
— binasal, 193
— bitemporal, (*Fig.* 4) 192–3, 194
— homonymous, (*Fig.* 3) 192, 194, 200, 204
— in migraine, 189
— quadrantic, (*Fig.* 5) 193–5
Hereditary optic atrophy, 211
Herpes febrilis of cornea, 35
— ophthalmicus, 37–8, 199
— zoster causing retrobulbar neuritis, 97–8
Hess's operation for ptosis, 147
Heterochromia, 55
Heterochromic iridocyclitis, 58

INDEX 273

Heterophoria, 84
von Hippel's syndrome, 211
von Hippel–Landau's disease, 82–3
History of patient and family, 2
Hodgkin's disease, ocular signs, 199
Homonymous hemianopia, (*Fig.* 3) 192, 194, 200, 204
Hordeolum, 143
Hormone therapy, ocular side-effects, 216
Horns on eyelids, 148
Horner's syndrome, 206, 211
— — pupillary reactions, 205
'Horse-shoe rents', retinal, 88
HPK bodies, 16
Hudson–Stahli line, 251
Hurler's disease, 200, 211
Hyaloid artery, persistent, 106–7
— — remains of, 253
Hydrocortisone, 245
Hyperadrenalism, ocular signs, 200
Hypermetrope, glaucoma in, 122
Hypermetropia, 164–5
— axial, 164
— squint in, 180
Hyperphoria, 184
Hypertelorism, 211
Hypertension, ocular changes in, 200
— in renal retinopathy, 73
Hyperthyroidism, ocular signs, 200
Hyphaema in diabetes, 198
— iritis, 49
Hypophoria, 184
Hypoprothrombinaemia due to drugs, 223
Hypopyon, 27
— complicating corneal ulcer, 28–9
— — iritis, 49, 51, 52
— in dacryocystitis, 156
— erythema nodosum, 199
— toxocara infestation, 207
— typhoid, 209

Illumination, oblique, in bright daylight, 4
— — with lamp, 4
— in slit-lamp examination, 250–1
— — — diffuse, 250
— — — direct focal, 250
Implants in cataract, 226–7
— vitreous, 91
Inborn metabolic errors, ocular signs, 200
Infantile epiphora, 157–8
— glaucoma, 129, 131
— iritis, acute, 53
Infections, ocular, 237
— — organisms of, 8–12 *passim*, 14–15, 242
— — response to chemotherapy, 237, 238
— — — sulphonamides, 238
— — spread of, 26

Infiltrating phlycten, 31
Infiltration(s) of cornea, 32–5
Inflammation(s) of choroid, 62–4
— eye, acute, differential diagnosis, 59
— eyelids, 142–5
— lacrimal passages, 155–7
— ocular, 237
— — chemotherapy for, 237, 243
— — steroid therapy for, 245
— optic nerve, 97–8, 201
— retina, 76–9
Infra-orbital (sphenomaxillary) fissure, 132
Injuries (*see* Trauma, Wounds)
Insomnia in miners' nystagmus, 187
Interstitial keratitis, 33–5, 50, 76
Intracranial tumours, ocular signs, 200
Intra-ocular neoplasms, 159–63 (*see also* Tumours)
Iodides, ocular side-effects, 216
Iridectomy, 231
— peripheral for glaucoma, 124–5
Iridencleisis in glaucoma, 125, 230
Iridocyclitis, 56–60, 199–204 *passim*, 209
— acute, differential diagnosis, 59
— diabetic, 198
— due to herpes ophthalmicus, 37
— heterochromia due to, 55
— heterochromic, 58
— keratic precipitates in, 235
— secondary glaucoma due to, 128
— sympathetic, 234–6 (*see also* Sympathetic ophthalmia)
— — steroid therapy for, 236, 247
— — treatment, 57–8, 235–6
Iridodonesis, 5, 129
Iridotomy, 231
Iris, anatomy, 45, 48
— arterial circle of, 46
— atrophy of, 5, 55, 123, 250
— bombé, 49, 54, 128
— clip implant, 227
— coloboma of, 61
— colour, in albinism, 61
— congenital abnormalities in, 54–5, 201
— cysts of, 55
— degenerations of, 55–6
— diseases of, 48–54
— essential atrophy of, 55–6
— examination of, 5–6
— — slit-lamp, 252
— melanoma of, 159–60
— 'muddy', 48, 49, 59
— nodules on, 5, 50, 160
— prolapse of, 30, 41
— red, in polycythaemia, 203
— rubeosis of, in diabetes, 198
— tumours of, 159–60
Iritis, 45

274 INDEX

Iritis, acute, 48–54
— — causes, 49, 52, 53, 200, 209
— — complications of, 48
— — differential diagnosis, 59, 123
— — treatment, 52–4, 247
— in ankylosing spondylitis, 51
— diabetic, 51, 115, 198
— due to focal sepsis, 50–1
— gonococcal, 50
— implants, complicated by, 226–7
— infantile, aftermath of, 163
— purulent, 30
— rheumatic, 51–2
— in scleritis, 94
— slit-lamp examination of, 252
— steroid therapy for, 247
— syphilitic, 50
— tuberculous, 34, 51
Iron foreign body, 108
Irritants, conjunctivitis due to, 18–19
Isihara's test for colour-blindness, 190
Isoniazid, ocular side-effects, 217

Juxta-papillary choroiditis, 63

Keyser–Fleischer ring, 39, 251
Keratic precipitates (KP), 5
— — after eye injury, 235
— — in iridocyclitis, 56–7, 58
— — sarcoidosis, 60
— — slit-lamp examination, 252
Keratitis, 201–4 *passim*, 209
— allergic, 248
— disciform, 33
— exposure, 32, 146, 200
— filamentary, 35
— infiltrating, 32
— interstitial, 33–5, 50, 76, 200
— mustard gas, 219
— neuroparalytic, 219
— profunda, corneal, 32–3
— punctata, 252
— sclerosing, 94, 208
— steroid therapy for, 247
— superficial punctate, 36–7
Keratocele, 29
Keratoconjunctivitis sicca, 19–20, 153 202
— TRIC agents, 38
Keratoglobos, 40
Keratomalacia in vitamin A deficiency, 222
Keratome incision for removal of foreign body, 109
Keratoplasty, 227–8
Koeppe's nodules, 60
KP (*see* Keratic precipitates)
Krause glands, 153

Krönlein's operation, 139
Kuhnt's operation for ectropion, 146
Kveim test in sarcoidosis, 60

Lacrimal abscess, 156–7
— apparatus, diseases of, 153–8
— — examination of, 6
— canaliculus, blockage of, 157
— fistula, 153, 157
— fossa, 132
— glands, anatomy, 153
— — diseases of, 153–4, 202
— — drying up, 19
— papilla, 141
— passages anatomy, 154
— — diseases of, 154–8
— — inflammations of, 155–7
— — obstructed drainage of, 155
— — obstructions of, 157–8
— prosthesis operation, 231
— punctum, blockage of, 157
— sac, 154
Lacrimation, excessive, in pink disease, 203
Lagophthalmos, 147, 219
Lamellar cataract (discoid or zonular), 113, 253
— scleral resection and overlap, 90
Lamina cribrosa, 93, 101
Laser coagulation in angiomatosis, 83
— — detachment surgery, 90
— — Eales's disease, 69
— — melanoma, 161, 162
— — retinitis, 78
— — retinoblastoma, 163
— dangers of, 256, 257
— in ophthalmic surgery, 256–7
— ophthalmology, 255–7
— ophthalmoscope, 257
— treatment in diabetic retinopathy, 75, 256
Lateral geniculate body, lesions causing optic atrophy, 101
Laurence–Moon–Biedl's syndrome, 211
'Lazy eye', 98
Lead poisoning, optic atrophy due to, 102
— — papilloedema due to, 99
Leber's disease, 211
— — causing retrobulbar neuritis, 97–8
Lenses (*see* Contact lenses; Glasses)
Lens, acrylic, 226
— anatomy, 110
— biochemistry, 110
— changes in cataract, 111–12, 116, 128
— coloboma, 119
— congenital abnormalities of, 119–20, 163
— diseases of, 110–20

INDEX

Lens, dislocation of, 120
— injuries to, 120, 128
— and media, examination of, 6–7
— — — in cataract, 116, 118
— opacities in, 253
— persistent vascular sheath, 106, 107
— slit-lamp examination, 252–3
— subluxation of, 119
— vacuoles in, 253
Leprosy, ocular signs, 200
Leucoma(ta), 26, 28
Leukaemia, ocular signs, 197, 200
— papilloedema due to, 99
— tumours in, 138
Leukaemic retinopathy, 76
Levator insertion, 141
— muscle, 175
— paralysis, 147
Lichen planus, ocular signs, 200
Lids (see Eyelids)
Light coagulation for melanoma of choroid, 161
— — retinal holes, 91
— sensitivity to, 170
Lignac's disease, 39
Limbus, malignant papilloma of, 23
Lipaemia in diabetic retinopathy, 75–6
Lipoid histiocytosis, 82
Lipoma, orbital, 138
Little's disease, 211
Loupe, Bishop Harman, 66
— monocular, 4
— use for foreign body, 107
Lowe's syndrome, 212
Lupus erythematosus, ocular signs, 200
Lymphadenoma, ocular signs, 199
Lymphoma, orbital, 138
Lysozyme, 154

Macula, hole in, 78, 86
— oedema in photoretinitis, 78
Macular degeneration, senile, 65
— — Stargardt's, 65
— disorders, diagnosis by fluorographs, 257
— haemorrhage, 68
— region of retina, 67, 87
— star figure in retinopathy, 73, 74
Maddox rod and wing tests, 7, 185, 186
Magnetic and non-magnetic foreign bodies, 108–9
Malaria, ocular signs, 201
Malignant hypertension, papilloedema due to, 99
— — retinopathy due to, 73
— retinopathy, diabetic, 74
Malingering, blindness in, 191–2
— night blindness in, 190

Malnutrition, effect on eyes, 221–4
Marfan's syndrome, 212
— — subluxation of lens with, 119
Marginal atrophy of cornea, 38
— ulcer, 31
Marie–Strümpell's disease, 212
Mascara as irritant, 18
Measles, ocular signs, 201, 204
Medication, systemic, ocular side-effects, 215–17
Megalocornea, diagnosis from buphthalmos, 131
— and keratoglobos, 40
Meibomian cyst, 4, 143
Melanoma of choroid, 160–2
— — type of cell in, 161
— ciliary body, 162
— iris, 159–60
— — differential diagnosis, 160
— laser surgery for, 257
— malignant, fluorescein angiography in, 257
— — operation for, 231–2
Membrane, Bowman's, 16, 25, 38
— on conjunctiva, 11
— cyclitic, 56, 106
— persistent pupillary, 54–5
— retinal, 67
— in retrolental fibroplasia, 92
— vitreous toxocara, 207
Meningeal irritation, 58
Meningioma, 139
Meningitis, bitemporal hemianopia in, 193
— ocular signs, 201
— papilloedema due to, 99
— paralytic strabismus due to, 177
Meningocele, orbital, 138
Metabolic cataract, 114–15
Metal foreign body, 108–9
— heavy, therapy, ocular side-effects, 216
Metamorphopsia in choroiditis, 62
Methyl alcohol amblyopia, 85
— — optic atrophy due to, 102
Microblepharon, 150
Microphthalmos, 204
— with cysts, 7–8
Microscope, operating, 259–60
— slit-lamp, 250
Migraine, amaurosis in, 188
— visual disturbances in, 189
Mikulicz's syndrome, 212
MIMMS sterile eye drops, 26
Miosis due to drugs, 43
Mitral stenosis, retinal embolus in, 69
Möbius's sign, 136, 200
Moll's glands, 141
Molluscum contagiosum, ocular signs, 201
— fibrosum of eyelids, 148

Mongolian cataract, 115
Mongolism, ocular signs, 201
Mooren's ulcer, 31
Morgagnian cataract, 111
Morgnio's disease, 212
Motais's operation for ptosis, 147
Movements, ocular, anomalies of, 174–87
— — tests of, 7
Mucopurulent conjunctivitis, 9–10
Multiple sclerosis, nystagmus in, 201–2
— — ocular signs, 201–2
— — optic atrophy with, 102
— — paralytic strabismus in, 177
— — retrobulbar neuritis in, 97
Mumps, ocular signs, 202
Muscae volitantes, 104
Muscle, ciliary, fibres of, 46
— extra-ocular, anatomy and physiology, 174–5
— eyelid, 141
— intra-ocular, drugs affecting, 43–4, 46
— levator, 175
— transplant in sixth nerve palsy, 231
Muscle-balance tests, 7
'Mutton fat' appearance in iridocyclitis, 57, 60
Myasthenia gravis, ocular signs, 202
— — paralytic strabismus due to, 177
— — ptosis first sign of, 147
Mydriasis in subdural haematoma, 204
— tetanus, 206
— traumatic, 252
Mydriatic drugs, 43, 44, 171
— — dangers in hypermetropes, 122
— — use in examination, 6, 7, 43–4
— test for glaucoma, 123
Myomectomy, inferior oblique, 231
Myopia, 165–7
— aetiology, 166
— cataract with, 113, 116
— in diabetes, 198
— high, contact lens in, 219
— malignant, 165
— retinal detachment in, 86
— squint in, 180
— treatment for, 166–7
Myopic crescent, 66
— degeneration, 166
Myosis, 202
— spinal, 204
Myotica atrophica imperfecta, ocular signs, 200
Myotonic cataract, 115
Myxoedema, ocular signs, 202

Naevus(i), choroidal, 161
— of eyelids, 148
— pigmented, of conjunctiva, 23

Nasal sinus(es), relation of orbit to, 133
— sinusitis and ocular disease, 135–6
— — ocular signs, 202
Nasolacrimal duct, 154
— — blockage of, 157–8
Nebulae, 5, 26, 219
'Needling' for cataract, 113, 115
— in high myopia, 167
— indications, 229
Neomycin, 242
Neoplasms, intra-ocular, 159–63 (see also Carcinoma, Sarcoma, tumours)
— paralytic strabismus due to, 177
Neostigmine in diagnosis of myasthenia gravis, 202
Neuritis, optic, 202, 209
— — hereditary, 98
— retrobulbar, 97–8
Neuro-epithelium, degeneration in retinitis pigmentosa, 80
Neurofibroma, orbital, 138
Neurofibromatosis, 83
— of eyelids, 148
Neuromyelitis optica, ocular signs, 202
Neoroparalytic ulcer, 31–2
Neuroretinitis, papillitis with, 97
— renal, 77
— syphilitic, 77
Niemann–Pick's disease, 82, 212
Night driving, danger of dark glasses, 171
Night-blindness in retinitis pigmentosa, 79, 80
— in vitamin A deficiency, 190, 222
Nodular degeneration, 39
Nodules in erythema nodosum, 199
— on iris, differential diagnosis, 160
— in leprosy, 200
— molluscum contagiosum, 201
Notifiable diseases, 11
Nottingham research into electronic aids, 258
Nuclear cataract, 113
Nystagmus, 186–7
— congenital, 187, 201
— — education in, 263
— in Friedreich's ataxia, 199
— miners', 187
— in multiple sclerosis, 201–2
— syringomyelia, 206

Oblique eye muscle, inferior, 175, 231
— — — superior, 174, 177
Occlusio pupillae, 49
Occlusive treatment for squint, 180–1, 183
Ocular allergies (see also Allergy)
— damage in battered baby syndrome, 197
— infections (see Infections)
— inflammations (see Inflammations)

INDEX 277

Ocular movements, anomalies of, 174–87
— paralysis, 205–6
— side-effects of systemic medication, 215–17
— signs of general disease, 196–214
— syndromes, list, 210–14
— torticollis, 176, 178
Ocutron, 259
Oedema of cornea, 5, 27, 122
— eyelids, 144, 209
— gross, of extra-ocular muscles in exophthalmic ophthalmoplegia, 137
— of optic nerve, 98
— retina in retinopathies, 73, 77
Opacities, band, 38
— corkscrew, 253
— corneal, 26, 34, 200, 203
— crystalline, 253
— in Descemet's membrane, 54
— flat, 253
— in lens, 111–12, 253
— punctate, 253
— spiral, 253
— in vitreous, 77, 104–5, 209
Open angle glaucoma, 125–8
Operating microscope, 259–60
Operations, ophthalmic, 225–33
— for squint, 182–4, 232–3
Ophthalmia neonatorum, 10–11
— — chemotherapy for, 237
— nodosum, 19
— sympathetic, 107–8
Ophthalmic operations, 225–33
— practice, recent advances in, 255–60
Ophthalmoplegia, exophthalmic, 136–7
— hereditary, 203
— ocular signs, 189, 202–3
— in subarachnoid haemorrhage, 204
— syringomyelia, 206
Ophthalmoscope, 6–7
— to detect floating bodies, 104
— in retinal examination, 68, 87
Optic atrophy, 100–2, 204, 206
— — causes, 80, 82, 85, 98
— — classification, 100–1
— — due to general diseases, 197–206 *passim*
— — — lesions between globe and lateral geniculate body, 101
— — primary and secondary, 101, 205
— disc, congenital holes in, 103
— — lesion, 101–2
— — regions of retina, 67
— foramen, 132
— nerve, anatomy of, 96, 132
— — atrophy of, 126
— — congenital abnormalities of, 102–3
— — degenerations of, 100

Optic nerve, diseases of, 96–103
— — head, oedema of, fluorograph, 257
— — inflammations of, 97–8, 201
— — injuries to, 103
— — sclerosis of, in glaucoma, 126
— — tumours of, 138–9
— — — exophthalmos in, 139
— neuritis, 202, 209
— — hereditary, 98
— oedema in subarachnoid haemorrhage, 204
Optical anomalies of the eye, 164–73
— treatment for squint, 180
Ora, 207
— serrata, 45
Oral contraceptives, ocular side-effects, 216
Orbicularis muscle, 141
— — spasm of, 145
Orbit anatomy, 132
— bony, relations of, 132–3
— diseases of, 132–40
— exenteration of, 161, 163, 229
— injuries of, 139–40
— — in childbirth, 139
— removal of, in cancer of eyelid, 149
— tumours of, 137–8
Orbital cellulitis, 135
— fissures, 132
— periostitis, 134–5
— — diagnosis from cellulitis, 135
Orthoptic treatment for phorias, 186
— — squint, 181, 183, 184
Osteogenesis imperfecta, ocular signs, 200
Osteopetrosis, 210
Osteosclerosis, ocular signs, 200
Otosclerosis, blue sclerotics in, 95
Oxygen respiration, vitamin C effect on, 223
— therapy, danger to premature infants, 92
— — ocular side-effects, 217

Paget's disease, ocular signs, 203
Pain in eye in mumps, 202
— — subarachnoid haemorrhage, 204
— — sudden acute, in glaucoma, 122–3
— temporal in arteritis, 206
Pannus, 5
— degenerativus, 38
— phlyctenular, 31
— trachoma, 15–16, 17, 27
Panophthalmitis, causes, 30, 62, 204, 209
— metastatic, 106
— risk of, in operation, 156
— wound causing, 42, 79
Papillitis, 97–9
— in cerebrospinal meningitis, 201
Papilloedema, 98–100, 101, 201
— causes, 99, 100, 198, 200, 204
— diagnosis from papillitis, 97, 98

Papilloedema, fluorescein angiography for, 257
— in malignant hypertension, 73
— unilateral, 99
Papilloma(ta) of conjunctiva, 23
— eyelids, 148
— malignant, of limbus, 23
Para-amino-salicylic acid (PAS) for tuberculous infections, 239
Paralysis, muscular, 200–3 *passim*
— nerve, causes, 177, 199, 200
— ocular, 205, 209
Paralytic strabismus, 176–8
Parasympatholytic drugs, 43
Parasympathomimetic drugs, 43
— — ocular side-effects, 217
Parathyroid cataract, 115
Parinaud's syndrome, 19
Parker's disease, 212
Pars plicata, 45
Partial cyclectomy, 231–2
— sight, classification of, 263
— — education, 263
— — occupations, 263–4
— — social aspects of, 263–4
Pemphigus, 20
— ocular signs, 203
Penicillin, hypersensitivity to, 239
— local administration of, 239–40
— spectrum, 239, 242
— treatment, 239
'Pepper and salt' fundus, 76
Perforation, corneal, 29–30
— of ulcer, 114
Perimetry, 7
Periphlebitis retinae, 68–9
Perivasculitis, 201
Pertussis, ocular signs, 203
Phaco-emulsification for cataract removal, 227
Phakomatosis, 82–3
— differential diagnosis, 83
Phenothiazine, ocular side-effects, 217
Phlycten, 12–13
— infiltrating and multiple, 31
Phlyctenular conjunctivitis, 12–13, 208
— — steroid therapy for, 247
— disease, types of, 31, 248
— ulcer, 31
Phorias, 184–6
Photocoagulation by laser, 257 (*see also* Laser)
Photophthalmia, 13
Photophobia, severe, in pink disease, 203
Photopsiae, 192
Photo-retinitis, 78
Phthisis bulbi, 47, 82
Pia, 96

Pigment changes in retrolental fibroplasia 92
Pigmentary retinal dystrophy, 79–81
— retinopathy, 100, 101
Pigmentation in Batten–Mayou's disease, 82
— retinitis pigmentosa, 80, 81
Pinguecula of conjunctiva, 21–2
Pink disease, ocular signs, 203
— eye, 9, 59
Pituitary gland, ablation in diabetic retinopathy, 75
— — disease, bitemporal hemianopia in, (*Fig.* 4) 192–3
— — dysfunction in retinitis pigmentosa 80
Pleoptic treatment for squint, 181–2
Plexiform neuroma of eyelids, 148, 150
Poisoning, cataract due to, 118
— optic atrophy due to, 102
Polaroid lenses, 170
Pollen sensitivity, 248
Polyarteritis nodosa, ocular signs, 203
Polycoria, 55
Polycythaemia, ocular signs, 197, 203
Polymyxins, 241, 242
Polyopia, 176
Port-wine naevus, 83
Posterior capsular cataract, 114
— lenticonus, 120
Post-neuritic optic atrophy, 101
Potato tumours in Bourneville's disease, 83
Prednisolone, 245
Prednisone, 245
Pregnancy, toxaemia of, retinopathy in, 76
Presbyopia, 167–9
— increase in glaucoma, 125
— premature, 165
Priscol test for glaucoma, 124
Prisms for phorias, 186
Probing, dangers of, 158
Projectorscope, 182
Prone position test for glaucoma, 124
Proptosis, 133, 202, 209
Prostigmin in diagnosis, 147
Protanopes, 189
Protein shock treatment in iridocyclitis, 58
Pseudoglioma, causes, 106, 163
Pseudotumours, orbital, 138
Pseudoxanthoma elasticum, 81
Pterygium of conjunctiva, 22
Ptosis, 147
— bar, 147
— in malaria, 201
— myasthenia gravis, 147, 202
— subarachnoid haemorrhage, 204
— sudden, in encephalitis lethargica, 199
— — syphilis, 206

INDEX 279

Ptosis, in Weil's disease, 209
Punctate cataract, 114, 201, 253
Punctum, 154
— blockage of, 157
— patency test, 6
Pupil, Adies's myotonic, 204–5
— Argyll Robertson, 204–5, 252
— effect of drugs on, 43–4
— examination of, 5
— — dilatation for, 6
— normal in hysterical amblyopia, 189
— occlusion by hypopyon, 28
— pink, in albinism, 61
— reactions of, differential diagnosis, 59, 98, 205, 206
— Wernicke's hemianopic, 205
Pupillary ectopia, 55
— membrane, persistent, 54–5, 252
— reactions, abnormal, 205, 206
Purpura haemorrhagica, ocular signs, 203
— ocular signs, 197
Purulent conjunctivitis, 10
— iritis, 30
— meningitis, 201
— retinitis, 79
Pus in vitreous, 106
Pyorrhoea causing iritis, 51

Quadrantic hemianopia, (*Fig.* 5) 193–5
Quinidine, loss of vision due to, 216
Quinine amblyopia, 85
— derivatives, ocular side-effects, 217

Radiation cataract, 115–16
Radon seed treatment of melanoma, 161
Raynaud's disease, amaurosis in, 188
Reading in myopic children, 167
— word blindness and, 191
von Recklinghausen's disease, 83, 129, 148, 212
Rectus muscle, external, 174, 177
— — inferior, 174
— — internal, 174
— — superior, 174
Refraction, errors of, 164–73
— examination of, 6
Refsum's syndrome, 79
Rehabilitation, 262
Reiter's syndrome, 20, 212
Relapsing fever, ocular signs, 203
Renal retinopathy, 73–4, 78
Resection and recession for squint, indications, 232–3
— scleral, 90
Residential courses for blind and partially sighted, 262, 263
Rete mirabile', 77

Retina, anaemic amaurosis of, 71–2
— anatomy, 67
— angiomatosis of, 82–3
— arterial obstruction in, 69–70
— — spasm of, 69
— atrophy of, 70
— — lesions causing, 64, 100–1, 206
— coloboma of, 60–1
— detached, 86–91 (*see also* Retinal)
— — cataract in, 116
— — diseases causing, 58, 73, 78, 82
— — laser surgery for, 257
— diseases of, 67–92
— glioma of (*see* Retinoblastoma)
— pigmentation due to choroid lesion, 64–5
— raspberry tumour on, 82
— relation to choroid, 60
— traumatic lesions, 85–6
— venous thrombosis in, 70
— — — glaucoma due to, 128
Retinal affections, classification of, 67–8
— degenerations, 79–82, 86, 166
— detachments, 86–91 (*see also* Retina)
— — causes, general, 86–7, 166
— — examination for, 87–8
— — simple and malignant, 160
— — sudden, 161
— — surgery for, 88–9, 257
— — tear in, 160, 166
— epithelial cysts, 55
— granulomata, 207
— haemorrhages, aetiology, 68
— — causes, 70, 78, 201, 204, 209
— holes, 88
— oedema, traumatic, 86
— rupture, 86
— thrombosis, 201
— vascular lesions, 68–72, 101, 206, 209
— venous congestion, gross, in polycythaemia, 203
Retinitis circinata, 77, 81
— degeneration of neuroepithelium in, 80
— exudative, 78
— night blindness in, 190
— pigmentosa, 65, 79–81, 100, 101
— — associated characteristics, 79
— — cataract in, 116
— proliferans, 69, 75, 77–8, 105
— — laser surgery in, 257
— punctata albescens, 81
— purulent, 79
— syphilitic, 76–7, 78
Retinoblastoma, 78, 162–3
— diagnosis from glioma, 139
— — — pseudoglioma, 106
— treatment, 163
— 'white pupil' in, 162

280 INDEX

Retinopathy, 72–6, 206, 209
— arteriosclerotic, 72–3
— central, diagnosis by fluorographs, 257
— diabetic, 74–6, 78
— — laser surgery in, 257
— hypertensive, 200
— nutritional, in prisoners of war, 221
— leukaemic, 76
— pigmentary, 100, 101
— toxaemic in pregnancy, 76
— vitreous haemorrhage in, 105
Retrobulbar neuritis, 97–8
— — causes, 97
— — differential diagnosis, 98
— — in multiple sclerosis, 201
— — nutritional retinopathy, 221
Retro-illumination in diagnosis of malignant tumours, 161
— in slit-lamp examination, 250, 252, 253
Retrolental fibroplasia, 91–2, 163
Rheumatic fever, ocular signs, 203
Rheumatism associated with acute iritis, 49, 51–2, 53
— — — scleritis, 94
Rheumatoid arthritis, ocular signs, 203–4
Riboflavin deficiency, ocular signs, 222–3
Ridley implant, 226
Rieger's malformation, 54–5
— syndrome, 212
Riley–Day syndrome, 212
Ring synechiae, 49
— ulcer, 31
Rod and cone layer of retina, 67
— — — — degeneration in Batten-Mayou's disease, 82
Rodent ulcer of conjunctiva, 23
— — eyelid, 149
Romberg's syndrome, 213
Rönne's step, 125
'Rosettes' in retinoblastoma, 162
Rubella, material, abnormalities with, 113, 114, 204
Rubeola, ocular signs, 204

'Sago grains', 15, 16
Salicylates, ocular side-effects, 217
Salzmann's nodular degeneration, 39
Sarcoid of conjunctiva, 21
— uveitis, 57
— — steroid therapy in, 247
Sarcoidosis, 58, 60, 208
— causing acute iritis, 49
Sarcoma of choroid, 87, 234
— conjunctiva, 23
— eyelid, 149
— iris, 50
— orbital, melanotic, 138
— — round-cell, 138

Scars, of cornea, 5, 26, 35, 37
— — ectatic, 29
Scheie's operation for glaucoma, 230
Schilder's disease, 213
— — ocular signs, 204
Schlemm, canal of, absence of, 129, 131
— — obstruction of, 121, 122, 126
Schüller–Christian syndrome, 213
Sclera, anatomy of, 93
— ectasia of, 94, 95
— examination of, 5
Scleral buckling, 90–1
— resection, 90
— staphyloma, 95
Scleritis, 94–5, 199
— steroid therapy for, 247
Scleroderma, ocular signs, 204
Scleromalacia perforans, 95
Sclerosis of optic nerve in glaucoma, 126
Sclerotic(s) blue, 95, 200
— jaundice of, 209
— perforation, in tuberculous choroiditis, 64
— scatter in slit-lamp examination, 251
Scotoma, central, in alcoholic amblyopia, 85
— in areolar atrophy, 65
— Batten-Mayou's disease, 82
— migraine, 189
— papilloedema, 99
— retrobulbar neuritis, 98
— tobacco amblyopia, 84
— choroiditis, 62
— in photo-retinitis, 78
— retinal detachment, 87
— — venous thrombosis, 70
— ring, in retinitis pigmentosa, 79
Sebaceous adenomata in tuberous sclerosis, 83
Seclusio pupillae, 49
Seidel's sign, 125
Senile cataract, 116–18
— — maturity of, 116
— — treatment, 117–18
— macular degeneration, 65
Sensation, loss of, in cornea, 5
Sepsis, focal, causing choroiditis, 62
— — — iritis, 49, 50–1
— — — retinal venous thrombosis, 71
'Siderosis' due to iron foreign body, 108
Sinusitis, frontal, 135
— nasal, 135–6
— sphenoidal, 135
Sjögren's disease, 213
— syndrome, 19–20, 153, 204
— — contact lenses for, 20
Skin treatment for acne rosacea, 32
Slit-lamp examination, 7, 54–5

INDEX 281

Slit-lamp examination of cornea, 5
— — for foreign body, 107
— — in glaucoma, 123
— — iridocyclitis, 57
— — of iris, 5, 160
— — in vitreous haemorrhage, 105
— — microscopy, 250–4
— — — magnification in, 251
— — — technique, 250–1
Snellen's sutures for ectropion, 146
— tables, 4
— test types, (*Fig.* 1) 3–4
Snow blindness, 13
Soframycin, 241–2
Sonic aids, 258
Spaeth's operation, 150
Specks (*see also* Opacities)
— in cataract, 111
— floating, in myopia, 165
Specular reflection in slit-lamp examination, 251
Sphenoidal disease, bitemporal hemianopia due to, 193
Sphenomaxillary fissure, 132
Splenic anaemia, ocular signs, 197
Spring catarrh, 17–18, 248
Squint (*see also* Strabismus)
— alternating, 183
— apparent, 179
— in concomitant strabismus, 178
— convergent, 179–80
— divergent, 183–4
— in hypermetropia, 164
— latent, 184–6
— Maddox tests for, 7, 185, 186
— in myopia, 165–6
— operations for, 182, 183, 184, 232–3
— sudden, in retinoblastoma, 162
— treatment, 180–6 *passim*
Stallard's operation, 157, 227, 230
Staphyloma(ta), 5
— anterior, 30
— ciliary, 94
— in myopia, 166
— posterior, 166
— scleral, 95
Stargardt's disease, 65, 82, 213
Stellar dust, 253
Stellwag's sign, 136, 200
Steroid therapy in allergic conditions, 249
— — contra-indications, 245
— — effects of, 245
— — **general, indications, 247**
— — local, indications, 246–7
— — method of treatment, 245–6
— — in sympathetic ophthalmia, 236
Stevens–Johnson syndrome, 213
Still's disease, 213

Stone as a foreign body, 108
Strabismus (*see also* Squint)
— concomitant, 178–86
— paralytic, 176–8, 199
Streptomycin, 240, 242
Sturge–Weber's syndrome, 83, 129, 148, 213
Stye, 143
Subarachnoid haemorrhage, ocular signs, 204
Subdural haematoma, ocular signs, 204
Subluxation of lens, 119
Substantia propria, 25
— — in trachoma, 16
Sulphacetamide, 242
Sulphonamide drugs, administration of, 239
— — suitable in ophthalmology, 238–9
— therapy, ocular side-effects, 217
Superficial punctate keratitis, 36–7
Superior orbital fissure, 132
Suppression of image, psychological, 178–9
Suppuration, acute, of uveal tract, 47
Suture cataract, 114
— of lens, 110
Symblepharon, 11
— in pemphigus, 20
— prevention in burns, 24
— — by contact lens, 220
— treatment, 24, 151–2
Sympathetic ophthalmia (*see also* Iridocyclitis)
— — due to foreign body, 107, 108
— — prophylactic treatment, 235–6
— — steroid therapy, 247
— — theories of causation, 234–6
Sympathizing eye in sympathetic ophthalmia, 234–6
Sympatholytic drugs, 43
Sympathomimetic drugs, 43–4
— — ocular side-effects, 217
Synchesis scintillans, 104–5
Syndactyly, ocular signs, 204
Syndromes, pathology and signs of, 210–14
Synechiae, 5, 252
— anterior, 30, 60, 128
— peripheral anterior, 49, 122
— posterior, 34
— — in iridocyclitis, 56
— ring, 28, 49
— syphilitic, 50
Syphilis, acute iritis due to, 49, 50
— bitemporal hemianopia in, 193
— cerebral, ptosis due to, 147
— choroiditis due to, 62
— congenital, stigmata of, 34
— of conjunctiva, 21
— eyelids, 144–5

282 INDEX

Syphilis, ocular signs, 204-6
— orbital periostitis due to, 134
Syphilitic iritis, acute infantile, 53
— — congenital and acquired, 50
— ophthalmoplegia, 202-3
— optic atrophy, 101, 102
— papilloedema, 99, 100
— paralytic strabismus, 177
— retinitis, 76
— scleritis, 94
— staphyloma, 95
— tarsitis, 144
Syringomyelia, ocular signs, 206

Tabes, optic atrophy in, 101, 102
Talking books, 259, 262, 264
Tarsal cysts, 143
— glands, 141, 145
Tarsitis, syphilitic, 144
Tattooing of cornea, 233
Tay's choroiditis, 65
Tay-Sach's disease, 81-2, 213
Tears, fluid, 154-5, 156
— — secretion and drainage of, 155
Tears (rents) in choroid and retina, 166
Teeth, hypoplasia of enamel, 113
Telangiectasis of eyelids, 148
Temporal arteritis, ocular signs, 206
— — steroid therapy for, 247
Tension of eye, differential diagnosis, 59
— intra-ocular, in buphthalmos, 129
— — glaucoma, 122-3, 126, 130
— — relief of, 129
Tetanus, ocular signs, 206
Tetany in cataract, 115
Tetracycline, 241, 242
Third-nerve paralysis, 177, 198
— — in migraine, 189
Thromboangiitis obliterans, ocular signs, 206
Thyroxine in exophthalmic ophthalmoplegia, 137
Tobacco amblyopia, 84-5, 98
Tonography, 7
Tonometry, 7
— in glaucoma, 123-4
Torticollis, ocular, 176, 178
Toxaemia of pregnancy, retinopathy in, 76, 206
Toxic amaurosis, 188
— cataracts, 188
— paralytic strabismus, 177
Toxocara canis, ocular signs, 78, 163, 206-7
Toxoplasmosis, acute iritis due to, 49, 52, 53
— choroidoretinitis due to, 79, 207
— ocular signs, 198, 207-8
Trabecular surgery for glaucoma, 230

Trachoma, 15-17
Trauma (*see also* Wounds)
— blockage of nasolacrimal duct due to, 158
— vitreous haemorrhage in, 105
Traumatic cataract, 118-19
Travel sickness drugs, ocular effects, 217
TRIC agent(s), 16
— — keratoconjunctivitis, 38
Trichiasis, 4, 145, 219
Trifocal lenses, 169
Tritanopes, 190
Trochlea, 174
Trochlear fossa, 132
Tuberculin for Eales's disease, 69
Tuberculosis, acute iritis in, 49
— of conjunctiva, 20-1
— iris, 34
— ocular signs, 208
— orbital periostitis in, 134
— PAS treatment, 239
Tuberculous choroiditis, 63-4
— iritis, miliary and conglomerate, 51, 53
— scleritis, 94
— staphyloma, 95
Tuberous sclerosis, 83
'Tubular vision', 126
Tularaemia of conjunctiva, 21
— ocular signs, 209
Tumours, 159-63
— bony, 138
— cerebral papilloedema with, 100
— of conjunctiva, 22-3
— of eyelids, 148-9
— intracranial, ocular signs, 200
— intra-ocular, causing glaucoma, 129
— 'mixed', of lacrimal gland, 153
— optic nerve, 138-9
— orbital, 137-8
— in phakomatoses, 82-3
— pigmented in skin, 83
Tunnel vision, 126
— — blindness in, 261
Turk's line, 252
Twenty-foot table, 4
Typhoid, ocular signs, 209
Typhus, ocular signs, 209

Ulcers in blepharitis, 142
— buccal in Behçet's syndrome, 52
— conjunctival, 24, 209
— — rodent, 23
— corneal, 5, 27-32
— — allergy in, 248
— — complications, 28-30
— — in dacryocystitis, 156
— — recurrent, 145
— — staining of, 28

INDEX 283

Ulcers, corneal, in trachoma, 16
— dendritic, 35–6
— — steroids contra-indicated in, 247
— fascicular, 31
— marginal, 31
— Mooren's, 31
— neuroparalytic, 31
— perforating, 114
— phlyctenular, 31
— ring, 31
Ulcerative colitis, acute iritis in, 49, 52, 53
— — ocular signs, 209
Ulcus serpens, 30–1
Ultrasonography, 7
Ultrasound in ophthalmology, 255
Ultraviolet light (UVL), exposure to, 13
Urticaria, 248, 249
Uveal inflammation, 47–54, 56–65
— — chronic, 48
— tract, acute suppuration of, 47–8
— — — — treatment, 48
— — anatomy, 45
— — blood supply, 46
— — diseases of, 45–66
— — nerve supply, 46
Uveitis, 202, 208
— anterior, 34, 208
— — complicating scleritis, 94
— antibiotics for, 48
— bilateral, leading to detached retinae, 58
— chronic, 248
— endogenous, 64
— granulomatous, 57
— non-granulomatous, allergic, 57
— posterior, steroid therapy for, 247
— sarcoid, 57
Uveoparotid fever, 58, 208
— — lacrimal glands enlarged in, 153

Van den Hoeve's syndrome, 214
Varicella virus in herpes ophthalmicus, 37
Varilux lenses, 169
Vascular lesions, paralytic strabismus due to, 177
— — of retina, 68–72
— sheath of lens, persistent, 106, 107
Vascularization, circumcorneal, 222–3
— corneal, 26–7
Venous thrombosis in retina, 70
— — — complications, 70–1
Vertigo in diplopia, 176
Virus diseases of cornea, 35–8
Vision, binocular, and diplopia, 175–6
— — phorias affecting, 184–5
— blurred, in hypermetropia, 164
— central, deterioration of, 65, 84
— gross diminution in central areolar atrophy, 65

Vision, loss of, in papilloedema, 99
— — retinitis proliferans, 69
— — sudden, 206
— severe impairment, 59, 98
— — — in glaucoma, 122, 123, 125
— — — mumps, 202
— tunnel, 126
Visual acuity, (Fig. 1) 2–4
— — in cataract, 113
— — optic atrophy, 102
— — papilloedema, 99
— — recording in squint, 180
— — reduced by macular haemorrhage, 68
— — — in migraine, 189
— changes in intracranial tumours, 200
— disturbances, subjective, 188–95
— failures due to malnutrition, 221
— fibres, course of, (Fig. 2) 193
— — lesions of, (Fig. 2) 193
— fields, disturbances of, (Figs. 3–5) 192–5
— — involvement in glaucoma, 130
— — spiral contraction in amblyopia, 188
— judgement, inaccurate, 176
— purple, 190
— sensations, disturbances of, 188–92
Visuscope, 179
Vitamin A deficiency, 190, 222
— B deficiency, 222–3
— B treatment in amblyopia, 216
— C deficiency, 223
— deficiency, ocular effects, 221–4
— K deficiency, 223–4
— K therapy, 105
Vitreous, anatomy of, 104
— aspiration, dangers of, 105–6
— diseases of, 104–9
— floaters, in 62, 166
— 'fluid', 105, 166
— foreign body in, 107
— haemorrhage in, 77–8, 105–6, 203, 206
— — in diabetic retinopathy, 75, 198
— — syphilitic retinitis, 77
— injuries involving, 107–9
— loss of, 107
— posterior, slit-lamp examination, 253
— pus in, 106
Vogt–Koyanagi's syndrome, 214
Vogt–Koyanagi–Harada's syndrome, 58 235
Vomiting in cellulitis, 134
— diplopia, 176
— glaucoma, 59, 122
— migraine, 189
— papilloedema, 99
VY operation for ectropion, 146

Waadenburg's syndrome, 214
Water-drinking test for glaucoma, 123–4
Weil's disease, ocular signs, 209
Welders' conjunctivitis, 13
Werner's syndrome, 214
Wernike's hemianopic pupil reactions, 205
— — — slit-lamp examination, 252
'White' pupil in retinoblastoma, 162
Wilson's disease, 39, 214
Wolfram–Tyrer's syndrome, 214
Wool-matching test for colour blindness, 190
Word-blindness, 191
Wounds, conjunctival, 23–4
— corneal, 41–2
— of eyelids, 150

Wounds of lens, cataract due to, 118–19
— sympathetic ophthalmia due to, 234–6

Xanthelasma, 148
Xanthomatosis, 213
Xerophthalmia, 222
Xerosis, 222
— night-blindness in, 190
— in pamphigus, 203
X-ray treatment, protective contact lens in, 220

Zeis's glands, 141
Zeiss gradual lenses, 170
— umbramatic lenses, 171
Zinn, annulus of, 174